MORE
SECRETS
FROM THE
SUPER
SPAS

MORE
SECRETS
FROM THE
SUPER
SPAS

BY EMILY WILKENS

Publishers • DEMBNER BOOKS • New York

To my wonderful children
and all the special people the world
over who made this book possible

Dembner Books
Published by Red Dembner Enterprises Corp., 1841 Broadway,
New York, N.Y. 10023
Distributed by W. W. Norton & Company, Inc., 500 Fifth Avenue,
New York, N.Y. 10110

Contents

INTRODUCTION

The spas are like the stars, ever-changing. That's why I never worry when I come down with a case of spavelitis. I know that, depending on my particular symptoms, I'll find a cure for it at one of the world's great health, beauty, and revitalization resorts. There is always something new being added that complements the old tried-and-true treatments and makes a spa visit as refreshing as a sip from the Fountain of Youth.

My most recent case of the blahs—that old feeling that I needed to trim this, firm or flatten that, put myself in the hands of experts who'd pamper or pummel me as needed—sent me spinning the globe. I traveled more than 100,000 miles researching my first book, *Secrets from the Super Spas*. Where should I head this time?

My antennae had been picking up signals of innovative treatments at some of the spas I'd visited many times over the years. I'd also been hearing good reviews on several of the new spas in the "super" category. It was time to see for myself—review the changes (for this new book) and revitalize (for me). As I was to discover, revitalization is the new spa catchword. It's a one-word slogan that stands for: forever young, forever fit.

When it comes to spas, you may have one conveniently nearby; you may prefer the freedom and escape of a spa in a totally different part of the country, or even halfway around the world; or you may have the itch to set up your own spa in the privacy and comfort of your own home. It all depends upon your own tastes and personality. There is a spa solution for everyone.

For many, a spa is the most dramatic possible change from humdrum, toxic living habits.

Others find it the surest way to lose weight painlessly—or even enjoyably.

A few go for what the Germans call an ENTSCHLACKUNGSKUR—a thorough scouring of all the pipes.

Some go to repair the devastation of holiday over-indulgence.

Increasingly, women go for new beauty and youthfulness as well as health.

A lot of people go simply to find sleep and rest.

But almost all who try a Super Spa find that they have sharpened their senses, reposed their bodies and minds, and restored their senses of humor.

Several years ago I was afflicted with spavelitis. It knocked me for a loop. I did what I have done so many times: I dropped everything and headed west for a blissful smog- and hassle-free stay at one of my favorite spas.

The day I got back, a friend said, "You can't fool me, Emily. I can tell you've been away having your face lifted."

She was wrong—but LIFTED was precisely how I looked and felt. My lift had been a spa—two weeks of royal care during which I'd been massaged daily, oiled to shimmering softness, bathed in fragrant exotic liquids, and steamed like a clam. My muscles had been roused to twitteration by lithe Amazons who cajoled me to move ever faster, to stretch ever farther, to reach that unreachable toe. My excess poundage was drained from my frame with cunning meals that looked and tasted delicious. A private room with a crackling log fire soothingly carried me off to a deep, refreshing sleep every night. A cool aquamarine pool splashed new life into every tissue of my body. Skilled technicians had fussed over me to make me relaxed, comfortable, and more beautiful.

My spavelitis was cured—at least for a while.

You can cure your own spavelitis by visiting a spa or by setting up your own spa regimen in your home. This book is designed to help you to do either or both. In my years of writing and reporting on beauty secrets, I have visited all of the most famous spas, as well as many of the lesser-known ones. A part of this book is intended as a spavelogue, an introduction to the hundreds of spas—at home in the United States or abroad in Europe and Asia—that you have to choose from. But perhaps more important, I will also introduce you to many of the secrets of the spas so that you can incorporate their regimens into your daily life. Many of the exercises mentioned here will bear the name of the spas where they originated or of the instructors at the spas. These names will become more familiar to you in Part II.

Visiting a spa is like having your shoes custom-made—a luxury you grow to cherish and, finally, NEED. But so much depends on your first visit. Unless you have a clear idea of what you're in for, it can be a distinct disappointment. Here are a few categories you'll want to explore before you board your plane:

CLOTHES: Estimate carefully what clothes you will need. Some spas feature an active social life that requires informal evening clothes. Others require no more than a bathing suit and a toothbrush. But find out BEFORE you leave! If the spa does not supply any of the following, you'll need at the minimum: shower cap, bathing suit, morning robe, leotard, tights, unstructured bra, plus a sweat suit for chilly days and serious exercising.

Experienced spa-goers also tote exercise sandals, walking shoes, a warm sweater, scarves, a turban, a washable wig, sandals, caftans, and a pants suit or two.

Absolutely DO NOT take laces, ruffles, lamé, or frills of any kind.

MONEY: Although often the "service charge" of 15 percent is added to your bill, it's extremely helpful to be able to press a dollar or two into the palm of an exceptionally considerate staff member. Especially abroad, a bit of lucre not only insures promptness, but promptness when you want it.

MISCELLANEOUS: A few other things you might find useful would be a travel alarm clock, notebooks for jotting down tips and thoughts, needlework, portable radio, books, your favorite cosmetics (occasionally difficult to come by), your own hair coloring if you feel you'll need it, and a tape recorder.

Many people have the impression that spas are only for the wealthy and for older women. It is true that a beautiful woman's early years do tend to be gloriously insouciant; growing old is something that happens to OTHER people. Then, suddenly, she is ambushed by time. Something happens—it may be the trauma of bearing her first child, or her second. It may be a divorce. In one awful, panicky moment, she is made to understand that she is no longer a girl. And formerly, it WAS only women of wealth and leisure who were interested in spas.

But now everybody is interested—men and women, young and old—and just about anybody can find a spa within a suitable price range. Sure, it's a magnificent experience to have platoons of uniformed nymphs and naiads arranging your meals, serving you, steaming you, helping you melt away the excess pounds, and it sounds like it's frivolously expensive. But, even if you are the sort who feels guilty at the slightest hint of luxury or hedonism, you can believe me when I say that you can have more fun and enjoy longer-lasting results by beautifying yourself through your own efforts.

In the final analysis, it's not what they do for you at a spa that's so important. It's what you learn to do for yourself—and that's what you will discover in this book. There are some treatments that can't be duplicated at home. There are many others that can be—and they are the ones I'm sharing with you in this new book.

Chemists aren't the only ones who can compound beautifying formulas. As I discovered at the super spas, beauty aids can be created with ingredients you'll find in your refrigerator (milk, eggs, mayonnaise, beer, cucumbers, avocados, lemons), on your pantry shelves (oatmeal, apple cider vinegar, powdered milk, herb tea, mint leaves, coarse salt, olive oil, corn oil, corn meal, spices, potatoes, bananas), and in your bathroom, medicine chest or on your beauty shelves (petroleum jelly, mint-flavored milk of magnesia, castor oil, witch hazel, rose water, vitamin E capsules, baby oil, epsom salts, cocoa butter, lanolin alcohol).

You can try the newest approaches to diet, trim inches with the most effective exercises, borrow the luxury touches for which the spas are famed, and pamper yourself at home.

I've had fun re-visiting spas that I discovered years ago. It was exciting to uncover new resorts in the "super spa" category. At each and every stop I learned something new. You will too as you read on. Don't just turn pages—turn over a new leaf and begin your very own spa program today.

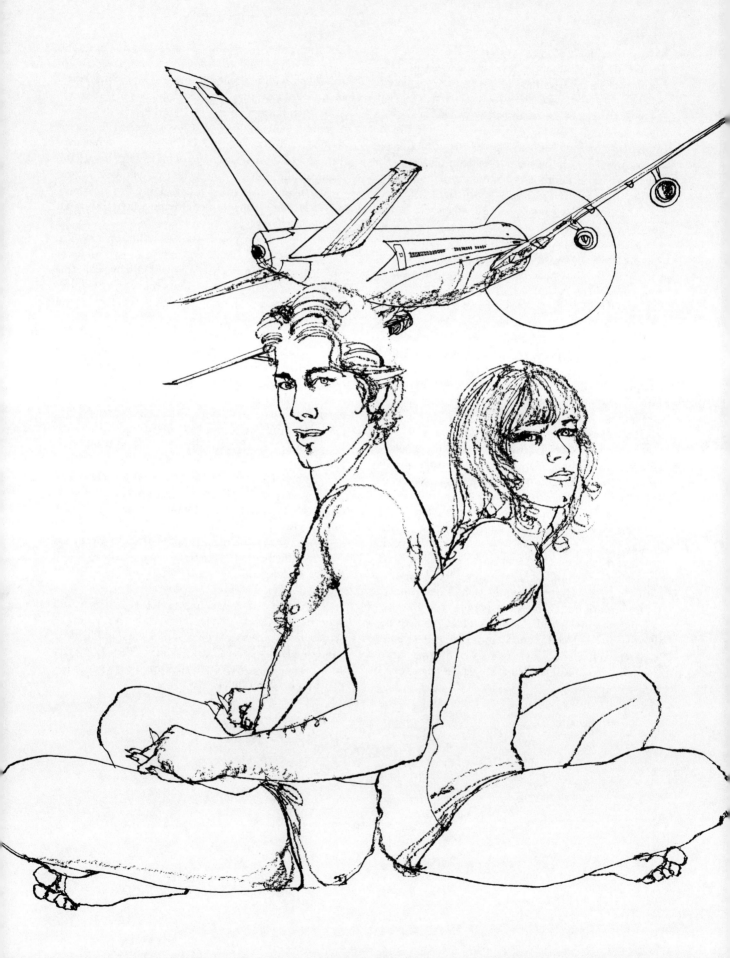

Part One:
The Emily Wilkens
Home Spa

1
Setting Up Your Spa

A week at a spa is the most luxurious, mind and body pampering experience I know of. It feels so self-indulgent that it seems almost sinful, yet a stay at a spa is one of the greatest health presents you can give yourself. In addition to the invaluable beauty tips and routines you will learn, the atmosphere at most spas is sure to strengthen your resolve to maintain that wonderful, newly-found feeling of fitness.

A spa visit should be the launching pad for self-care habits you can stick to, for a happier, healthier lifestyle. There is no reason why you should abandon the benefits you reaped from the Toni Beck exercise sessions you enjoyed at the Greenhouse, or the double-hairbrush method of scalp circulation you picked up at Arden's Maine Chance, or the Happy Feet Therapy you discovered at Rancho La Puerta, or the famed Palm-Aire Salt Glow that smooths you from toe to top.

If you visit a spa and take home just one helpful nugget to incorporate into your lifelong beauty- and health-care program, you'll have gotten your money's worth.

And whether or not you ever get to visit a spa, you can make use of spa techniques in your own home, even turn part of your home into a mini-spa.

The secrets I offer here are natural. Natural beauty to me is more than avocado facials and lemon hair rinses. It's a way of looking and feeling better by working WITH nature rather than against it; by learning to accept (and maybe even learning to like) what can't be changed about yourself.

You can learn how to become sensitive to your own beauty potential. You can become aware of how it feels to look terrific.

I don t mean to demean the value of paint, powder, perfume, and a good hair stylist. I don't recommend abandoning them now. But you can condition your hair to a NATURAL body and shine, instead of disguising its failings under a nest of teasing and spray. You can trim your thighs with exercise instead of squeezing them into latex shackles. The best makeup can't hide a complexion that has been coarsened by neglect or sallowed by french fries. The most expensive girdle can't give a flabby body its long-gone youthful grace. The most elaborate facial can't banish wrinkles or discontent and boredom. But once you're in the best possible physical and mental shape, you can look fantastic with half the effort! Every stroke of lipstick and every hair roller will perform to the maximum. TO SHOW YOU HOW, I'M READY RIGHT NOW TO SHARE THE SECRETS I'VE LEARNED FROM MY FAVORITE SPAS ALL OVER THE WORLD. Making the most of your home spa program can be most rewarding. Make every day count, and let's start working right now!

That Spa-like Atmosphere

SATISFY YOUR FIVE SENSES

Seeing

At the Greenhouse in Texas, the first thing that strikes you is the color of plants and flowers—indoors! Gorgeous greenery encompasses you when you first open the doors to this greenhouse for "wilted women." In your home spa room, or corner if you're cramped for space, hang pots of ivy or ferns from the ceiling. (One greenthumb trick I learned from an indoor Greenhouse gardener is to "water" hanging plants by adding a couple of ice cubes to each basket every few days.) Aside from the lovely, refreshing spring-like look plants give, they also give back oxygen to the air, a health plus for you!

The colors you use in your home spa can help nourish your soul as you go about the business of self-care. Always remember that color can truly influence how one feels. Elizabeth Arden personally loved pink. (She named her special shade Arden Pink—it's still in evidence on her original packaging.) Arden thought pink was the color most flattering to all her clients. At both her Maine Chances you were surrounded by crystal and mirrors and Arden Pink everywhere.

Mirrors are important for taking a long honest look at oneself. I don't believe that someone need be skinny-skinny to be attractive. In fact, over forty, and DEFINITELY over fifty, there are advantages on your side if you have a little flesh. Men like it—and you'll look better and feel better. (And if you need models to bolster being able to live with a few extra pounds, look at Ava Gardner and Christina Ford. Neither are model thin. Both are beautiful.) But your body should be in alignment; those extra pounds count too much if they're all huddled around your middle or your seat. If you look like a pear, or a banana, or even something not edible, start working. Everything is possible.

Hearing

At every spa—be it the Golden Door, the Greenhouse, Maine Chance, Palm-Aire, La Costa, the Ranch—music to exercise by stays in your head long after you've returned home. A good mix of José Feliciano, Burt Bacharach, Bert Kaempfert, Peggy Lee, Grover Washington, as well as Frank Sinatra (or German-style um-pah-pah), gets you in or out of a mood.

I've too often been tempted to tape the familiar music during the exercise sessions at Arden's Arizona Maine Chance. (In fact, when I did just that not too long ago, the cassette was taken away from me in front of the whole class—at Arden's taping IST VERBOTEN!)

Many spas have exercise cassettes available to take home, the Greenhouse and Palm-Aire leading the parade. If you're ambitious, you can tape your own series of cassettes of whatever music turns you on.

Smell

Incense is one lovely way of sparking up your home spa. I remember the first time I visited famed yoga teacher Indra Devi at her magnificent domicile in Tecate, Mexico. The special fragrance she brought back with her from her many visits to India was very much in evidence throughout. I recall feeling as if I were in another beautiful world after ten minutes.

One can find incense in one form or another at import-export shops in every big city. Many department stores sell it as well. Experiment until you find the smell that turns you on.

Don't forget that flowers are another way of catering to the sense of smell, as are such fragrant additions as eucalyptus or other scented leaves. It's simple enough to place bowls of POTPOURRI around the house, and especially in your spa center. (Gloria Vanderbilt does.) Save the petals from any flowers you grow or buy, spread them all out, and let them dry in the sun. Collectively, they have a faintly sweet and sexy smell. (Rose petals mixed with cinnamon and nutmeg is a good combination.) For your closets you can make pomander balls by sticking an orange all over with whole cloves, and hanging it from a ribbon. The scent of the orange and cloves melds for a freshly sweet result. (Replace pomanders every six months or so.)

Feeling

You'll never be a beauty unless you "feel" like a beauty. There's little pleasure in working out on a rough-surface rug or exercise mat. Try a fluffy terry velour or even a glove-like plastic, like the white Atlas exercise mats they have at the Golden Door.

When it comes to health and beauty preparations, let your sense of touch play a role in pleasing your skin, hair, nails, etc.

Taste

You'll read all about it further along in the diet section. I know (as I'm sure you do) that no one has made much progress in health or good looks by eating things they hate—or by using products and preparations for self-care that smell as if they taste horrible.

The Equipment You Need and How to Organize It

Now that we've established a delightful atmosphere, we have to get down to the nitty-gritty and talk about what you need to operate your beauty spot. Some people can work well with nothing more than an exercise mat or towel, a watch or clock, and determination! At the other extreme are those who can only thrive if supplied with every spa-like convenience or device. Here's the whole gamut of home spa equipment. Choose what you think you need and can accommodate.

Exercising Equipment

SLANT BOARD: This secret, which I first discovered at Maine Chance, allows you to lie in the beauty angle (feet twelve to fifteen inches higher than your head) while you relax or exercise. You can buy a slant board (which handily folds up for easy storage) in most department and sporting goods stores, fitness shops, and by mail order. If you're of normal height, the board should be about six feet long and eighteen inches wide.

Gaylord Hauser says the board should never be higher than one foot at the feet end—at least that's the magic angle he got from Greta Garbo. But I'm comfortable with it a mite higher. Ann Delafield said it brings the spine and viscera into balance, lifts falling faces, mitigates the baleful effects of gravity on the abdominal muscles, reverses the pull on vital body fluids, straightens out the spine, and enhances circulation to the hair and entire upper torso. My unscientific opinion is that it probably does a lot of good for your thought processes and memory. You can pad it with foam rubber or polyurethane, then cover it with canvas or plastic.

If you don't want to buy one, improvise a beauty board with a leaf from your dining room table (with beach towels for cushioning) or the ironing board tilted against your bed. Make sure it's strong enough to support your weight.

EXERCISE MAT: If store-bought exercise mats don't suit your fancy or your décor, make up your own exercise mat about three feet wide by six feet long. Either buy three-fourths- to one-inch-thick urethane foam cushioning (easiest to work with) or use cotton wadding. Make the cover of terry towels or another fabric that feels nice to you (and is washable), sew it, or if you're a lazy seamstress, safety-pin it together. If you have storage problems, roll up the mats so they become floor pillows when they're not being used for exercise. If you don't care about the aesthetics, simply exercise directly on your bedroom carpeting or use a quilted mattress cover in double bed size.

TWIST BOARD: A twist board is a nifty little device that really works on the waist and hips. (Most notions departments carry them, and they're quite inexpensive.) All you do is stand on the board and do an old-time twist motion, moving your hips or your shoulders from side to side with your legs firmly planted on the swiveling board. It's only about twelve by twelve inches and a really worthwhile beauty investment.

EXERCYCLE: If you have room for one, an exercycle is an excellent way to keep legs in beautiful shape. If you have the space, but lack the funds, several nationally known mail-order houses carry a device that transforms an ordinary bike into a stationary exercising cycle for about ten dollars.

JUMP ROPE: Two minutes a day jumping rope is a marvelous way to keep trim. (The Golden Door suggests that each of its guests take one home.) You can buy one with weighted handles for extra slimming benefits.

BALLS: A couple of brightly colored rubber balls (the same size as tennis balls) can be held between the palms of your hands and squeezed, then released, becoming a beautiful isometric exercise recommended by Maine Chance for firming the upper arms (a good safeguard against that aging flab) and the pectoral muscles. When the balls are pink or red or green, they're conspicuous and conducive to picking up during the day for ten quick squeeze-releases. If you work up to ten times a day, that's a hundred squeezes and a terrific boost for your arms and bosom area.

WEIGHTS: Strap-on weights or small barbells add to the effectiveness of many exercise programs. (La Costa's exercise classes use them.) If you don't want to buy the weights, hold a book in either hand instead. But if your problem is building shaplier legs, I suggest you buy the strap-on weights and wear then on your ankles while doing leg exercises.

EXERCISE STICK: A discarded mop or broom handle can be used for routines of stretching, bending, and posture-building. Palm-Aire has an entire exercise routine using a simple stick.

BALLET BARRE: If you simply cannot obtain a ballet barre (every Super Spa has one), a towel rack is very helpful for support in other bending and stretching exercises.

MASSAGE TABLE: A massage table is important so that loving hands can knead out all those kinks, knots, and maybe even some "cellulite"—and so that you can return the favor with what is justifiably called "the loving touch."

APPAREL: A leotard and/or a sweatsuit—or whatever makes you feel good while you're exercising—is necessary. It's nice to have a special outfit, and it's also more efficient. Anything sloppy or too tight will impede your movements. I like the leotards with a scoop neck and long sleeves. While long tights are fine if your exercise room gets cold, they're hardly necessary. If you want to wear them, get the kind with no feet for less constraint. If you're modestly proportioned on top, you won't need to wear a bra while exercising, but for those who need some support, a soft stretch bra will do. This is a meeting between you and your body, and the more fluid your clothes, the better. So no tight waistbands or collars; just a nice, easy knit—anything that can be thrown into the washing machine.

While the minimum in clothing provides maximum ease during exercising, there are cases where wearing more can mean more results. At many spas, the theory is that the body area that needs slimming down should be covered because the perspiration and lack of air helps work off the bulges. At the Golden Door for example, you're given a sweatsuit to wear for the morning walk. If you're top-heavy, you're given TWO sweat shirts. If you're bottom-heavy, they make sure you are doubly covered up in the leg area, with undershorts as well.

A hair covering—band, hat, or scarf, whatever suits you—is also important. Long floppy hair gets in the way while exercising, and all that movement does your hairdo no good. All the spas include special headgear to wear during workout sessions. I especially like the adjustable white terry turbans at The Greenhouse, but you may prefer a simple scarf or headband.

A washable, casual robe to wear while relaxing, before bathing, or while lying on the beauty board is also suggested.

For Beautiful Bathing

Aside from the tub and shower, you'll need and/or enjoy:

Bath oil, bubble bath, herbs for scented bath
After-bath splash-on cologne and talc
A Loofah mitt to scrub away dead skin cells
Body oil or lotion
A bathtub tray, handy for holding pumice, manicure implements, other grooming aids you'll want to use while combining a relaxing bath with self-care chores
A luxuriously big and fluffy bathtowel or a terry robe
The prettiest shower cap you can find because you hope you won't be taking all your showers alone.

These are everyday needs everybody can include in a home spa. Here are four delightful extras that maybe you'll have to wish on for a while.

A JACUZZI WHIRLPOOL, attached to your tub, to swirl and whirl the water for the most relaxing hydrotherapy you can have this side of one of the big spas. There are Jacuzzi dealers in every major town, eager to quote prices and give information.

A NEEDLE-SPRAY ATTACHMENT for your shower if you really want to wake up feeling zingy. You don't need a plumber to attach these special shower heads, and they're available in department stores and bath specialty shops as well as through many mail-order sources.

A HOME SAUNA, which can vary from a specially built model to transforming your existing bathtub into dual use as sauna and tub. This is a fairly recent addition to the home comfort field. Such manufacturers as Am Finn Inc., Haddon Ave. and Line, Camden, New Jersey, will send you details and prices.

A HOME STEAMBATH, excellent for soothing those aches and pains, is simply installed in your tub or shower. (For details, write ThermaSol, Ltd., ThermaSol Plaza, Leonia, N.J. 07605.)

THE ENVIRONMENT, a new concept, a new dimension in living. A special unit built into your home provides a synthesis of our natural environment. Using an exterior control, you can select the elements of nature you want to enjoy—Baja Sun, Tropic Rain, Jungle Steam, and Chinook Winds. This *pièce de résistance* is expensive, but well worth the price if you can afford it. (For details, write Kohler Company, 6 Corporation Park Drive, White Plains, N.Y. 10604.)

Facial Care Equipment

This will run the gamut from witch hazel for astringent to fresh fruit and eggs for natural facials, and such implements as tweezers for eyebrow grooming. An important category includes items for dental hygiene, from a toothbrush and toothpaste to a water-pik to keep gums healthy, breath sweet, and ultimately, those teeth cavity-free. Makeup, moisturizers, creams, and any other skin-care products also fit into this category, and the most important point is that they should be well organized and easily accessible. If you don't have a dream bathroom with many nooks, crannies, and drawers in which to store each and every need, think about using hatboxes or other portable cases for grouping specific products together so that you don't have to go searching for what you need.

The same organization is needed for HAIR-CARE EQUIPMENT. If you can't store them conveniently in your bathroom, pack all hair needs in a hatbox or wig case or whatever you fancy, stash it in your closet until you need it, and then pack it away again. Your kit should contain an ace bandage or hair band to protect hair and keep it away from your face during facials, a comb and natural-bristle brush, shampoo, conditioner, setting lotion, rollers, clips.

A portable kit also works well for products that take care of HANDS, FEET, and LEGS, including emery boards, orange sticks, cuticle remover, pumice or Pretty Feet lotion, nail polish, polish remover, cotton and/or cotton swabs, depilatory, hand and foot lotion, bed socks and short cotton gloves (to wear while giving hands or feet cream treatments), castor oil and white iodine (for nail building). While you may not want to include these in your special kit, exercise sandals are great for your feet and should be worn while you're working or just walking around the house.

Miscellaneous Niceties

One nice thing about an at-home spa is that you can keep improving it as you get into the swing of things by adding items as you can afford them. One special extra I would love is a mini-refrigerator planted in my bathroom or spa corner to hold a supply of healthy foods and beauty preparations. Creams keep better and longer when refrigerated, witch hazel works best and feels loveliest when chilled, and ice cubes are handy for toning skin.

Other extras that are not as costly might include a bowl to hold fresh fruit for snacking, an electric juicer to make fresh fruit and vegetable juice on the spot, and a facial sauna or skin machine for skin-care treatments.

Plan to wash your hair, do your nails, and give yourself a facial at a specific time each week. Your exercises and complexion care should be performed daily at a fixed time. If something important comes up that must have priority over your home spa time, set your alarm ahead one hour to provide time THAT DAY.

Not every beauty or exercise ritual will be for you. Try the ones you think will be fun, the ones you can stick with, the ones YOU need. Then figure out your program and mark it down on your special home-spa calendar. You will need to reserve at least ten minutes a day for exercises, and twenty minutes for beauty rituals—that is, twenty minutes over and beyond your customary cleansing, toothbrushing, bathing, etc.

2
Fabulous Feet
and
Lovely Legs

Like most people, you probably spend pitifully LITTLE time on your BEST beauty booster—happy feet.

Your feet can make or break your whole beauty effort. When your feet hurt, YOU hurt—all over. They carry your entire body. When you walk, your whole weight pounds down on each foot with every step. If feet are cramped into badly fitted shoes or too tight stockings, they can become very bitchy. Feet need air as well as room. When your feet hurt, you're less inclined to walk—and the less you walk, the dumpier your figure becomes. Tired feet telegraph their discomfort in frown lines on your face. The nerve endings of every vital organ in your body relate to a spot on the bottom of each foot, according to zone therapists (sometimes called acupressurists). Deep massage of the feet can alleviate many body conditions.

Feet should feel free and cool and comfortable —even with shoes ON. Take a look at the shoes you "live" in. Are they narrow of toe, too high of heel, too generously platformed? High heels bend your foot so that most of your weight is forced forward onto your toes. Usually they carry far too much weight. They thrust forward so that every step is off-balance. When your body is pitched forward at a forty-five-degree angle, there's no way you can stand or walk gracefully. High platforms imprison the feet and breed injuries ranging from twisted ankles to backaches.

Every woman, in my opinion, needs a pair of wood-and-leather exercise sandals. Most drugstores carry them. True to their advertising claims, they DO massage your leg and foot muscles with every step. I wear mine in the house instead of bedroom slippers.

15

How Clean Is Clean?

Of COURSE you wash your feet. But the soap-and-rinse routine of a bath or shower doesn't clean your feet. To remove ground-in dirt accumulated during a hard day's walking, you need a sturdy brush. You can use your old nailbrush, but you're more likely to remember to scrub if you keep a special foot brush with your bathing gear. Soap the brush very well to get those gray areas around your toenails and heels really clean.

Now, how do you get rid of the ugly crevices and calluses themselves? A wet pumice will plane them down smoothly if used every time you bathe. (Or, when your feet are dry, work on calluses with the fine side of an emery board).

Every time you bathe or shower, use your scrub brush and pumice stone and then dry each toe thoroughly. It may take a week or so to get your feet flower pretty, but you can be sure they will improve. (Don't expect any treatment to remove calluses or corns permanently if your shoes fit badly. Calluses "defend" your feet against pressure. As long as the pressure exists, they'll come right back.)

Solutions for Smoothing, Coddling, Sensualizing Feet

Are your feet truly smooth to the touch? Not yet? Okay, now is the time to slather on the smoothers —commercial products especially for feet. For feet that need a crash course of coddling, massage well with vaseline or corn, safflower, or baby oil. Then put on a pair of white socks for the night. One week of this nightly ritual often brings about spectacular results.

If your feet are perpetually rough and scaly, you might try a secret I picked up at the Ranch. Summon a few wheat-germ oil or vitamin E capsules to the rescue; puncture each capsule with a pin; squeeze out the oil; rub well into your feet and toenails nightly.

Baby or foot powder can absorb the moisture that often leads to irritation and blisters. Sprinkle it all over your feet, especially between the toes, and in your shoes. If your feet are already blistered, use cornstarch instead.

In the summertime—or whenever you're slinking barelegged and barefooted around the house—add twenty grains of menthol crystals or one ounce of spirits of camphor to a pint of unscented rubbing alcohol. When blended with baby powder and massaged well into the feet, this will give a luminous glow to the skin.

Baths That Revive or Relax

How many times have you found yourself just too tired to face a dinner or party that's only an hour or two ahead of you? When that happens to me, I have a great remedy I learned at Bircher-Benner! I sit at the edge of the tub and let hot water run over my feet. The water is as hot as I can bear it. I let it run for a minute or two, then switch to cold water. I alternate hot and cold streams over my feet for about ten minutes and —magically—I come alive all over.

More Footbath Tips
To assure restful sleep after a long HOT day, place a handful of mint leaves (mint tea bags are fine) in a basin of hot water, then soak your feet for ten minutes.

Following a long COLD day, use a cupful of Epsom salts in a basin of hot water to soak your feet.

If you ever have to show off your feet, soak them in a strong solution of ordinary tea. This tints the heels healthily and seems to prevent calluses.

16

A terrific footbath for tired feet is made by simply throwing a couple of spoonfuls of baking soda into hot water. If you follow the soaking with an alcohol rub and massage, you've got the perfect foot-resuscitating formula.

Massage alone relaxes and revitalizes your feet, but the more sophisticated can affect quite distant areas of the body by using zone therapy. At Maine Chance, the masseuse in zone therapy stimulates the left foot, for example, to affect the left side of the body. The tops of the toes are said to relate to sinuses, the area between the big toe and the next toe to eye tension, and so forth.

You can become your own therapist and relieve general bodily tension while getting your feet in tip-top shape. Here's how they do "Happy Feet" at the Ranch:

Happy Feet
Begin by sitting on the floor, one foot crossed over the thigh of the opposite leg, the bottom of the foot facing up to you and start working, first on one foot, then the other, in the following steps·
Grab the big toe and squeeze, rotating in large circles in both directions with much pressure. Follow with

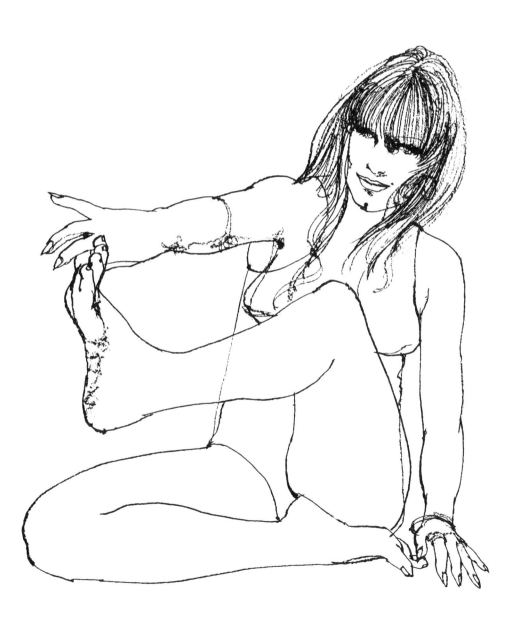

17

each successive toe, counting 1—2—3—4 as you "swing" them around.

Use your thumb behind the ball of the foot, forcing toes forward and then backward. This gives a definite lift to circulation generally.

"Dangle" one foot by lifting it up and holding on to one toe at a time—a form of traction permitting the toes to stretch out completely.

Now lean back, shake out your hands, flex feet, point toes. With legs straight before you, circle both feet one way, then the other—and take several deep breaths.

Return to first step. Insert fingers of one hand between toes, squeeze hand and toes with the other hand to exert as much pressure as possible.

Pretend your foot is a wet towel and wring and twist. Twist HARD!

Relax, then repeat this routine with the opposite foot, finally "slapping" both legs all over, bottom to top. Lie down, stretch out, and take a few deep breaths while you enjoy the reward of your labors: a fresh flow of energy from head to toe.

When you only have time for a simple massage, using your thumb or fingers (or the eraser end of a pencil) press firmly over the entire sole of the foot. Do this once a day if you can, spending two or three minutes on each foot. It feels particularly good when you've just taken off your shoes after a day on the job. Follow by one of the lovely footbaths cited above.

Maine Chance's Malaysian Foot Remedy
Fill a pair of shoes (low-heeled Oxfords would be ideal) with dried peas or round beans (such as soybeans). Get into the shoes, and walk around as long as you can bear the pain. The beans will massage every part of your sole.

Now that your feet are limber, clean, and smooth, it's time to pretty them up with a pedicure. Before you reach for the polish, a major complaint women have about their nails is constant dryness and splitting (this goes for fingernails, too). Remember, the cause is often old polish. Never, ever keep your toenail polish or

even base coat on longer than two weeks. If possible, let them live for a day or so without polish now and then. Help avoid dryness with a nightly oiling with baby oil, even if you're skipping the entire foot-smoothing.

Here's a professional five-point program, just as I learned it from the pedicurist at Tonfoni, that will give you the most perfect pedicure—and the prettiest feet—you've ever had.

The Perfect Pedicure

GET READY TO GO: Line up your implements. Keep a separate set from the ones used for fingernails, since feet can carry bacteria. You'll need a supply of fresh emery boards, a good pair of nail clippers, an orangewood stick, cotton, baby oil, a pumice stone (or pumice in stick form), a basin large enough for your feet, and a few soft towels.

CLEAN UP FIRST: Remove all nail polish. Then, file or trim toenails straight across. Use the scissors initially, followed by an emery board for smoothing. Leave corners exactly straight; rounding them encourages in-grown toenails. Then, soak feet in warm, soapy water (to which you've added a handful of baking soda or sea salt) for a few minutes. Use a pumice stone to smooth out calluses on bottom of the feet or any thickened skin areas on toes.

MASSAGE AND "FEEDING": Next, dry your feet and massage nails with either baby oil or petroleum jelly. Follow by working a dampened cotton-wrapped orangewood stick all around the cuticle gently to clean nails. This removes soap, cream, and other matter that tends to accumulate. Use cuticle scissors to remove any hangnails.

FINAL SUDSING: Now, plunge your feet back into the soapy water and scrub thoroughly with a nailbrush. After drying feet, use the fine side of an emery board to make sure no rough spots remain that may snag hose.

POLISH UP: To prepare for polish, separate toes with strips of tissue or cotton for easier application. Initially, apply a base coat. Then apply one or two coats of enamel. (Incidentally, it's considered just a bit tacky to match your toenail polish to your fingernail shade.) A final coat of sealer will help your pedicure remain intact.

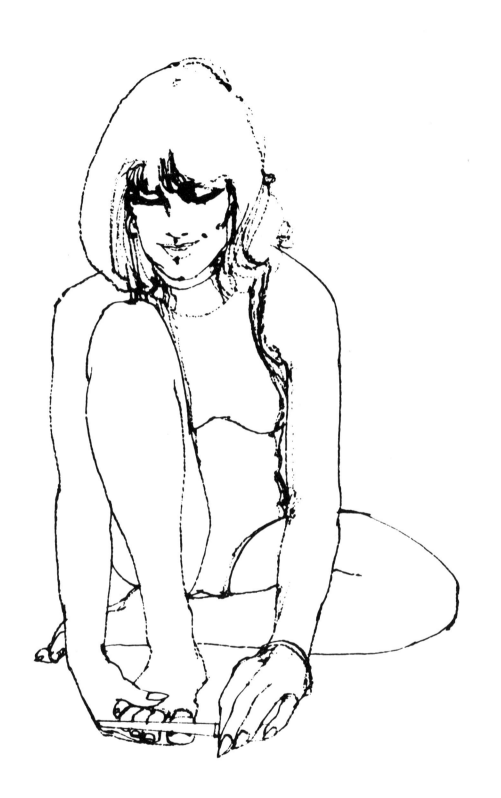

Your Legs Are Showing

Can they stand the scrutiny? Can they pass the tests of touchability and visibility? The shape of your legs depends on old Mother Nature and that little old exerciser—you. The touch test is something we have to settle right now, in the privacy of your home spa.

It isn't a complex problem, really. Look-again legs are the result of one major characteristic—smoothness. Your legs should be silky-smooth to touch, as soft as a baby's and as free from calluses, rough spots, scaly patches, AND hair as a baby's.

One major enemy of smoothness is a skin condition with a very homely name: "housemaid's knees." You're not a housemaid and you don't think you have it? Check your knees. Are they rough and grayer looking than the rest of your legs? You don't have to spend half your life on your knees for them to get that way (just as you don't have to hang out in bars to get "barmaid's elbows," a similar condition). Knee and elbow skin is constantly being stretched, leaned on, abraded. Even daily wearing of nylon hose can cause the knee skin to appear all dried out.

Here's a super treatment from the Golden Door to "recondition" your knees and keep them soft:

Soft Knees

BEFORE BEDTIME, apply a combination of cocoa butter thinned out with olive oil and rub into the problem area. Then soak for five minutes in a hot tub of water to which you've added a handful of baking soda plus two handfuls of unprocessed bran (available at health food stores). Using a rough terry washcloth, massage knees with the hot water, working in the oil and cocoa butter. Don't use soap. Dry lightly after bathing, reapply cocoa butter and oil mixture, and bandage knees lightly with cheesecloth for the night.

THE FOLLOWING MORNING, use hand lotion or baby oil or lotion on your knees before dressing. The second night, follow the same procedure, but massage knees in hot tub with coarse salt (instead of washcloth). This type of salt is widely available in supermarkets. Finish after-bath "treatment" as described above.

THE THIRD NIGHT, repeat the same routine, then use a mixture of cornmeal and oatmeal as a scrub instead of the salt or washcloth. By this time your knees should be looking very much better.

YOU MAY DISCONTINUE THE "BLITZ" PROGRAM after the third day, repeating one phase of it once or twice weekly as necessary. Keep up the cocoa butter and oil applications at night and use lotion by day. Between times, rub knees with the cut side of a cucumber to keep the skin extra soft.

Now I come to the hairy part of the smoothness story. While some European and South American countries still hold to the idea that body hair (I should say leg, arm, and underarm hair), is very sexy, most American men prefer to see their women's legs and arms free of those short, dark wisps. Until you get an Italian or Brazilian lover, better face the fact that you'll have to get rid of that excess hair. Choose your weapon:

SHAVING is not the solution for all women: the regrowth may get stubby from shaving steadily over the years. Others find there's no change in the quality or quantity of the hair. Always shave after a bath; always work up against the grain for closer results; should ingrown hairs occur, reverse direction and shave down. Most experts agree that you shouldn't shave the downy hair above the knee. This should be camouflaged by bleaching, or removed by using a depilatory or wax preparation.

DEPILATORIES must usually be repeated about every two or three weeks. They aren't as messy or smelly as they used to be, but for speediest clean-up, step into a lukewarm shower afterwards.

WAXING lasts the longest, from four to six weeks. This method—especially at first—is best handled by professionals who employ hot wax, honey wax, or cloth wax strips. The most daring variation of leg waxing used to be the bikini waxing to take care of leg-torso hair revealed by a brief bikini. This has been superseded by the string waxing, a result of the new bathing suit look that really brings your legs into sharpest focus. You can wax it yourself with commercial preparations (available at beauty counters), but they're a little tricky to use, and it's easier if a friend helps you.

3
The Body Beautiful

All About Bathing and Grooming

A beautiful body is, first of all, clean! The daily bath we take for granted was a luxury a century ago, when a lady had to make do with her china pitcher and wash-basin. A beauty bath can be soporific or energizing; a beautifier of body or a beautifier of the psyche; it can be spartan or luxurious. The "baths" produce all these effects and more, thanks to extraordinary muds and minerals.

In your home spa, you have to work with the water supply you have on hand, usually hard water. If you can't manage a water softener for your entire water supply, at least consider investing in one for your bathroom supply. If that is impossible, add commercial softeners to your bathwater. Hard water leaves a drying, irritating film on the skin—definitely not a best

friend of beauty. Only lavish rinsing will get rid of this.

Soap is a crucial consideration of your bath. Any soap will get you clean. But if you care about your skin you'll choose the right one for you. For DRY SKIN (very common in the United States), super-fatted soaps (containing cold cream, coconut oil, lanolin, or even cocoa butter) are best; OILY SKINS are better off with non-fatted glycerine or "soapless" types; blemished or sensitive skins respond to medicated soaps. After age thirty, however, it's best to use soap only two or three times a week and a liquid cleanser the rest of the time.

Once you're squared away with your soap and your water, you'll need a LOOFAH for scrubbing dry skin and reviving circulation, a shower cap, and bath oils, bubble bath, dusting powder, and body lotions.

Fountain of Youth Bath Secret

Wrap equal portions (a spoonful of each will do) of dried lavender flowers, rosemary, thyme, and dried mint in a large handkerchief or double cheesecloth. Place into the tub and pour very hot water over the bag, let it steep for 10 minutes. Then finish filling the tub and soak away! (This is a pleasant switch from bath oil and bubbles.)

Nero's wife Poppaea filled her tub with gallons of asses' milk, thus endearing her to both her admirers and the local dairies. The milk she used was said to have been enriched by an herbal diet. Here are some modern versions of Poppaea's milk bath that I've collected from spas all over the world.

Skim Milk Bath

Measure a cup each of powdered skim milk, oatmeal, and laundry starch into a handkerchief or double cheesecloth bag. Swish the bag around in the bathwater. Then scrub your body with it, soak for about twenty minutes, and you'll emerge with soft, smooth skin.

Luxury Milk Bath

Beat or blend a half-cup of corn oil into one quart of whole milk. Add it to a warm bath.

Oatmeal Bath

Tie a few fistfuls of oatmeal (instant oatmeal, please) in cheesecloth and add to your bathwater. Make a paste of some of it to apply vigorously to any rough spots—such as the knees, elbows, feet. (You may also use the paste on your face.) Let it harden awhile, then rub it off with a washcloth.

Sunburn Mollifier Bath

This will not only make your sunburn hurt less, but will also make you feel more alive. Fill the tub with tepid water and add two cups of cider vinegar. If you just need perking up, but haven't time for a whole bath, just add three tablespoons of vinegar to four cups of water and use the mixture for sponging.

Wake-Up-And-Go Bath

The greatest energizer I know is a proper bath. Yet few people know how to take a warm-up-and-go bath. You simply fill the tub with lukewarm water, soap up, and then rinse from the shower with alternating hot and cold blasts.

A bath can help you get to sleep, as well as wake you up. Try a luxurious, bubbles-overflowing, fragrant bath, with the water about two degrees above body temperature, with soft lighting and your favorite romantic music in the background.

After your bath, follow through with perfume and talcum powder. You can make your talcum powder even silkier (and your skin feel silker, too) by adding cornstarch. Especially good if you're using expensive talc.

Best Grooming

Good grooming is an umbrella term covering having clean and unwrinkled clothes, keeping your hair neat and your make up flawless. Here I want to cover only those grooming chores that involve the body. It's no more feminine to be so antiseptically unsweaty that you come off as a neuter than it is masculine to smell as if you hadn't changed your T-shirt in a week.

Your personal odor is a unique way of establishing individuality. My generation of Americans was conditioned to be perpetually anxious about offending with their "b.o." We blocked or masked personal smells with a bevy of deodorants and anti-perspirants, plus perfumes, colognes, and toilet water.

I'm not suggesting that you MUST throw out your anti-perspirant and perfume. I am suggesting that you let the real you come through a little more. For example, avoid mixing different cover-up fragrances. Buy UNSCENTED hair spray, deodorant, soap, or hand lotion. Or, buy a scented variety that will not clash with your favorite perfume. A lemon-scented body lotion and an earthy, musky cologne don't go together. Settle for one or the other.

Be careful about the scent you choose. Every person has distinctive differences in body oils, and those differences may make Chanel wonderful on Charlotte, but absolutely wrong on Charlene.

Judge by the reaction you get. If he loves it, lavish it on; if he is vaguely hesitant, keep searching till you get a definite "ummmmmm" or "Yummmmmm!" out of him. Remember, too, smoking, boozing, and certain medications can annihilate the effect of your perfume. A little perfume goes far. Just because YOU can't smell it doesn't mean others can't.

If the man in your life doesn't smoke, the irritation caused by the foul odors and tastes of your tobacco is quadrupled. Hair and wigs get a funny, musty smell, and so do clothes—not to mention your hands. Smokers should be extra vigilant about airing out, washing, refreshing—whatever is needed to deodorize smoke.

Typically, perfume is applied to the pulse spots—behind the ears, at the wrist and crook of the elbows, and behind the knees—where warmth helps the perfume to develop. Try different spots, or a little in several, until you get the right combination.

Deodorants and anti-perspirants are probably an improvement on our grandmothers' baking soda, but there are people who cannot use the popular products because they're sensitive to the anti-perspirants' aluminum chloride or chlorhydroxide. There are, however, hypo-allergenic products. Those who use anti-perspirants should have a smooth, unbroken skin surface. The combination of a rough shave plus the alcohol in the anti-perspirant can seriously irritate the skin.

You may be perfectly happy with your choice of deodorant until it loses its effectiveness. Your body gets used to a certain product and it no longer counters the perspiration. Change to another brand for several months. then you can switch back.

4
Holdable Hands
and
Fabulous Nails

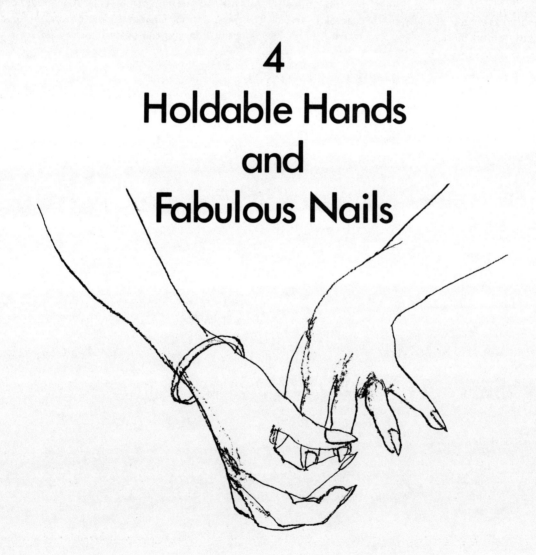

Your hands can be the surest giveaway to your age and your personality. Makeup can hide facial flaws, and a figure can be kept in shape for years. But hands that are neglected tell time and show toil all too well!

It's too bad we can't keep our hands in "cold storage," unveiling them only on special occasions. All day long, your hands help make the world go round. They rest only when you're asleep.

Hands

Here are some minute-taking, long-range effective ways to keep your hands young-looking.

Work Hand-in-Glove

This is a definite must. Collect a wardrobe of rubber gloves for the bathroom, the kitchen, the laundry room—any room where your hands may be exposed to water and/or chemicals. It may seem awkward at first to work "under cover," but if you develop the habit of wearing gloves ALWAYS, you'll enjoy smoother-looking, unworn hands.

Lavish on Lotion

Since skin gets thinner as the years go by, "wash" your hands with lotion rather than with soap and water when possible. Daily use of soothing baby oil, castor oil, lanolin thinned with oil, or softened cocoa butter maintains softness. In fact, castor oil helps guard against those dreaded brown ("liver") spots that can make your skin look so old. Remember to work the oil into your arms and up to your elbows, too. And speaking of lotion, don't put ANYTHING on your hands that you wouldn't put on your face!

Fight Red

A rub of fresh lemon helps bleach out redness on hands (or feet). For sweet results, try this secret from the Golden Door: Mix juice of one orange with a spoonful of honey and apply to hands to combat red-rawness.

Use the lemon or orange halves as little cups to rest your elbows in for five minutes (a good bleacher-smoother).

Crash Course

When hands are especially rough, the Greenhouse recommends mashing a ripe banana with a little olive oil. Smooth on, massaging well, then rinse off with lukewarm water and follow with hand lotion.

Fingertips

Keep your fingers flexible (and bump-free) by massaging for one or two minutes daily. Pretend you're putting on a tight pair of gloves and work from fingertips down to palm. Conclude your routine by gently "pulling out" each finger and shaking vigorously. Any task that involves manual dexterity is a youthifier, too. Playing the piano, knitting, typing, even weeding the garden, all help encourage joint flexibility and prevent aging rigidity.

When you want your hands to look luxuriously pale, raise them up in the air for a few seconds several times a day. This helps dispel the blue-veined look.

Cultivate Graceful Gestures

How you USE your hands is important, too. Follow the lead of famous actresses who develop graceful, elegant motions to give weight and drama to their words and motions. Stand in front of a mirror and practice.

And Now, About Nails

The vogue for longer-than-ever nails is stronger than ever—a trend frustrating to those who never seem to get all ten nails uniformly long and keep them that way. Nail beauty can be yours, however, if you com-

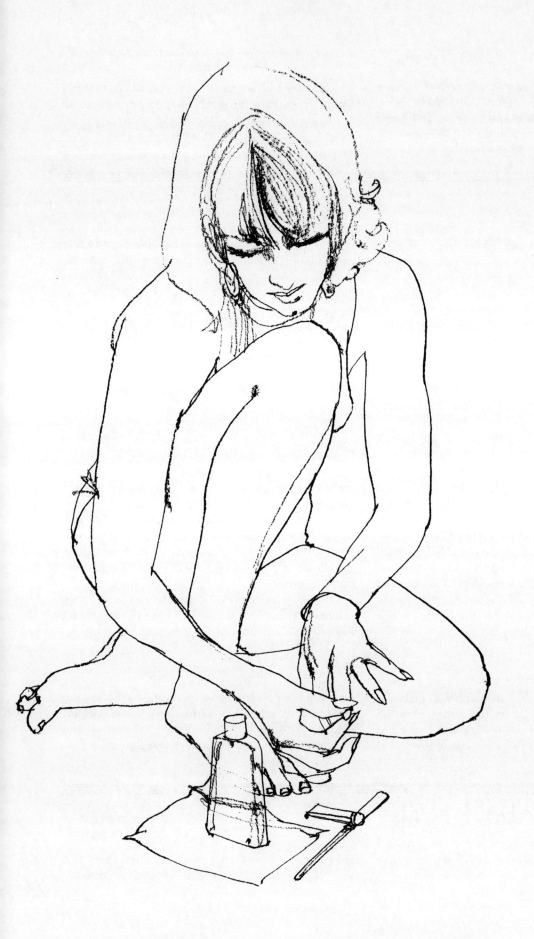

bine time, patience, and know-how with the right nail-care products and keep yourself in optimum general physical shape.

It's hard—no matter what you apply to them—to keep nails pretty if you're not in good health and eating right. There is also a hereditary factor to contend with.

The ridges, scalings, or differences in natural nail color are often a barometer of your condition. To your doctor, pale pink nails, for example, may suggest anemia, since they indicate the blood color. He may advise adding iron-rich foods (such as liver, raisins, beets, dried apricots, spinach, eggs, orange juice) to your diet. Nail softness is often a sign of thyroid imbalance.

Gelatin has long been thought of as a nail-enhancer, but calcium may be better still.

Milk and skim milk products are particularly helpful. Your doctor may recommend a calcium supplement containing di-calcium phosphate, calcium gluconate, plus vitamin D, and these seem most effective when taken with breakfast.

That's the inside story. Now here are protective and strengthening tips for the outside.

I've always believed that long, lovely nails—like healthy plant seeds—have to be kept warm to grow well. Try this Golden Door "nurturing" routine for a while:

Nail Nurture

Nightly, apply a mixture of castor oil and white iodine to the nails all around the cuticle. Ask your pharmacist for an applicator-type of bottle. Then massage in petroleum jelly and don a pair of thin, cotton gloves. If possible, wear the gloves all night when you sleep. If you have time during the day to repeat this procedure, do so. And if the iodine—castor oil routine seems too onerous for you, use hand lotion or baby oil. Remember that healthy cuticles are the secret to healthy nails.

To toughen your nails, try this secret I learned at Renaissance:

Dr. Popov's Nail Toughener

Wash an egg and cover it, shell and all, with fresh lemon juice. Let it bubble away for two hours at room temperature (the acid will dissolve the calcium in the shell) and then store in the refrigerator. Strain the mixture through a piece of cheesecloth; dilute and sweeten the juice with honey to make a calcium-packed lemonade. If you drink this daily your nails will, within a week, begin to grow stronger and lovelier.

Dr. Popov also has a solution for those brown "liver spots" on your hands:

Dr. Popov's Aging Spots Eliminator

Just rub the cut side of a juicy onion half over the spots and cover with castor oil. Leave the mixture on at least two hours (preferably while you're alone).

Don't expect overnight results. It takes four to six months to replace a new nail and the average growth is about one-eighth of an inch per month. Nails grow faster during the summer, and they also grow faster if you play the piano or type or if you bite your nails, but THAT defeats our whole program. Use your knuckles or the pads or sides of your fingers—or better, a tool—for finger work.

A good manicure not only protects your nails, but also calls attention to those newly-long nails and beautifully soft hands and rewards all your patience.

If you observe the following Maine Chance ritual once a week, your chance for exquisite nails is almost guaranteed:

Beautiful Nails

First, clean your nails carefully with polish remover.

File nails softly with the fine side of a worn emery board (rub one board against another to wear them down), keeping sides MORE SQUARED THAN TAPERED because this provides additional support for the new nail growing in.

Heat corn or castor oil in a Pyrex cup, and soak nails for five to ten minutes.

Wash with soapy water and cotton pads (NOT a brush). Dry carefully with a soft towel and push cuticles back gently. Use cuticle remover if necessary. Take care of hangnails with a sterilized cuticle-nipper or scissors (dipped in alcohol). Buff nails in one direction only, with either a chamois buffer or the heel of one hand working against the nails of the other.

Now you have ten sparkling nails smiling back at you. You are ready for careful application of these nail preservers:

1. A clear liquid base or protective conditioner, which can be compared to a prime coat before painting and acts as a buffer between polish and nail.
2. A milky base, of a creamy consistency, with hardener included.
3. TWO coats of your favorite polish. First apply under the tips of your nails and then do the "face" side. Be

sure to use a full brush. Wait at least ten minutes between coats.

4. If you insist on a pearlized finish, the third coat can be frosted. I advise against it on problem nails.

5. A coat of sealer, first underneath the nails, then on top, as a finale to your manicure and every few days thereafter to give you firmer nails than you ever thought possible.

Always allow several hours for drying this super manicure, and stay away from hot water (even with gloves on) since anything hot will soften the layers. To speed hardening, soak your nails in a bowl of ice water for twenty minutes.

Breakage

Now, what if you break a prize nail? You do NOT have to cut the rest of your nails down to matching size. You can repair the damage professionally by following these steps.

First remove the polish from the "fractured" nail, preferably with non-oily remover. Next, cut a strip from a fine linen hankie, a little longer and wider than the wounded nail. Squeeze a bit of glue—either the kind used for false nails or a heavy-duty contact cement—onto both the linen and the nail surface. Wait till the glue is tacky. Then place the patch over the damage, smooth it out with an orangewood stick, and remove any excess glue from around the patch with polish remover.

To create a smooth edge, tuck the overlapping part of the patch cleanly under the nail wherever possible. If near the base, carefully snip off excess with a cuticle scissors. You now have a fresh surface for applying your base coat, nail hardener, and polish. You may still use the nail fix and paper for added security. You will have to allow at least several hours of drying for this type of manicure.

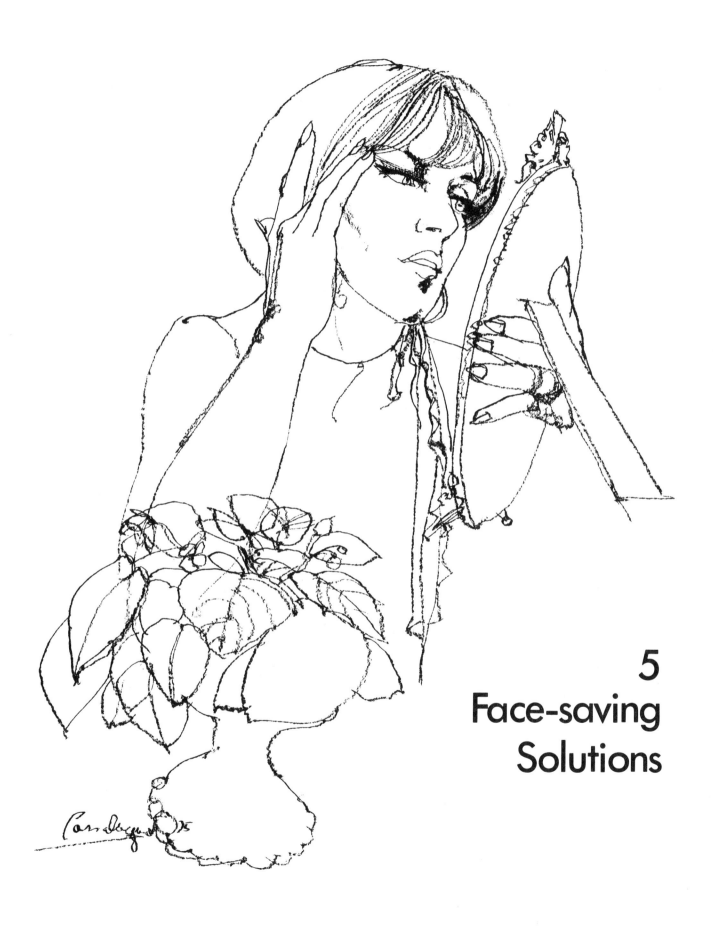

5
Face-saving
Solutions

What makes a woman look beautiful? It's that skin you love to touch. No makeup, no hairdo, no fashion can match the feminine, translucent, velvety glow of healthy skin.

No lotion or potion can take the place of good old-fashioned self-care—the kind of care your mother lavished upon you as an infant. Nutritious food and vitamins, proper rest and sleep, fresh air and sunshine, play and exercise, and most important, love and laughter—none of these is expensive. But we make them so hard to come by.

If the perfect complexion comes from dedication, the problem complexion usually comes from neglect. And I consider reliance on cosmetics and ignorance of true skin care the most appalling neglect.

Each period of a woman's life is distinguished by special problems. During adolescence the onrush of hormones excites physical and emotional problems. The sebaceous glands often produce more oil than the skin can cope with, which results in blemishes, blackheads, whiteheads, and acne.

Young adulthood is the most productive, usually happiest time. The girl blossoms as a woman. Unfortunately, she still has to cope with the legacy of her adolescence—often telltale scars, pits, and the like —which may disturb an otherwise poised adult. While hormone activity is usually more stable, occasional blemishes (particularly before the menstrual period) are bound to crop up. Add to this the tiny lines and wrinkles appearing for the first time—particularly for chronic dieters, sun worshippers, and midnight-oil burners—and you will realize why the "summertime of life" requires complexion assistance.

The years from forty-five on are a woman's prime. The "fabulous forties" are the best age for a woman to be—FOREVER! But they can seem like terrifying stretches of deterioration. Add the threat of discolorations that become permanent, the crinkles that become wrinkles, and you'll realize why dedication to a self-care program AT ANY AGE is so vital!

Do you think you can atone for the signs of neglect or the afflictions of bad genes or poor health with clever cosmetic camouflage? I assure you that you cannot. In fact, cosmetics may be compounding your problems. Notwithstanding all the propaganda for skin peelings, dermabrasions, silicone injections, face-lifts, miracle makeup, rejuvenating creams, hormones, and the like, the best answer is to treat your skin like the precious possession it is—always working from the inside out! This means proper diet, the right vitamins, brisk outdoor exercise, and sound sleep to stimulate the body functions.

Undoubtedly you've tried a multitude of commercial products that produced less than spectacular results. While you experiment with one, it seems that five more are introduced to take its place in a costly and frustrating cycle. If you've tried the rest, now try the BEST (and the CHEAPEST).

Aside from its role as a protective covering, the skin is an "organ" of the body with special functions. It responds to care just as your heart and stomach do. It is vital to maintain the skin's balance of acidity and alkalinity. In choosing any skin-care product, be sure to check the pH. A pH below 7 is acid; above is alkaline. Alkaline tends to destroy your acid mantle.

One scientific fact should make you optimistic: the cells of the skin are shed and replaced every twenty-seven days by a process called "keratinization." Anyone can refresh a complexion with fabulous results within one month.

The Rules of the Skin Game

1. NUTRITION. Greasy foods and high-carbohydrate concoctions are your enemies; high-protein meals, fresh fruit, and vegetables are your allies. Vitamins A, the B complex, C, and D are all skin beautifiers.

2. WATCH THAT WEIGHT. Excessive weight loss means accelerated wrinkles. Drastic dieting stretches the skin, leaving lines almost impossible to erase. Try not to lose more than one or two pounds a week, especially after age forty.

3. WONDERFUL WATER. Water is a beauty aid more precious than you might think. If you drink six glasses of water per day for one week, you'll see results more convincing than words. There's no better way to put a moist look from inside out on older skin and help clear up a blemished complexion.

4. ELIMINATION IS ESSENTIAL. If you don't get rid of wastes, the results will show on your skin. If necessary, eat more bulk foods such as WHOLE grapefruit

(the pulp counts), a WHOLE orange, leafy greens such as spinach, dandelions, and cabbage. Dried prunes are good. (So are the six daily glasses of water.)

5. FRESH AIR. A daily walk does wonders for your face and figure and feeds your face some precious fresh air.

6. SUN SAVVY. Twenty minutes of this natural source of vitamin D is fine, but excessive sun exposure can be disastrous.

From the thirties on, the sun brings out fine lines that never quite disappear. Later on, the sun encourages brown spots, permanent freckles, and spider veins. Sunscreens help, but if your skin tends to drink them up and break out from too much lubricating, sun-control products—which get baked into the skin—are almost worthless.

7. SERENITY. There's no substitute for tranquility. Worry etches its havoc into your face. So work for inner calm. Regular rest and adequate sleep are crucial.

8. VICE IS NOT NICE. Research has proved beyond question that smoking and excessive sun are the chief enemies of youthful skin. Too much alcohol can eventually puff up the face and slacken the skin and elasticity. If you must, smoke a little and drink a little—but THINK a little, too!

9. THAT BEAUTIFUL ANGLE. You'll enjoy a bonanza of benefits to the circulation and the complexion when you rest with your feet twelve to fifteen inches higher than your head. This creates the "beauty angle." Ann Delafield, who popularized it, often enjoyed facials in this feet-up, head-down position. So did Elizabeth Arden. All emollients, masks, and beauty treatments work better in the beauty angle. It is a face-saver that defies both gravity and aging. If you only remember one thing from this book, remember to lie in this position for ten minutes to half an hour every single day!

The nuts and bolts of skin care are cleansing, toning-firming, moisturizing, and lubricating.

Super Cleansing

The first step to lovely skin is to come clean with one of these soaps:

FOR NORMAL OR COMBINATION SKIN:	**Camay** or **Dove** (both gentle and non-drying) **Neutrogena,** coconut oil, or glycerine soap, **Basis.**
FOR OILY SKIN:	**Kirkman's, Physicians and Surgeons.**
FOR DRY SKIN:	**Castile Soap, Hershey's Cocoa Butter Soap,** yogurt- or lanolin-based soaps
FOR BLEMISHED COMPLEXIONS:	Sulphur, mud, oatmeal, or brown laundry soap.

Wearing rubber gloves, splash the face with hot water. Work up a lather, massaging well into the chin and nose areas. Fill the sink with hot water and a few drops of cider vinegar. Rinse with at least thirty splashes of the water-vinegar solution. The rough surface of the gloves stimulates facial circulation, especially in lined areas.

Baby oil is a soft-touch way of removing your makeup. Apply with tissue or cotton wads; then use an old terry towel for mopping up. If you prefer cleansing cream, apply all over face, then remove by pressing a tissue flat against your face. Smooth over the creamed areas and let the tissue absorb the excess. Peel off, starting with the cheeks, then the forehead. Use the cream-soaked tissue to massage (upward, always) your neck.

Another good makeup remover (especially for blemished skin) is a combination of milk-of-magnesia and mineral oil. You ought to spend as much time taking off makeup as you do putting it on. Yesterday's cosmetics breed tomorrow's skin problems.

In addition to daily cleansing, you'll need to know special clean-up techniques for coping with blemishes or scrubbing off dead skin. Try these champion cleansers:

Commercial Scrub
Various cleansing grains (such as Brasivol): for scrubbing blackheads, twice weekly, instead of the soaping routine, moisten the scrub with water, apply to face, rub the areas where blackheads pop up, and rinse off with lukewarm water, finishing with chilled witch hazel or ice toning (see below).

31

Cornmeal-Oatmeal Scrub

Mix equal quantities of cornmeal and regular (NOT instant) oatmeal with hot water to make a paste. Apply while still warm. Leave on ten minutes. Rinse off with cool water. For extra cleansing and tightening, add a few drops of camphor spirits to the rinse water.

To dry up pimples, wage war with one or several of the following:

Blemish Banishers

1. Calamine lotion with 1 percent phenol
2. Spirits of camphor, used on a cotton swab
3. A mild solution of boric acid, applied with a cotton pad
4. Lotion Alba, a soothing preparation available through your pharmacist
5. Unperfumed talc
6. Milk of magnesia (mint flavor), especially helpful on oily areas.

Moisturizing Magic

More and more beauty experts are stressing the fact that dry skin looks like old skin. Two vital beauty stratagems are MOISTURIZING (which maintains or increases the water content of the outer skin) and NOURISHING or "lubricating" the skin (by adding oil or other skin enhancers).

SUPER MOISTURIZING TREATMENT: Moisturizers protect your skin from outside attack, including cosmetics. They should be applied in the morning each and every day.

1. Apply baby oil to your face and castor oil beneath the eyes and on your neck. Work the oils round and round, up and out with your fingertips. Dot any blemishes with calamine lotion plus phenol. You should not ever use any type of oil or cream on blemished areas.
2. Try the Rag Doll Shake to bring the blood to your face. Bend down with head and arms dangling toward floor and sway from side to side, doing a few bounces to the left, a few in the middle, and a few on the right side. When finished breathe deeply.
3. Follow through with your soap-and-hot-water routine. Complete with vinegar rinse and witch hazel toning.
4. Next, take an ice cube in each hand and massage entire face. Finish with chilled witch hazel or astringent.

MOISTURIZING MASKS: Masks are the newest commercial beauty fad and the oldest skin treatment. Mudpacks were discovered by Egyptian slaves who found that washing clothes in a river day after day made their hands and feet beautifully smooth. So they tried the mud on their faces, and that worked too. Through the centuries, women have found that slapping natural ingredients on their faces—from mud, honey, and fruit to oil and milk—enhanced the complexion.

The general procedure for applying a mask is as follows:

Pat castor oil (or baby oil or eye cream) around the eyes. If your skin is VERY dry, oil or cream the neck, too. Then apply mask to the rest of the face AND the neck. Whenever possible, rest in the beauty angle for ten or fifteen minutes while you wear the mask. Remove with cool water and follow with chilled astringent.

Greenhouse Dry Skin Pleaser

To make this mask at home you simply mix avocado oil with a little skim milk powder to thicken. Follow general procedure.

Safety Harbor Oily Skin Pleaser

Mix fresh grape juice (white grapes are best) or fresh tomato juice (if you have a juicer) with skim milk powder. Follow general procedure.

Toning, Firming, Tightening Up Your Face

All skins respond to toning, freshening, and firming. My favorite toner is that all-time winner, witch hazel—nicest and most effective when chilled. It restores vitality to your complexion by refining the pores and sustaining a glow. An astringent should be the finale for any special beauty treatment, whether cleansing, moisturizing, or nourishing.

Maine Chance Quick-Result De-Pouching Procedure

Following a really deep cleansing of the face, apply an unsaturated or Vitamin E oil. Then take a large thin piece of absorbent cotton and form a mask large enough to cover the whole face. Poke holes for eyes, nose, and mouth. Soak the mask with astringent (I use witch hazel), then cover your face with it, patting well so that it fills in all the hollows. Then lie in the beauty angle position for twenty minutes. When you get up (which, I guarantee, you'll do reluctantly), remove the cotton and wipe off the excess cream.

La Costa Facial Skin Balancer

This technique can give drab, lusterless faces a marvelous healthy glow. Just pat buttermilk (or a cup of whole milk with a teaspoon of lemon juice) over the face, let dry, and then rinse with cool water. This restores the normal acid-alkaline skin balance and acts as an effective astringent.

Warmbad Villach Ice Toning

Keep a special small-cube tray of ice cubes made of spring or distilled water to cap your morning wash. If your skin is dry or sensitive, cover ice cubes with thin cotton or tissue and rub lightly to tighten pores and dispel tiny lines. Rubbing the ice lightly around the eyes reduces morning puffiness. (If wrinkles are a problem, apply castor oil first.)

Vinegar Winners

If your face feels tight after a soap-and-water wash, use a teaspoon or two of apple cider vinegar in a basin of cool water for a final rinse. (Five or six drops of fresh lemon juice on a dampened cotton pad will also help restore pH and cut down excess oiliness.) Barbershops and salons in spa areas often use a commercial vinegar lotion for refreshing. You can make your own toner (and avoid smelling like salad dressing) by adding a good amount of mint, sage, lavender, rosemary, or a blend of spices to a quart of vinegar. Let it sit for two days, strain off the herbs, boil the solution with an equal amount of water, let cool, and then use as astringent.

Cucumber Wonder

For bleaching and toning bonuses, squeeze the juice from one cucumber with a juice extractor, add to an equal amount of milk (cream for dry skin; whole milk for normal; skimmed milk for oily) and pat on face. Remove with lukewarm water.

Renaissance Dry Skin Firmer

Mix two egg yolks, two teaspoons honey, one teaspoon rosewater, one beaten egg white until thick enough to hold. Add a little skim milk powder if it seems too runny. Follow general procedure for masks.

Dr. Lauda's Oily Skin Firmer

Beat two egg whites until stiff; blend in one-fourth teaspoon baking soda and one drop of spirits of camphor. Follow general procedure for masks.

Emily's Honey Mask

Beat the white of an egg until stiff; fold in a teaspoon of honey. Follow general procedure for masks. To tighten and super-clean, mix a handful of oatmeal with water and a little honey. Apply to face; let dry and rinse off with cool water. (This is a good scrubber for backs and shoulders, too.)

Palm-Aire Cucumber Cure

Put a cucumber through the blender; mix pulp with a beaten egg white, add a few tablespoons of baby cream to the mixture. Chill several minutes and follow general procedure for masks.

Special Renaissance Tightener

The membrane that lines eggshells can help dispel wrinkles. Remove carefully while still moist, apply to clean skin. Smooth over forehead frown lines and along nose-to-mouth furrows, as well as over crinkles at sides of eyes. Relax face completely. Lie in the beauty angle, and—after ten minutes—remove egg with warm water. Massage skin lightly with castor oil.

How to Give Yourself a Face-saving Facial

Facials are different from masks, which usually work quietly on their own without any further help from you until it's time to remove them. You can enjoy glowing results with a do-it-yourself home facial by using any of the creams or oils (or a combination) that I talked about above.

Home Spa Facial as Taught at the Ranch

Start with an ultra-clean face. Make a paste of oatmeal and water (or buttermilk), rub all over face except the eyes. Let dry for a few minutes; rinse off with cool water.

Prepare your face food. Warm your chosen oil or cream in a Pyrex cup until it's pleasantly warm, not hot. Tie back your hair, sit in front of a mirror. As you work on each area, dip your finger in the cream or oil.

Using your right hand, start at the left side of your throat just under the COLLARBONES and sweep the cream up toward your CHIN. Follow with the left hand on right side, and keep alternating hands as you work across your NECK from left to right, from collarbone to chin —about six strokes to each of the three places for each hand.

Hold your left ear taut with left hand. Swing right hand under the chin from left to right. Repeat movement from right to left, holding right ear with right hand. The backs of your hands work well for this step.

Place both forefingers on either side of the NOSE, and draw them down from the bridge of the nose toward the cheekbones. Then slash off under cheekbones toward each ear.

Using index fingers of each hand, work firmly up the NOSE BRIDGE, on to the FOREHEAD over the EYEBROWS, and out toward the TEMPLES (smoothing over each line or imaginary line).

Rest your elbows on a tabletop, close your eyes, and massage your TEMPLES with the middle fingers, rotat-ing backwards with slight pressure five or six times. (You must be relaxed for this movement.) From the temples, work down the SIDES OF THE FACE past the earlobes, using a slight vibrating motion. Continue down the cords of the NECK and taper off at the back of the neck.

Concentrate on the area between your lip and nose next, using your index finger with a bit of pressure to massage those little lines (or lines to be) round and round.

The EYES are last. Starting at the temples, use forefingers and follow the bone structure of the eyes, working in toward the nose with butterfly pats under the eyes, since this is non-contractile skin. When you reach the inner bridge of the nose, switch to pressing and rotating movements up and under the eyebrows, lifting up and out.

Repeat each step several times with a definite rhythm. Once you've mastered the art, it should take no more than ten minutes to achieve face-saving results.

Here's a facial I learned at Bad Gastein:

Facial à la Marianne

Mix an egg yolk with a tablespoon of cottage cheese. (Marianne uses eggs in most of her recipes. The whites, she feels, are best for young skins with large pores that need tightening. The yellows are particularly nourishing for mature skins.) Add a few drops of fresh lemon juice, the contents of four (100 I.U.) vitamin E capsules (simply pinprick, squeeze out the oil, and throw away the gelatin capsules), a half-teaspoon of honey and a half-teaspoon of water. (Too much honey makes the mask "pully.") Mix well and apply to the face, leaving it on for ten minutes. When you feel the skin tightening, wash it off with lukewarm water.

Then sponge off the face with cool rosewater.

Super-Rich Masks

Emily's Magic Mask

The eyes: Before donning your mask, pat castor oil around your eyes, which get special treatment after the mask is applied to the rest of your face and neck. Try the mask and eye treatment while reclining on your slant board. The eyes are revitalized by filling two gauze bags with grated raw potato, which you leave on your eyes while you're resting.

The face: Mix a handful of oatmeal with water and 2 teaspoons of honey, forming a thick paste that you will use to cover your face. After it dries, massage it off and rinse with cold water. (As an alternative, mix equal parts of cornmeal and oatmeal with hot water to make the paste.) The rest of the mask is removed by rinsing first with warm water, then cool water, followed by chilled witch hazel.

Apricot Ace
For a rich facial plumper, soak a cup of dried apricots in water; then mix with a handful of grapes and a little skim milk powder, and whirl in a blender. If you don't eat this luscious concoction first, follow through with general procedure for masks.

Avocado Wow
Halve and peel an avocado, place in a blender with a bit of skim milk powder. Follow general procedure.

Banana Bonanza
Mash half a ripe banana with a fork or potato ricer. Add a little skim milk powder. Follow general procedure.

Berry Beautifier
Mash one-half cup of fresh strawberries with a fork until the berries are puréed. (Or mix in blender.) Stir in skim milk powder to thicken. Follow general procedure.

Miscellaneous Specials to Help You Save Face

Wrinkle-Fighting Exercise
Guard against droopy lines and wrinkles by CHEWING SUGARLESS GUM (in PRIVATE, of COURSE). Chewing relaxes facial muscles, helps tone them, and prevents those lines. Another good exercise is chewing the honey cappings (wax) from a jar of natural honey.

Dr. Lauda's Blitz Mask
In a hurry for a facial mask to work? Remove the hood from your portable hair dryer, and turn the temperature to warm. In less than five short minutes, you're dry and ready to rinse off the mask. This shortcut works well when you're on your beauty board (as you should be after applying a mask). Simply place your board near an outlet and let the drier do its work while you relax and enjoy it. Incidentally, smile whenever you have a mask or makeup on.

Mountain Valley Fresh Face Finish
Fill a spray bottle with mineral, spring, or rainwater. After completing your makeup, mist face lightly, blot with tissue. This avoids an overpowdered look and leaves face looking fresh. (Use the rest of the water to give your plants' leaves a treat.)

Eye Beauty

Eye-Doers
If commercial eye creams make your eyes swell, switch to castor oil—effective and non-allergenic. Plastic surgeons recommend it. Apply the oil gently and finish by lifting each eyebrow up and out. Blot oil off after ten minutes.

Banish Bags
Erase temporary wake-up bags, crybaby eyes, fatigued or allergy eyes with a cold water pep-up straight from the faucet or refrigerator, or use cracked ice wrapped in a handkerchief. For SUPER results, place chilled wet tea bags on eyes for five or ten minutes to reduce puffiness. Another spa secret: Grate half a potato and wrap in a dampened gauze square. Leave on eyes for about five minutes.

Pillow Talk
If puffiness seems chronic, try sleeping on an extra pillow.

6
Hair Care

Every woman knows the appearance of her hair is more important than her makeup, or even her dress. Millions of dollars are spent each year on hair care. But ironically, the luxurious, thick mane so admired on the Gibson girl has become a memory. Salon hairdos, artificial drying, detergent shampooing, teasing, spraying, coloring, and over-processing have damaged hair and created a host of problems.

If you get to know your own scalp and hair, you can get better results at the salon. All top models are expert with their hair, since shining locks and with-it styling are musts for them. They know outer control and styling as well as the diet and care needed to maintain that glorious sheen.

Hair responds to care. You can improve its texture and thickness, brighten its color, increase its body and manageability. Know-how is crucial. Happily, many of the best treatments use everyday, inexpensive ingredients.

Typecasting: Necessary Know-how

First you must determine your hair type.

DRY HAIR looks dull, feels brittle, breaks and splits at ends, is limp and generally hard to manage. Improper diet, exposure to sun and wind, and over-processing can be the culprits.

FINE HAIR has little body or curl, is hard to set, straight, and often dry. The condition is sometimes inherited, sometimes diet-caused.

COARSE HAIR is usually limited to brunettes, redheads, and those with naturally curly hair; it tends to be busy and unmanageable. External aids, including oil shampoos and conditionings, will improve it, as will a good layered cut.

OILY HAIR looks stringy and separates easily, even a day or so after shampooing. It may be caused by glandular changes (adolescence or pregnancy) or a diet over-rich in carbohydrates and animal fats.

Dandruff often accompanies oily hair. Shampooing too frequently with strong soap can be a factor; illness is often at the root of the problem.

Hair reflects your general health. Since hair is nourished by the bloodstream, it weakens when body resistance is down. Italian, Spanish, and Oriental women have lovely, luxurious hair—which is why the best wigs are made from imported hair. Their secret is the use of unsaturated oils (olive, sesame, soy) in daily cooking. While surface treatment of conditioning, massage, and shampooing can smooth and strengthen hair strands, hair is actually fed from the inside out through proper diet. Vitamins A and D (found in fish liver oils) and the B complex are extremely important, along with a high-protein diet stressing iodine-rich fish, meat, poultry, eggs, fresh fruit and vegetables, and dairy products.

Hairbrushing

Triple-treat your hair to brushing, massaging, and head-down exercising. Each increases circulation at the scalp while activating the oil glands of the hair shafts for elasticity and "bounce."

Maine Chance Two-Hairbrush Method of Increasing Scalp Circulation and Hair Luster

First, before washing, massage the scalp with a SMALL amount of cream or oil. Then, bending over from the waist to let the hair hang down freely, brush the hair thoroughly but GENTLY with two soft, natural-bristle brushes alternately. If your brush is a bit too "boarish," you can soften it by soaking it in hot water. Brush from the SCALP down. (It's not always necessary to brush a hundred times a day. For fine or damaged hair, this could be disastrous.)

Experiment until you find the amount of brushing that leaves your scalp feeling alive and tingling. Daily brushing helps control oil by removing the excess (cover your brush with cheesecloth or an old stocking for extra benefits). Since brushing stimulates the glands, it also helps dry hair.

The Carlsbad Dry-Hair Rectifier

Warm a half-cup of oil—olive, sesame, or corn oil —and add to it a teaspoon of cider vinegar. Section off your hair. Pat the oil over your entire scalp with a cotton pad. Now wrap your head in plastic or aluminum foil, followed by successive hot towels. The more hot towels you apply, the better the results you'll get. Leave the oil on at least two hours—or better, overnight—shampooing away the residue in the morning (using two or three soapings and a most thorough rinsing).

If hot towels aren't convenient, you can use a hair drier for ten minutes.

Mayonnaise, rich in eggs and oil, is an excellent alternative to any of the oils mentioned. After either a mayonnaise or oil conditioning, three soapings may be necessary to remove all the oil.

The Carlsbad Dry-Hair Groomer

Use the tiniest smidgen (size of your thumbnail) of a blend of lanolin (one part) and fresh castor oil or sesame oil (five parts) on the dry ends. Apply with your palms or brush bristles after shampooing.

Other conditioners are applied in the form of after-shampoo rinses or setting lotions.

Roland's Baden-Baden Beautifier

Mix two egg yolks with a half-cup of safflower oil or other unsaturated oil. Warm the oil before mixing. You can do this by placing it in a Pyrex cup over the hot water you're going to use for your shampoo. When it's lukewarm, but not hot, apply the mixture to your scalp and hair. Leave it on for two hours, wrapping it in aluminum foil and then a towel.

Afterwards, shampoo your hair three times, and set it with beer.

Shampoo Science

The best rule for shampooing is to wash your hair only when you feel that it needs it. Remember, that it's the SCALP that needs massage and soaping. Don't worry about the hair itself. The scalp must be liberated from dirt so that the oil glands can work properly and effectively.

La Costa Shampoo Strategy

When shampooing, massage scalp with your fingertips, never your nails. Two soapings are usually adequate (except after an oil conditioning), thorough rinsing is most important. A final rinse of cold water will make your hair shine and hold a set longer, too. Always rinse until your hair squeaks.

Emily's Special

Once a month, treat yourself and your hair to this feast. Separate two eggs, add the whites to your castile shampoo, and beat until foamy. Apply this egg-shampoo mixture to hair, massage well, rinse thoroughly, and lather again. Then massage the beaten egg yolks into the hair for a few minutes. Rinse first with lukewarm water, then cold.

Montecatini Secret

If you have dyed or tinted hair, be sure you've investigated the special shampoos for treated hair. After soaping, follow with a rinse of one egg beaten with a tablespoon of bay rum until foamy. Rub well into scalp and then rinse with cool water. Dandruff often responds to daily shampooing with a coal-tar or anti-bacterial shampoo; tincture of green soap improves excessively oily hair.

Emergency Shampoo

For oily hair, between washings, go over the scalp with cotton dipped in witch hazel or cologne.

When you can't shampoo, use cornmeal for a quickie clean-up: light cornmeal for light hair, yellow for dark. Rub into the scalp; then bend over the bathtub and brush out the cornmeal. Your hair will feel much cleaner.

Bad Gastein Rinse Hints

Add a tablespoon of vinegar to a cup of water as a final rinse. Blondes should use white vinegar; brunettes, apple cider.

Tea is another body-lender. Brew a mixture of one tablespoon of rosemary or camomile tea with one-half pint of water; simmer one hour; strain. Add three tablespoons of bay rum.

Stale beer adds protein to hair. Work into scalp. Rinse with cold water.

Gelatin is a source of pure protein. Mix half a packet of unflavored gelatin to a cup of water; work through hair; rinse as usual.

Setting Secrets

Before setting, hair should be smooth and untangled. Setting lotion tames the tangles and assures a good set. Many women do well with beer straight from the can or bottle as a setting lotion, applying it directly after shampooing and rinsing.

Another winner. Boil three-quarters of a cup of flaxseed (available in drug and health food stores) in one quart of water. Simmer ten minutes; strain through cheesecloth; cool and store in a glass jar.

Always rewet hair before applying setting lotion; apply to one strand of hair at a time, as you set it.

7
The Tiger-Woman Diet

This diet will do more for you than anything you can get at any spa, no matter how fancy or expensive. It can help you become thinner, livelier, lovelier, healthier—and stay that way. In short, you can become a beautiful tiger of a woman!

It includes the best part of diet plans from many spas. I've snooped around spa kitchens and interviewed spa chefs and learned a lot of spa-food tricks. My conclusion is that no spa offers you a workable plan for MAINTAINING YOUR OPTIMUM WEIGHT WHILE ENCOURAGING OPTIMUM GOOD LOOKS, VITALITY, AND HEALTH.

A spa visit is a CRASH COURSE, not a way of life—an interlude on which you build, not continue. You can lose a lot on a Shangri-La fast, or a Grayshott Hall water-and-grapefruit regimen. But you can't go on fasting-and-floating for the rest of your life.

Some spa-inspired diet "cheats" are marvelous and imaginative, and I've incorporated them into my home spa plan. For example, try serving just the crunchy, delicious vitamin-packed skin of a baked potato with a little sea salt and butter.

The serenity and pleasure of having a lifelong diet plan mapped out for you was brought home to me not so long ago by a glamorous friend. Gretchen and I had dinner together in Paris. She ordered grapefruit, salad, steak, and demitasse. A few weeks later I dined with her in Rome in a gourmet's paradise. She repeated the same menu. Some months later in Switzerland, seeing that her dinner choice was the same, I couldn't resist asking: "Don't you EVER eat any of these tempting delicacies?"

"Emily," she said, "I was very overweight once, and I worked extremely hard to get the figure I now have. I can't bear the thought of ruining it for a few moments' license. And what I eat, I enjoy. I really like grapefruit, salad, and steak!"

Gretchen's diet beautifies her body and nourishes her brain. Her daily plan consists of one orange or one-half grapefruit, two eggs, and a slice of whole-grain bread with butter and coffee for breakfast; cottage cheese, fish, poultry, or liver, a vegetable, and a fresh fruit for lunch; a mid-afternoon snack of skim milk, yogurt, or one-half cup of cottage cheese, two teaspoons of honey in tea or coffee; and her standard grapefruit-steak-salad (unsaturated oil and vinegar dressing) dinner.

My program is similar to Gretchen's in that it focuses on the positive aspects of eating FOR beauty, instead of flagellating you with warnings of what you SHOULDN'T eat in order to lose weight. Get in the habit of asking yourself what foods will do for you, and you won't go wrong.

The mainstay of the diet is protein, the tissue-builders found in fish, meat, poultry, dried beans, milk, milk products, legumes, nuts, and some vegetables. We all need a few teaspoons daily of fats, found in oil, butter, and cream, as well as some carbohydrates, which build energy. Carbohydrates are found in breads, cereals, honey, sugar, and ripe fruit and vegetables. But, for super beauty-building, you should emphasize the raw fruit and vegetables.

The portions given in the diet are moderate but satisfying. If you have to lose pounds, reduce the size of the servings. Have half a slice of whole-grain bread, a smaller lean hamburger, a little less unprocessed cheese. You'll still be eating beautifully.

Now, how do you work out this make-sense eating plan? Check with your doctor first to see if you have any special diet problems (vitamin supplements can be added, if necessary), then, follow me:

	Breakfast	Lunch	Afternoon Snack	Dinner	Bedtime
Monday	1 orange 1 soft-boiled egg 1 slice whole-grain toast 1 pat sweet butter 1 teaspoon honey Tea or coffee	1 cup vegetable soup 1 slice bread grilled with 1 slice Monterey Jack cheese 1 apple 1 glass skim milk Tea or coffee	½ grapefruit Tea with honey	1 glass tomato juice 1 lobster tail with 1 tbs. butter and lemon Tomato wedges Green salad Fresh fruit Macédoine Tea or coffee	2 sun-dried apricots 1 cup yogurt
Tuesday	½ grapefruit 1 poached egg on whole-grain toast, lightly buttered 1 cup skim milk Tea or coffee	1 cup cottage cheese Fresh fruit salad 1 small whole-wheat roll with 1 pat butter Tea or coffee	Carrot and celery sticks 1 cup milk	1 cup chicken broth Pot-au-feu (chicken with vegetables) Green salad 1 small slice chiffon cake Tea or coffee	1-inch cube of hard natural cheese 2 crackers
Wednesday	4 ounces fresh orange juice ½ cup oatmeal with 2 Tbs. cream + ½ cup skim milk Tea or coffee	Salad plate of hard-boiled eggs, cottage cheese, fresh vegetables; herb-flavored yogurt 1 serving berries or melon Tea or coffee	1-inch cube cheese 2 crackers	Fresh fruit cup Broiled sole Broccoli with lemon Scooped-out baked potato skin Baked pear Coffee or tea	1 cup yogurt with 1 tsp. honey
Thursday	4 ounces tomato juice 1 scrambled egg 1 bran muffin 1 pat butter 1 tsp. jam 1 cup skim milk Tea or coffee	½ avocado stuffed with chicken salad (1 Tbs. mayonnaise) Sliced tomato 1 serving sherbet Tea or coffee	1 cup potassium broth	1 slice melon Broiled calf's liver Mixed green salad Cheese Tea or coffee	1 apple 1 cup yogurt
Friday	½ grapefruit 1-inch cube of cheddar cheese, plain or grilled, on 1 slice whole-wheat bread 1 cup milk Tea or coffee	1 can salmon or tuna fish on lettuce with tomato and hard-boiled egg wedges (1 tsp. dressing) 1 pear Tea or coffee	½ cup cottage cheese	1 cup vegetable broth 2 broiled veal or lamb chops Spinach salad with mushrooms Baked custard Tea or coffee	1 baked apple 1 cup yogurt
Saturday	4 ounces orange juice MIRACLE-MILK-SHAKE (8 ounces)	1 grilled hamburger on rye toast ½ cup of peas 1 hot pepper Ice cream (small serving)	Tea with honey 1 orange	Crudités Veal marsala Baked eggplant Green beans vinaigrette Coffee Fresh fruit	1 glass wine or sherry

40

	Breakfast	Lunch	Afternoon Snack	Dinner	Bedtime
Sunday	2 screwdrivers or 2 glasses of champagne Fresh strawberries with ½ cup of half-and-half 2-egg omelet cooked in 1 tsp. butter	2 chicken livers sautéed in 1 tsp. butter Coffee or tea 1 croissant with 1 tsp. jam Fresh fruit	Cheese and crackers Milk	(restaurant) Petite marmite Trout almandine Petit pois Endive salad Lemon soufflé Espresso or fruit	1 glass fresh fruit or vegetable juice or yogurt

Occasionally A small slice of a light cake (such as chiffon), if you've been good about the bread and other starches during the day. On occasion, a "rich" dessert like baked custard is allowed if you haven't had eggs or more than 1 cup of milk that day.

Beverages ALL THE WATER YOU WANT. Hopefully, at least 6 to 8 glasses every day, preferably spring water.

COFFEE OR TEA with ½ teaspoon of sugar. (I prefer raw sugar.) Experiment with various teas—they are satisfying and soothing. Now and then try fresh hot coffee with a spoonful of real whipped cream for "dessert."

CARBONATED DRINKS. Skip the ersatz concoctions called diet sodas and try a naturally-carbonated mineral water like Perrier or Vichy instead. A glass of mineral water with a twist of lemon makes a wonderful prop at a cocktail party.

COCKTAILS. One drink now and then won't hurt you, but you won't find an allowance for a daily martini on this diet.

WINE. One glass of wine as a cocktail before dinner and a glass with dinner is civilized, relaxing, good for your appetite, and better for your beauty than liquor.

MILK. One or two glasses a day of milk, buttermilk, skim milk, or yogurt is important.

While I'm not including recipes for the sample menu suggestions (see chart), there are two special spa recipes you won't be able to find anywhere else:

Miracle Milkshake

16 oz. (1 pint) skim milk (or whole milk if not dieting)
4 Tbs. lecithin granules
4 Tbs. dry skim-milk powder
2 Tbs. wheat germ
2 Tbs. tupelo honey
1 or 2 raw egg yolks
(You may add 2 Tbs. of protein powder if you wish.)

Whirl in blender or shake in a closed jar; refrigerate. Drink 8 ounces as a meal substitute, or 4 ounces at a time for a snack.

Maine Chance Potassium Broth

10 qt. water, to which you add, well-washed:
1 bunch UNPEELED carrots
6 UNPEELED parsnips
2 large UNPEELED onions
1 bunch parsley
3 leeks
1 whole stalk celery

Simmer for 3 hours. During last half-hour, add 4 cubes of beef bouillon, Vega Sal to taste. Then strain through cheesecloth. When ready to use, clarify with 2 egg whites and strain through cheesecloth.

You'll enjoy my lifetime diet, and the people you live with will thrive on it, too. Too many diets exist in a vacuum, as if the dieter lives all alone, cooks for one, and eats by herself. This isn't so, of course, and starvation-type dieting is hard on everyone: the regular eaters feel guilty, and the dieter feels awful. My plan is flexible. If you've had a wonderful Saturday night, keep the mood going on Sunday with a long lazy brunch preceded by champagne or screwdrivers. (For brunch you can combine your allowances for breakfast and lunch and still come out ahead.)

My Special Water Fast

In my syndicated beauty column, I once mentioned a short water fast that many Hollywood stars and with-it people take from time to time. Until then, it had been a pretty well kept secret. But that single reference to my water fast brought in literally thousands and thousands of letters asking for the specifics.

So, here is the popular celebrity water fast. Many people follow it once a week, others for one week a month, and still others whenever they feel the need for a thorough catharsis. I use it after gastronomic holidays or whenever I've just emerged from a particularly harrowing business trip.

All you need for the fast is one day at home, a gallon of distilled or spring water, a few lemons, and honey. The lemons make the water taste better and help rinse out the toxins from your system.

Drink indulgently of the pure water, adding a teaspoon of lemon juice and a half-teaspoon of honey to each glassful.* I mix the water, honey, and lemon juice in advance—storing it in a glass jar that I keep in the refrigerator. I call it my Wonder Water.

You will be amazed to find that within a matter of

---

* This same lemon-juice-to-honey ratio, by the way, works very well with tea. When I'm at home writing, I alternate between English breakfast and herbal teas (peppermint being my favorite).

HOURS you will see yourself looking younger! Believe it or not, it's true.

Some people develop a slight headache, which is easily treated either by lying down for a few minutes or with an aspirin.

The only discomfort you might have is the increased frequency of bathroom trips. But then flushing out accumulated poisons is what this fast is all about.

You can try this fast in different ways: from breakfast through breakfast, or from dinner through dinner.

Rest is important. Just relax and think about all the good things you are going to do for yourself, now that you've taken this first big step. Think about a new you. If this sounds egocentric, I assure you that this new you will be a godsend to everyone close to you.

Breaking the fast properly is also important. Your first food should be a large salad of shredded cabbage and carrots. Squeeze the juice of one whole orange over it for dressing, and drink a cup of hot herbal tea. If you're very hungry, have stewed tomatoes, too. Peel and dice them before heating them to a boil. A few slices of whole-wheat toast—dry and melba-like—are also permitted.

The day after your water fast should be a strictly fresh-fruit-and-vegetables day.

By now you will be feeling like a million (uninflated) dollars. And this is the perfect time to start on a serious new everyday dieting program!

8
Exercise

I know a woman who runs her own Exercise-of-the-Month Club. First it's the Canadian Air Force Program. Then it's isometrics. Then it's yoga. Then it's aerobics. Then it's whatever her favorite women's magazine is featuring that month. She reads the books and articles avidly, draws up elaborate charts, buys herself a new pair of tights and another leotard, just for inspiration.

The first day is exciting. If the book tells her to repeat each exercise three times, she does six repeats. The aches and pains she suffers the next morning are pretty exciting, too: it hurts, so it must be working! Resolute, she goes through the motions, consulting the book and the chart between leg lifts and side stretches. Her protesting muscles are still protesting on the third day, so she lays off the exercise to let them rest. On Day Number Four, her leotard and tights are in the wash, so she can't exercise. On the fifth day, she just plain forgets to work out. And that's the beginning of the end.

Although exercising regularly isn't the world's easiest habit to form, once you've got it, you've GOT it! Once you know how well it makes you feel (not to mention how well it makes you look), it's hard to stop, even for a day or so. When I backslide, I feel it first in the back of my legs: they become kinked and uncomfortable. If I don't exercise for a week, I see it in my waistline and generally feel blah.

The question, of course, is how to acquire the habit. Spas and exercise classes help because no self-discipline is required, and you have the strong motivation of knowing you've paid for the program, so you had better participate.

An exercise routine you set up on your own will feel good and will be fun to do. Once boredom sets in, you're in trouble. If you've ever been to a beauty spa or belonged to a health club, you know that you respond to some exercises with pleasure and that others, no matter how proficient you become at them, remain despicable.

I'm not going to tell you that you'd better do your exercising my way or you'll go completely to pot. I know you won't do it—why should you, it's YOUR body! What I am going to suggest is several exercises for each specific body area or problem, as well as a selection of routines for over-all firm-up. Study these, try them out, along with those given in the spa chapters, and then develop YOUR OWN PROGRAM. If you follow that program every day, within weeks you'll be in much better shape than you are now. And you don't have to do the same ones every day, either. Your needs may change, your moods may change.

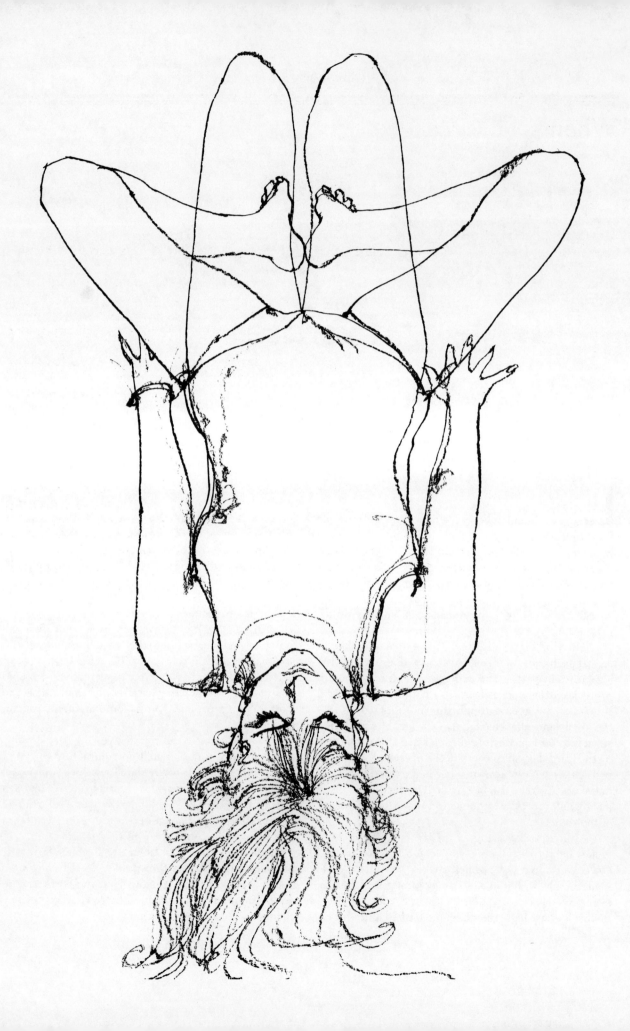

When to Exercise

Almost any time is the right time. The important thing is to try for the same time every day.

Some women like to exercise before breakfast every day. The "bouncy," active routines can be great waker-uppers, and the feeling is "Well, that's out of the way." If you're housewifing, try for an hour when the children are napping or at school. Take the phone off the hook, pull down the blinds, and go. If the neighbors think you're having an illicit liaison every afternoon at 2:00, let them—and let them gossip about your slender new figure, too!

If you can't exercise at the pre-ordained hour one day, for heaven's sake, don't skip that day! Find another fifteen minutes, somewhere, and get back on schedule tomorrow.

My one exception to the anytime-is-the-right-time maxim is before bedtime. Exercise is a great energizer. All that deep breathing and muscular activity fills your bloodstream with oxygen and gets the circulation stirred up. So you're stimulated, which isn't the best idea when you are about to try for a good night's sleep. (Incidentally, if fifteen minutes of exercising leaves you exhausted, you're not exercising properly—your movements are increasing tension instead of releasing it. Try the exercises again and find those that do not deplete you.)

Many experts suggest an hour of exercise two or three times a week. I think an hour is too long for most individuals to maintain interest, unless there's the motivation of an instructor around. Besides, who could remember an hour's worth of exercises? The Golden Door suggests that you alternate your household chores with four or five ten-minute exercise periods. This way you won't tire so easily and you'll have all the benefits of a long, exhausting workout. Fifteen minutes every day is easier on your time and better for your body. The good effects accumulate steadily instead of sporadically, and you're virtually guaranteed immunity against the aches and pains that can occur when you've been off exercise for three or four days. You'll also find that fifteen minutes goes by so quickly you never become bored or begin to resent the time you devote to exercising.

All experts recommend a brief warm-up period before beginning actual exercises. Without it, you might strain your "cold" muscles and cause unnecessary discomfort. Warming up is especially important if you're working out in the morning. At whatever time, have a window open so the oxygen you breathe is fresher than what's already in the room.

An idea I've taken from several spas is exercising to music, which helps keep your movements graceful and flowing and makes the exercise more fun. It also acts as a concentration device so that, when you exercise, your mind is full of exercise only, not what to fix for dinner or what to wear to work. The concentration definitely adds to the relaxing, rejuvenating effect. Most spas choose their music for the masses. But if the idea of listening to "pop-pap" music every day drives you wild, try some Chopin Etudes. Or the "Ode to Joy" from Beethoven's Ninth (that's enough to get anyone moving), or some hypnotic Indian sitar music, or Middle Eastern belly dance records. Or folk songs. Finish your exercise sessions with some running in place, jumping, or disco-dancing to very lively music. My favorites are "Chicken Fat" and Tom Jones' "Delilah."

NOTE: Some of the exercise routines given below work on more than one area of the body, so in some cases you can have two results for the price of one. Another two-for-one bonus: Apply castor oil to your neck and face (dry areas especially) before exercising.

Warm-up Exercises

Toni Beck's Lazy Girl Stretches
After waking, while lying in bed on your back, toss aside your pillow and stretch out tall. Stretch each arm, each leg, your head and neck; now once again, your entire body, and add a few good healthy yawns. Next, roll from side to side and STRETCH, releasing all the tensions of your sleeping position. Relax for a minute. Now, still on your back, push the right leg out from the hip joint without raising it off the mattress. Hold to the count of sixty; relax. Repeat with the left leg.

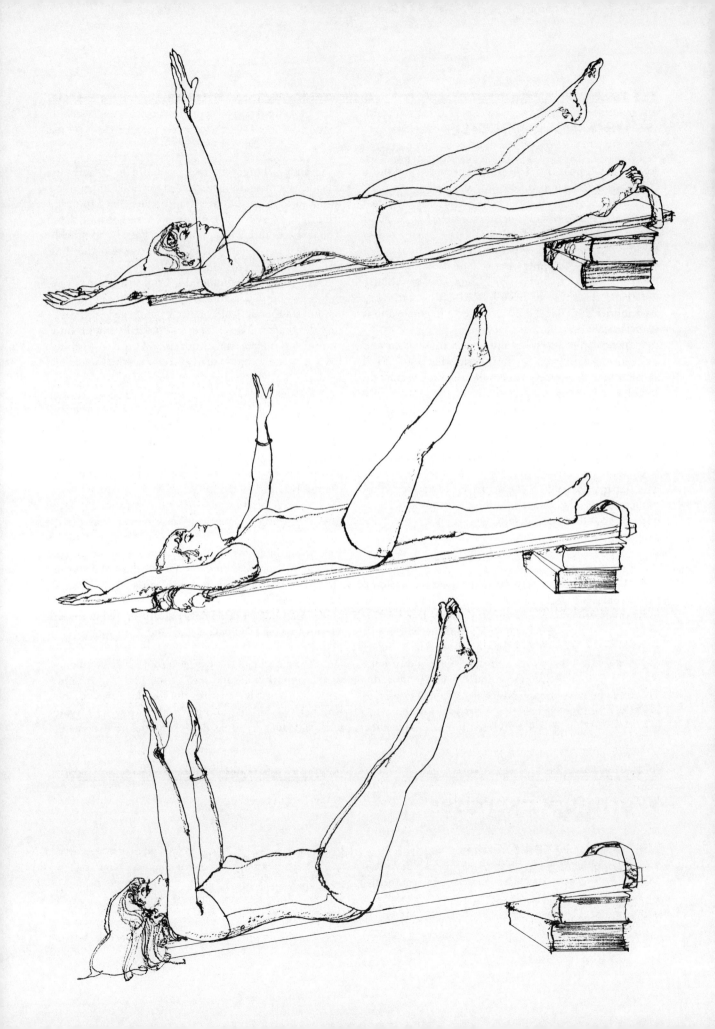

The Total Stretch

The exercise director at Bonaventure in Florida suggests: Lie on your back on your slant board, with feet free (not under the strap) and arms relaxed over head, stretch right arm and left leg. You should feel the pull through the torso and hips. Relax. Then reverse and stretch left arm and right leg. Repeat at least eight times. Next, stretch both arms and both legs simultaneously, pointing your toes. Relax. Now stretch arms and legs and FLEX the feet. Repeat at least eight times. (Inhale when stretching; exhale when relaxing.)

Marjorie Craig's Maine Chance Standing Start-Up

With feet a little apart, bend forward, letting your hands drop toward feet. Hold for a few seconds while exhaling. Then slowly, moving from the base of the spine, come back to upright position, tucking in your abdomen and inhaling. Keep your arms loose and at your side until your body is completely straight. Then lift arms out to sides and up over head. Don't tense or raise your shoulders; maintain a good posture. Exhale and bend forward again. Repeat ten to fifteen times.

Salem Baranoff's Safety Harbor Stretches

Stretch out on your back. Relax. Breathe deeply in and out through your nose. Bring your knees up to your chest, and hold onto your legs under the knees. Press your knees to your chest and relax (five times). On the fifth count, hold and breathe deeply for ten seconds.

Stretch out again. Bring right leg to chest (bent) and hold under knee. Circle bent leg toward the right ten times. Repeat with left leg (to the left).

The Butterfly: Bend knees and place both feet flat on floor (lying on back). Open knees and force apart slowly and pull back together ten times. On tenth count, force apart, press, and hold, breathing deeply for ten seconds.

Lying on back with legs straight out, alternate flexing and pointing toes ten times and then rotate feet (first in outward circles, then in inward circles) ten times.

Lying on back with legs straight out, tighten right buttock and pull right hip up. Release and do the same with left side. Alternate ten times without pausing between.

Do the bicycle exercise ONE LEG AT A TIME ten times each leg.

Bring bent legs to chest again, hands under knees. Now straighten legs up into the air and hold to the count of ten. Don't be disturbed if legs tremble; as they get stronger, the trembling will stop. Breathe deeply while holding legs up.

With hands clasped behind your head, raise chin the chest. (Putting elbows together helps to bring head up.) Do ten times.

Lying flat on back with arms stretched straight above head, stretch first arms, then legs, alternating sides. Do ten times.

Repeat from the beginning.

Face and Neck Exercises

Golden Door Rubber-band Bonanza

A large, sturdy rubber band will accomplish wonders for the lip and chin area and strengthen that around-the-mouth sag. First, slip the band over your head, under your ears and nose, and then, through expressions ONLY (no cheating with fingers), work it over your lips and chin. If it gets stuck between the lips, use your tongue, a few good neck stretches, and/or lip purses to move the rubber band on its way. If it sticks in your chin crevice, use your tongue (INSIDE your mouth) to release it. When the band slips down to your neck, you know you've had fun and a marvelous workout, too.

Golden Door Tongue Tune-up

First, stretch your tongue as far out as you can while exhaling. Then inhale through the mouth and move the tongue far inside, as if trying to touch your tonsils —straining to keep your mouth open as you do so. Exhale again, curl tongue up over upper lip. When repeated several times daily, this stretches the inner neck muscles and vocal cords. (A cure for laryngitis, too, as endorsed by a famous actress who was treated by several doctors and an equal amount of medication to no avail. This one exercise, carefully done, restored her voice.)

Indra Devi's Yoga Chin-chin

To prevent a double chin, press the chin tightly against the neck in the thyroid region. Squeeze tightly and raise the lower lip over upper lip four times. Relax neck completely. Again, move the bottom lip over the top one and raise head. Then, slowly attempt to touch the left ear to the left shoulder, the right ear to the right shoulder, four times on each side. Drop head back and raise four times.

Palm-Aire's Neck Knack
To have a neck like that proverbial swan, make like a turtle and slump your neck into your shoulders while you hunch your shoulders. Hold position to the count of ten; then pull your neck way up as if it's being pulled by a string attached to the top of your head. Your shoulders should go way down, as if someone is forcing them down. (This firms long muscles on side of throat; helps release tension in the shoulders.) Repeat three times.

Arm and Bosom Exercises

Because of the interplay between arm and chest muscles, all the following exercises work as both arm and bosom beautifiers.

The Super-Beautifier
Lie down flat on the floor. Stretch arms out to shoulder level. Holding a book (or a weight) in each hand, raise your arms up over chest until the books meet. Hold for a brief moment. Lower arms back to the floor SLOWLY. Start by doing this exercise five times; work up to twenty-five, increasing only as you feel up to it.

Criss Cross
Standing erect, hold a book (or two-pound weight) in each hand. Bend forward from the waist throughout this exercise. Cross your hands in front of you and raise arms up sideways as high as possible. Lower arms and recross in the opposite direction before raising them again. Do five alternately criss-crossing movements, then stand up and relax. Begin slowly; work up to five sets daily.

The Praying Set
There are three "acts" to this set:

Stand erect, hold hands in front of you, pressing one palm against the other, fingertips together and pointing upward (as if praying). Continue pressing hands together as you move arms slowly from side to side, resisting both ways.

Still standing erect, with hands in same praying position, raise arms up overhead as high as you can, continue pressing one hand firmly against the other all the way up. Come back to starting position. Relax.

Maintain praying position and lower arms in front of you as low as possible, continue pressing hands together firmly. Come back to starting position and relax.

Do each of the "praying" exercises once or twice at first. Work up to ten, SLOWLY.

Windmill Stretches
Using weights or books, stretch arms out at sides and rotate them in large, windmill-like circles, first forward, then backward, six times each way. Work up to twelve.

The Finger Pull
Stand erect, fold arms in front of you, place hands together so that fingertips of left hand are resting against the fingertips of right hand. Take a deep breath in through the mouth and tighten the abdomen as you attempt to pull your hands apart. Elbows are up. Pull HARD now—to the count of five—holding your breath all the time. Breathe out through mouth, relax completely, hands down.

Begin by doing ten times, work up to as many as you can do comfortably. (Incidentally, if you look straight ahead into a mirror during this routine, you won't be apt to get dizzy.)

Rancho La Puerta Ball Exercise
Use a volleyball or basketball or soccer ball to shape up. Hold the ball in front of you at chest level, standing with feet spread wide apart. With arms and back straight, reach forward and lower the ball to the floor in front of you. Bend your elbows and push forward, then push away by straightening the elbows. Do this a few times. It's excellent, especially for the upper arms and abdomen!

Dr. Lauda's Neck Drop
This finale is really a wonderful, rewarding routine to top off arm-firming exercises. Get yourself two five-pound weights. (If your arms are not very strong, you

may begin with 3-pound weights.) Lie across the bed on your back. Let your head and upper shoulders dangle toward the floor. Grasp weights in either hand, raise arms up, inhale deeply and hold your breath as you lower arms and weights toward the floor. Breathe out and bring arms straight back up. Repeat at least five times; work up to twenty-five. This will not only lift your bosom via strengthening your pectoral muscles, but will also tighten your tummy and help firm your waistline as well. (If you strap wraparound weights to your ankles you'll avoid the tendency to slip off the bed while doing the neck drop.)

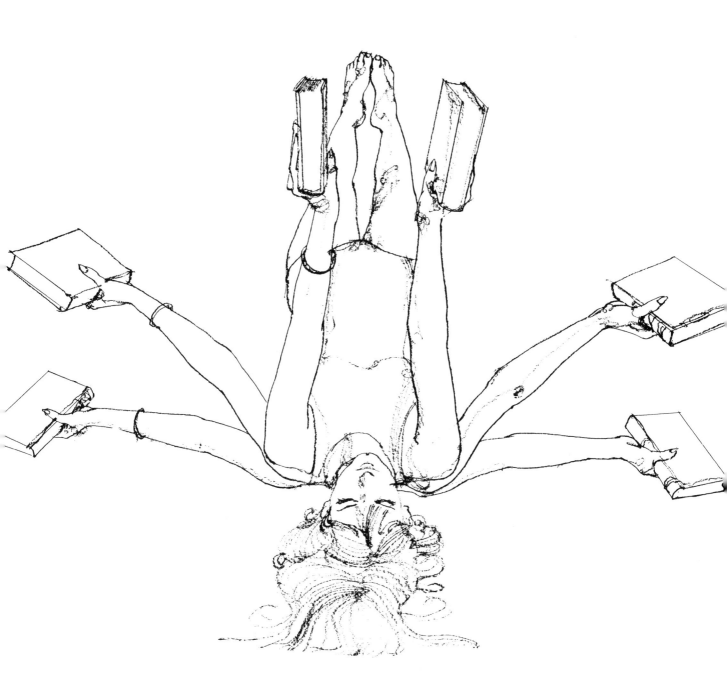

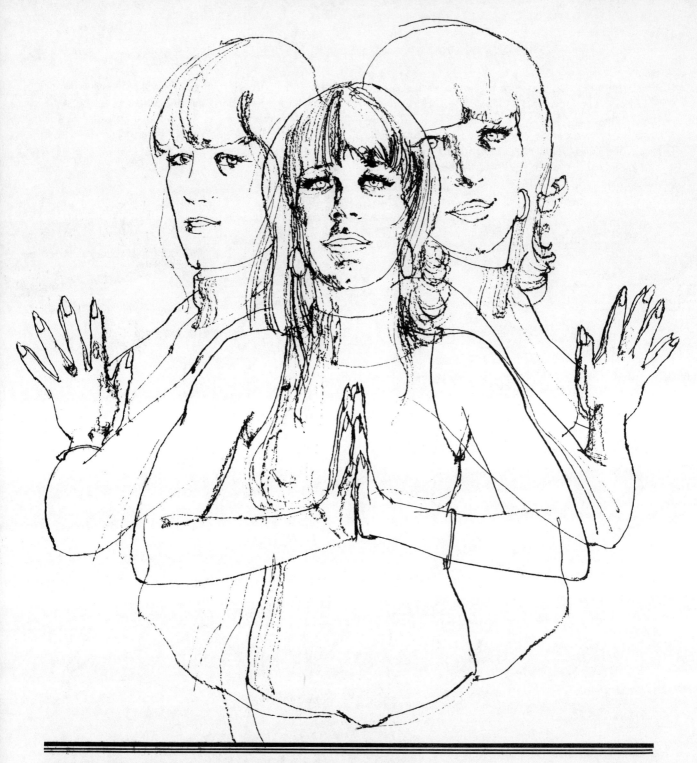

Midriff and Waistline Exercises

Emily's Midriff Slimmer

Use your exercise pole or a broomstick or mop handle. For each of the following movements, stand erect with legs about eighteen inches apart. Begin by performing each variation for one minute. Increase time until you're working out two minutes on each exercise.

Hold stick at arm's length in front of you at shoulder level, hands near the ends of the pole. Then twist from side to side (as far as possible), arms remaining taut throughout.

Hold the pole over your head, arms straight, hands holding the ends of the pole. Keeping arms stiff, bend

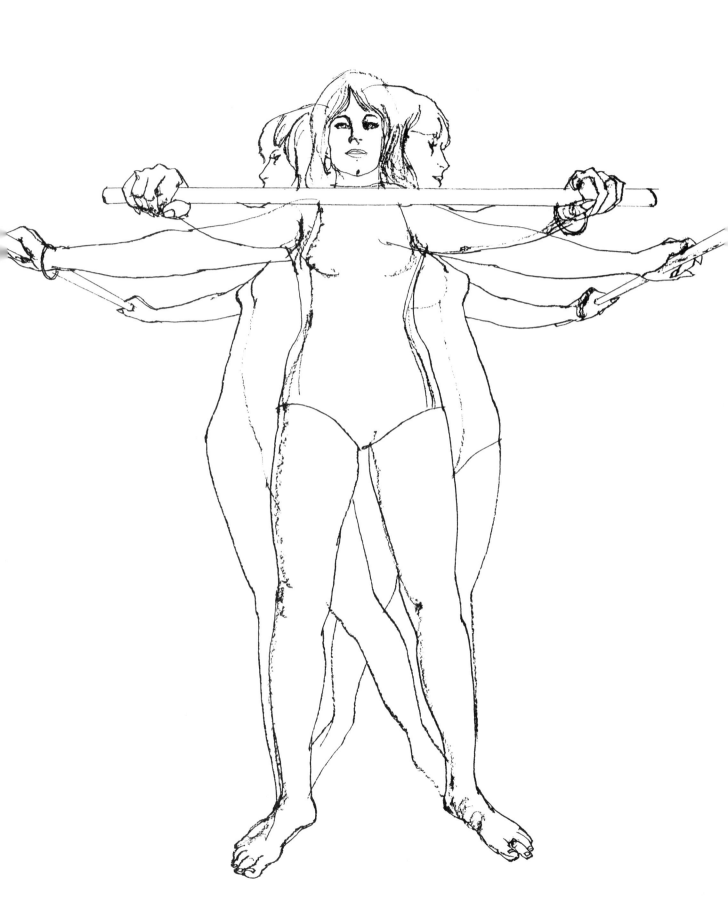

sidewards toward the right as far as possible without moving legs. Return to overhead position, repeat on left side. Work into a bend-return-bend rhythm, stretching a bit more each time.

With arms taut, hands near ends of pole, bend forward from the waist and swing body from side to side in rhythmic motion, making a half-circle with the pole.

During each of these routines, you should feel the pull in the muscles about your waist. After a week or two of daily workout, your midriff will be shipshape, taut and trim.

Maine Chance Exercise Secret

NEVER do waist or tummy exercises with your knees locked together. ALWAYS keep your knees relaxed and a little bent when doing sit-ups, toe-touches, and so forth. The stiff-kneed stance can easily damage the small of your back—and thus discourage you from exercising altogether. A rolled-up Turkish towel can serve as a buffer.

Maine Chance Waistline Special

For most effective results, it's important to tone up ALL the muscles that come into play at or about the waist. This favorite exercise is an excellent side stretch. Lie flat on your back, arms outstretched, palms up. Raise knees over your chest, then holding them together, drop as far right diagonally as possible, keeping arms and back flat on floor. With knees as close together as possible, pull them along the floor until level with your waist, swing them back across chest to original position, and drop them diagonally over to the left side without breaking the rhythm, simulating a figure eight. Repeat ten times; work up to twenty.

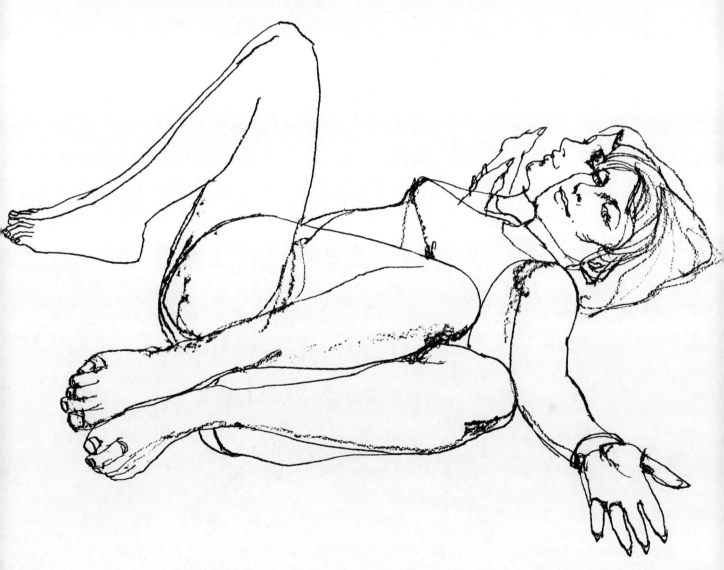

52

Maine Chance Side-to-side Roll

Lie flat on floor, arms outstretched, palms up, knees together and bent comfortably, feet resting flat on the floor. Contract abdominal and buttock muscles, simultaneously forcing the small of the back "into" the floor. Holding this contraction and keeping feet flat, let knees fall to the right. Return to center, then let knees fall to the left, and return to center, repeating in brisk, continuing rhythm and always reinforcing the abdomen and buttock contractions in center position. Do at least twenty times.

Golden Door Pendulum Stretch

Stand erect with legs about fourteen inches apart, arms in front of you, grasping the ends of a towel and spreading arms as widely as is comfortable. Keeping the towel taut, raise arms above your head; now bend straight to the right as far as possible, feeling the long stretch on your left side. Come up straight, repeat to the left. Knees should be slightly flexed. Repeat ten times on each side; work up to twenty. You'll find you can stretch a little more each day.

Abdominal Exercises

The Scissors

Lying on your back on a slant board or an exercise mat, bring both legs straight up about fifteen inches. Don't tense. Lower the right leg to board or mat; then raise again. The left leg stays up. Now lower the left leg and raise again while the right leg is up. Inhale as you move right leg down and up; exhale when moving left. Repeat twelve times with each leg; work up to twenty-five.

The Pelvic Tilt

Lie on your back on your slant board or mat with feet six to eight inches apart, knees bent, feet turned out. Breathe in deeply (feel the rib cage expanding), pull in the abdomen so you feel the lower back pushing onto the board, tighten the buttocks, and hold this position for a count of ten. Then exhale and relax abdomen, buttocks, and back. (Notice the difference in the position of the lower back when you pull in the abdomen and when you don't.) The shoulders should stay relaxed throughout. Start with twelve; work up to twenty-five.

The Firm-up

This is an isometric exercise that really works. Do it without fail at least once a day. (1) Lie flat on your back, feet together, toes pointing up. Rest hands on abdomen, elbows bent upwards. (2) Now lift head, pointing chin toward ceiling. (3) At the same time, raise legs about twelve inches from floor, heels pushed out. (4) Contract the muscles of your buttocks and stomach as tightly as possible, holding the position to count of twenty-five.

Repeat five times; work up to ten.

Abdominal Lift

This is a yoga routine that tightens and trims the tummy and firms abdominal muscles. (1) Sit in any comfortable position, hands on knees. (2) Exhale all breath from lungs through mouth (with a h-a-a-a sound). Hold breath out of lungs until you have completed one set of five lifts described in steps 3 to 5. (3) With breath held out, pull abdomen in and up briskly. You should see a hollow indentation in abdominal area, unless you're very overweight. (4) Push abdomen out again. (This pulling up, in, and "popping" out movement should take no longer than two seconds.) (5) Repeat movement of pulling abdomen in and up, then popping it out, five times. This is one set of five. (6) Take several deep breaths after completing each set. Start by doing one set of five. Increase by one set per week until you're doing five sets. (The abdominal lift should be done on an empty stomach; wait at least two hours after eating.)

Hip Exercises

Upper Hip Reducer

For the bulging side area just below the waist, lie on your back with arms outstretched and palms up, keeping knees bent over the chest. Roll on the superfluous padding of the hips as you move briskly from side to side. Be sure to keep knees together throughout. Remember your upper back must remain flat on the floor all the while. Start with twenty rolls; work up to fifty. The more you do, the slimmer your upper hips will become.

Over and Over

This is my favorite hip slimmer and a fabulous waist whittler as well. (1) Lie on your back, with legs straight, arms outstretched at shoulder level, palms facing floor, knees together and bent, feet flat on floor. (2) Now, holding shoulders flat throughout, snap knees over to touch the floor on the right side. (3) Bring them back to center, then repeat briskly on left side. Slap hips from side to side, over and over. Start with ten, work up to twenty-five slaps daily.

Hips Away

(1) Lie flat on your back, legs outstretched, arms at shoulder level, palms facing floor. (2) Raise legs to-gether until perpendicular to floor. (3) Lower toes to right side, trying to touch right hand. (4) Rise up to center; then lower toes to left side toward left hand. (5) Raise once more to center perpendicular, then return slowly to starting position. Keep shoulders flat on floor all during exercise. Work up to five counts on each side.

From the Greenhouse for the Hips

Lie flat on your back with your arms out to the sides. Bring your knees up to your chest. Keeping the legs bent, twist them to the right. With both hips remaining on the floor, return to the center. Now repeat the movement to the left. Keep both hips down so that you feel the tug in the upper thighs and hips.

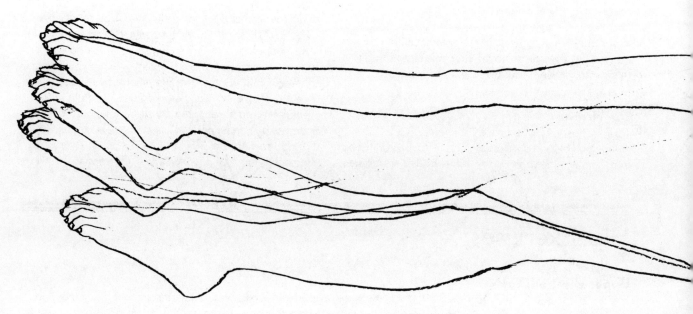

Buttocks Exercises

The Goosestep

Standing straight, slowly raise your right leg forward and up while you pull in abdomen. Keep body erect and toes pointed. If you have difficulty in maintaining balance, hold onto a chair or towel rack. Lower leg slowly. Using your buttocks muscles to "lift," flex right foot and swing it backwards. Keep your back straight. Slowly return to original position; relax buttocks muscles. Next, slowly raise right leg sidewards, lifting with outside upper thigh muscles. Return to position slowly.

Repeat twelve times with each leg; inhale when lifting; exhale when lowering.

The Fanny Walk

Sitting on a rug or smooth floor in an erect position, with arms raised and elbows bent at chest level, "walk" forward, using your elbows and heels to propel you. "Walk" on your buttocks at least fifty steps forward and fifty back, moving as briskly as possible. (Wear a leotard or pants; a skirt impedes your progress.)

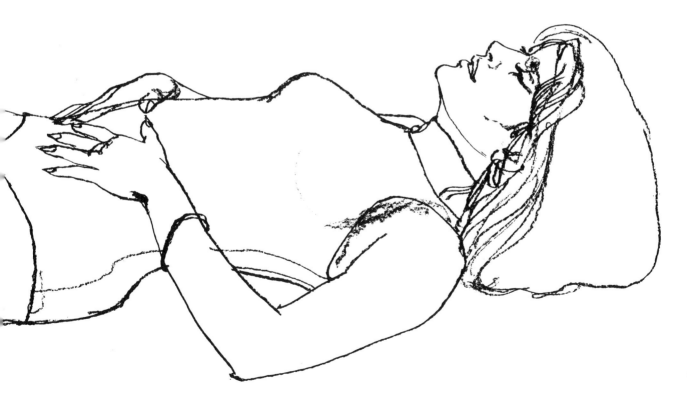

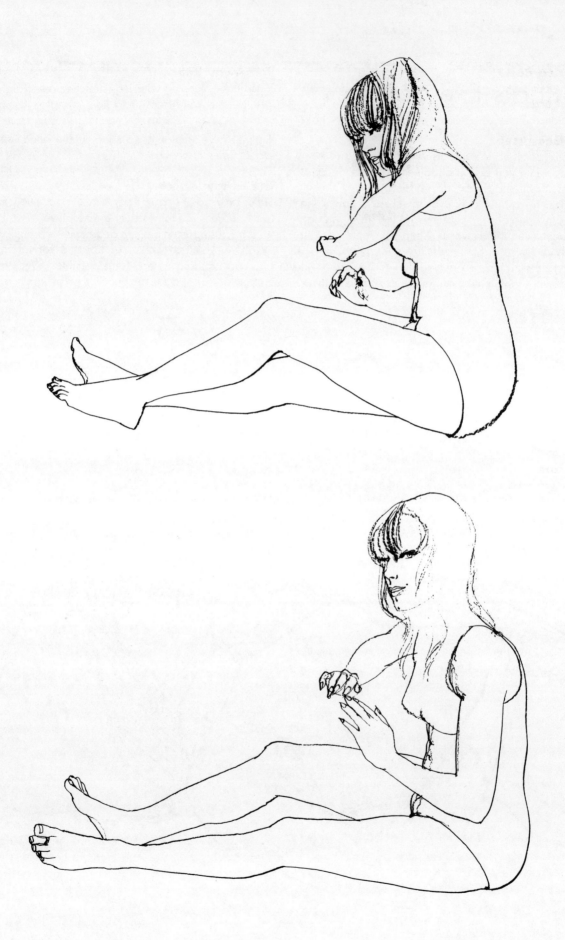

Side Leg Raise

Lie on your right side, your right hand stretched out straight under your head, left hand resting on the floor for balance. Raise your left leg as high as possible, hold to the count of five, then slowly lower to the count of ten back to starting position, forcing the heel out all the time. Roll over and repeat with right leg. Start with five lifts on each side; work up to ten daily.

Roll Away Rear

Sit on floor, keeping your legs stretched out straight in front of you. Roll from side to side, swinging the same hand over your head as the side that rises up from the floor. You will come down on the palm of your opposite hand. Push up again. For best results, this roll should be done very briskly and repeated from side to side at least twenty times.

Leg Exercises

Ever Trim Legs

Sit on the floor in a half-reclining position with knees straight, toes pointed, hands on floor behind torso with palms down and pointed forward. Breathing in, bend knees toward chest, keeping the toes pointed, chin up. Then, still breathing in, stretch your legs upward, tilt your head back. Breathing out, lower both legs to floor. Repeat five times; work up to ten daily.

Leg Parer

If your legs are heavy, you must avoid excessive exercise, which will develop them even more. Lie on the floor, place a pillow under the hips and raise legs straight up in the air slowly. Start inscribing circles in the air with both feet up, first one way, then the other. Repeat ten times each way—slowly.

Leg Muscler

The more you exercise (walk, run, skip, bicycle, dance, golf, always in the lowest of heels), the more developed your leg muscles become. So make walking, not riding, your way of life. Whenever possible (not only during regular exercising), try this builder-upper. Take off your shoes and hold on to a straight chair, feet about eight inches apart, toes pointing straight ahead. Keeping back straight, rise up on tiptoes and hold for a few seconds. Then, still on tiptoes, bend the knees until you reach a squatting position. Hold for a few seconds, rise up on tiptoes and repeat. Start with ten bends, work up to twenty within a few days, try for at least three repeats during each day.

The Thigh and Knee Trimmer

Sit on the floor, legs apart, back and shoulders straight, knees straight, toes pointed up, hands at waist. Breathing in, bend left knee, bringing leg inward so toes of left foot touch the right thigh. Breathe out and return left leg to starting position. Repeat movement with right leg. Alternating, repeat exercise with each leg five times; work up to ten.

From the Greenhouse for the Inner Thigh

Lie flat on your back, legs straight up, toes inward, hands placed under the buttocks to keep the lower back rounded. Open your legs to a wide position, still with toes facing in; then bring legs back together. Repeat sixteen times.

From the Greenhouse for the Outer Thigh

Lie on your right side, with your left hand in front to keep you on your side and with your right arm propping the head. Raise your left leg high, flexing the heel and keeping the knee forward; then lower the leg. Lifts should be fairly brisk and uninterrupted. Remember to keep legs straight and not to roll over onto your back.

Then try the reverse, lying on your left side, raising and lowering your right leg. Repeat sixteen times.

Inner Thigh Firmer

Sit on a volleyball with legs apart and about twelve inches in front of you, feet flat on the floor. Roll forward on your toes, then back on your heels; twenty-five times, at least once a day.

Another winner for inner-thigh tightening: Lie flat on your back, arms outstretched at sides. Raise the right leg up and out toward the sides, then slowly lower it to original position. Repeat with the left leg, remembering to lower very SLOWLY. (Strapping a three-pound weight to each ankle helps make this exercise more effective.) Alternating, repeat each exercise with each leg five times; work up to ten.

Hollow Thigh Filler

Hollow thighs are hard to correct, but it's definitely possible if you practice this routine daily: Lie on the right side, head resting on outstretched right arm, bracing yourself with left hand in front of you. (Abdomen and hips are under you as far as they can be.) Raise the top leg about twelve inches off the floor. Hold. Now pull the under leg up to the top leg and hold to the count of ten. Lower SLOWLY. Repeat on the other side. Alternating, repeat each exercise with each leg five times; work up to ten.

Back-strengthening, Posture-improving Exercises

Backaches are probably (next to headaches) the most common complaint of men and women. A backache can make you feel miserable, look worse, and louse up your love life. While all backaches are not caused by poor posture, some are. The following exercises will strengthen your back and improve your posture.

The Reverse Spinal Roll

Lie on your back, hands at sides, palms down, knees bent, feet flat on the floor. Roll up slowly from the base of your spine, one vertebra at a time until you are resting directly on the base of the neck. Inhale and exhale, then push up just a little bit more until you feel the stretch behind your ears; roll head from side to side to loosen tensions. Finally, roll down slowly, one vertebra at a time until your back is flat on the floor. Relax for a moment; repeat several times.

The All-over Stretch

Lie down on your back. Stretch every which way, always remembering to flatten your back against the floor. It's an ideal time to bend the knees, hands at sides, palms up, feet flat and roll up, vertebra by vertebra, until the back of your neck is pressing hard against the floor. Breathe in and out deeply and lower back slowly, stretching out fully as you return to original position. Do this once or twice.

The Reposer from La Costa

Roll over on your tummy and crouch on your hands and knees, raise your back like a cat getting ready to fight. Lower your head and stretch your back out once or twice.

Remaining on your knees, fold arms in front of your chest, rest head on arms—your body will "fold" into place. (Incidentally, this knee-chest position is recommended by many physicians after pregnancy. Keep it in mind as an ideal way to rest during any exercise session, since a few deep breaths while in this position will relax and revive you in short order.)

Dr. Lauda's Standing Special

Stand about four inches from the wall, feet apart, and attempt to press the back of the neck and small of the back into the wall. Bend the knees (turn out slightly) and dig the waist into the wall. Your pelvis will tilt upward. Now, slowly push yourself up against the wall until your legs are practically straight. Lift chest toward ceiling. If you put a book on top of your head at this point, you'll be able to balance it as you step out bravely—walking with dignity and grace and, at the same time, helping greatly to improve your posture.

The Shoulder Roll

This exercise is especially effective at eliminating any tendencies toward that aging "dowager's hump." Lie flat on the floor or on a firm mat, clasp hands behind head, raise head up slightly. All during this exercise, legs should be apart, with heels "dug" into the floor for anchorage. Your hips must remain firmly planted on the floor the whole time. Now, roll from side to side briskly, purposely concentrating on the fatty spots. Start out doing about twenty rolls; then gradually increase the number, working up to fifty.

The Back and Leg Stretch

This is a marvelous routine that reduces flabbiness in the derrière while strengthening the entire back area: Sit with legs straight out in front of you, knees straight. Raise arms slowly. Slowly bend backward and stretch arms up. Slowly stretch arms and upper body forward and grasp calf, ankle, or foot (whichever is most comfortable). Do not bend knees. Gently pull upper body down as far as you can, trying to touch it to legs. Don't strain, tug, or pull. Drop head and neck. Hold for five seconds. Let go of legs and slowly straighten upper body. Uncurl spine as you slowly move up to sitting position. Raise head last.

Perform exercise three times. Increase holding time by five seconds each week until you can hold the stretch comfortably for a count of twenty.

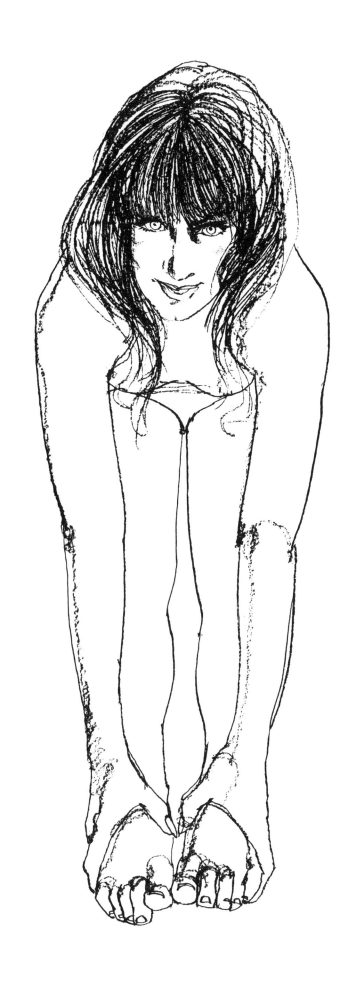

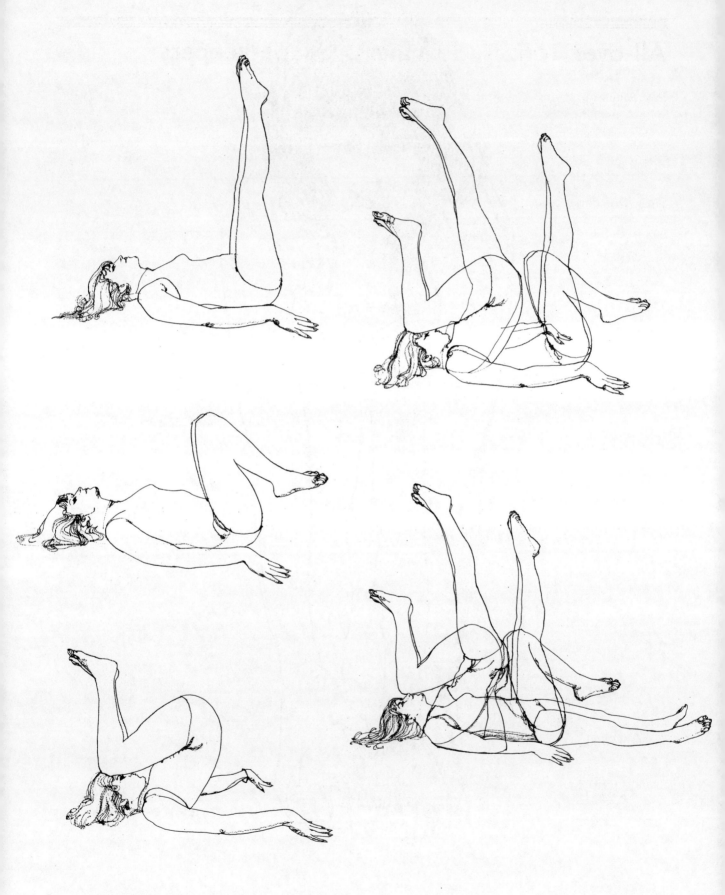

All-over Toners, Trimmers, Shape-keepers

Five minutes of any exercise program should be devoted to keeping your entire body in top shape, not only for cosmetic effects but also to get all your muscles moving, your heart and lungs working a bit harder, your whole body revved up.

Side Arm Fling

Stand with feet apart, raise bent arms up, elbows out, and make fists with your hands. Holding tummy taut, fling arms out to the sides at shoulder level. Swing arms back to the original position. Repeat exercise five times, with force.

Front Arm Fling

From the same "wing" position (with arms bent, elbows out, hands making fists), force arms forward at shoulder level. Tummy should be tensed. Hold five seconds with arms about twelve inches apart. Fling fists back to original position. Repeat five times.

Overhead Arm Fling

From starting position, fling arms (fists tight) straight up over your head (they'll spread apart), remembering to keep abdomen muscles taut all the while. Fling back to original starting position; repeat five times.

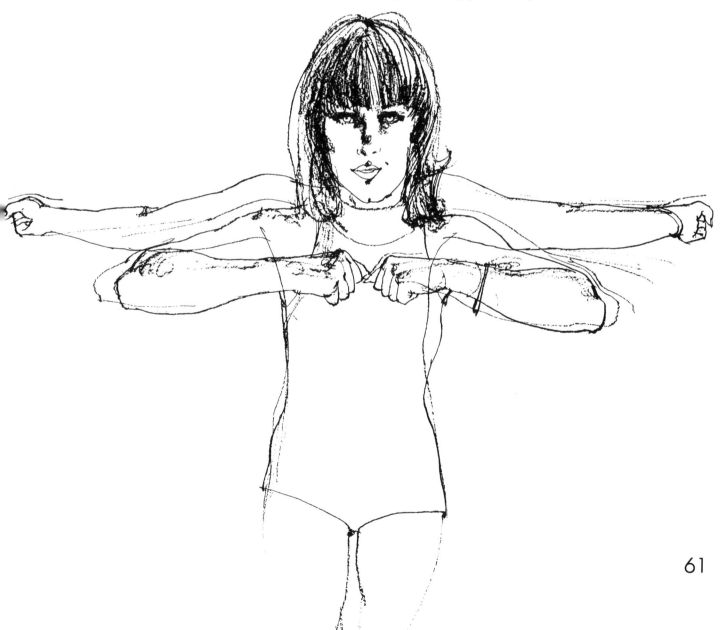

Arm Circles

With arms straight overhead, make fists; then swinging arms down in front of your body, cross them in front of you and come up swiftly to the starting arms-overhead position, like a windmill. Repeat this fling briskly five times, coming back up to original overhead position each time. (Don't forget to breathe and keep your tummy taut all the while.)

The Rope Trick

Standing straight, with feet slightly apart, imagine that you are going to pull down a rope from above your head until it touches the floor in front of you. Reach high up to the right side (stand on tiptoes) over your head and, grabbing the imaginary rope in two places, start dragging it down, knees bending as you do, until the "rope" is in front of you. Then let the rope "go up" the other side. Now reach up the left side over your head, and drag the rope down once more. Repeat five times on each side.

The Yoga Rock

Sit on a rug or mat with your hands under your knees. Draw your knees up, put your head down, and —keeping your spine rounded—swing back and forth like a rocking chair. Rock back and forth several times; eventually your toes will swing over your head and touch the floor behind you. Repeat twice.

Line Up

Right after awakening, stretch out on the floor, keeping back flat. Clasp your hands over your chest, elbows bent upward, and pull one hand against the other and raise your chin toward the ceiling simultaneously. Hold this position to the count of thirty; relax. Work up to sixty seconds.

Rock

Sit up straight, arms stretched out in front of you. Keeping arms in this position, quickly roll back, with legs coming up perpendicular to floor (arms flinging back over your head). Then, speedily sit up, touch your toes. Repeat backward roll. As you go faster and faster your feet will eventually go back over your head and reach your outflung hands. Start with thirty "rocks"; work up to sixty.

And Roll

Lying on back, clasp your knees together with your hands and roll from side to side, over and over and over. Do thirty times; work up to sixty.

The Sportive Life

Choose one sport to become a fiend about. Swimming is marvelous, of course, if you can get to a pool two or three times a week and if you spend an hour or so breast-stroking or crawling lengths. Meditating on the ceiling while you float on your back counts as meditation, not swimming.

Tip

Wherever you do your swimming, remember that fifteen minutes or a half-hour of a long, smooth sidestroke will do more for your figure than frantic, off-and-on speed swimming. The point is to stretch every muscle. This way you'll become pleasantly tired, not tense and exhausted.

Tennis is terrific, too. Golf is all right, but you should play it without cart or caddy. If the whole idea of sports bores you, walk.

Walking is the greatest exercise of all. But you must WALK—not stroll or amble. I once watched Greta Garbo walk down Park Avenue, and it was beautiful —long legs striding purposefully, arms swinging loosely and easily. She made it look like a graceful dance. Don't wear high heels or constricting clothes when you walk.

Let your arms swing in rhythm with your legs. Let your legs swing out their full length. Walk with your knees unlocked—don't look as if you're on parade duty. You'll probably be the only woman on the block who's REALLY walking. People will look at you, yes. Smile at them! Breathe deeply. It's fun to move and it gets you where you're going—beautifully!

The Supreme Exercise—Relaxing

The best rejuvenation secret I know is a series of techniques for taming tension I learned from Indra Devi. Age alone isn't the thief that robs our youthful good looks. It's the everyday tasks and troubles, stresses and strains, worries about money, husbands, children, homes, meals, laundry, pets, automobiles, even taking care of OURSELVES, that takes its toll on appearance. Surgery, pills, hormones, clothes, make-up, money, are totally ineffectual unless one has learned to let go and develop inner serenity.

Whenever you feel tired, world-weary or simply put-upon, use this method to deal with your cares. This very minute, begin to unwind and RELAX from head to toe. Read the following twice, then get out of your chair and down onto the floor.

First, close your eyes and stretch, tensing your body as hard as possible. Tighten each and every muscle; then give them each an extra burst of tension. Squeeze your eyes, your fists, toes, buttocks, shoulders, as you hold your breath and count to five. Next, let go, feel yourself growing very, very limp all over.

You are sinking into complete oblivion. Your head feels so heavy, it's sinking right into the floor. You can almost hear that tight, tense neck creak as you let go. Your shoulders follow. Pretend you're leaning back in luxuriously warm water, a lovely scented bath. Let your entire spine relax, your arms, even your elbows.

Now for your hands. Allow every single finger to go limp by first making a fist, then relaxing the hands completely. FEEL the difference. Back to your spine: it continues sinking down, down, down through the floor. Feel your buttocks simply melting away; your thighs feel loose, and your legs limp. Each of your toes has been liberated.

You are a cloud, a beautiful soft white cloud, floating in the vast blue sky—very light, very carefree, floating over a green valley, over a peaceful meadow. You can almost hear the rustling of the treetops, and smell the grass and the wild flowers.

Now it's time to return to the land of the living. Stretch out completely. Yawn. Turn to one side and arch your back and stretch; turn to the other and stretch and yawn. Then open your eyes and sit up SLOWLY.

More Tension Tamers

If you can't take time out for the complete relaxation method, there are some good calmer-downers that can be done quickly while standing.

Edith Risch's Bircher-Benner
Facial Relaxation Exercises
Sit on a chair, close your eyes, and stretch your head from side to side. Now place the third and fourth finger-tips on your eyebrows, touching only the hairs, and relaxing your eyes simultaneously.

Repeat this twice more; the third time, touch the skin below the brows as well. To enhance the relaxing effect, tense all the facial muscles tightly. Cover your face with your hands, sensing the warmth of your face. Now relax completely, slowly removing your hands from your face.

Now cup your hands over your face again, eyes closed, feeling for the cheekbone joint. (If there's tension in the face, that's where you'll feel it strongest.) Remove them, as before.

Let your lower jaw hang loose, and feel your tongue as a lump in your lower jaw.

Do-it-yourself Massage
To relax a stiff or tense neck, place your hands in back of the neck, thumbs down, and work round and round, pressing harder in the sore areas. Release the pressure, work up back into the base of the scalp, up behind the ears, round and round, pressing and releasing as you go. Then, in front, massage the ear area, move up to the temples, across the forehead and finally, under the eyebrows. (As your hands get tired, shake them out.)

63

Eye-easer

A quickie for relaxing strained eyes, anytime, anywhere. Squeeze eyes tightly closed, then open them very wide. Again, squeeze tightly, open very, very wide. Repeat five or six times.

Tongue-twister

Believe it or not, your tongue needs relaxing, too. Stick it out as far DOWN as you can. "Retreat" and relax the muscles in your neck. Third, stick it out pointing UP toward your nose. Repeat each movement three times.

Head and Shoulders

Pretend your head is a heavy lead ball. Really IMAGINE the WEIGHT of it. Let it drop forward, then pull up slowly. Let it fall back, and relax your jaw by opening your mouth. Pull this heavy head back up to center, then drop to the left side (left ear almost touching left shoulder). Bring your head back to center and drop over to the right, with the right ear reaching toward the right shoulder. Return to center and reverse the movements, beginning with the right side, and then repeating on the left.

Shoulder Shrug

Keep your arms and hands loose and limp and use your back muscles only to shrug your shoulders up and down. Attempt to touch your earlobes. Now go faster and faster, each time letting your shoulders "flop" down deliberately.

Forward Bend

Stand with your legs apart, knees slightly bent, and pretend that your head is so heavy it's pulling you forward. With eyes closed, let the weight of your head pull your arms, hands, entire body down. Your spine should feel completely loose, hips and thighs free, head relaxed and tucked into your chest, as you "melt" downward. When your hands reach the floor (if possible), bounce on your fingers, touching floor, then dangle there, making sure your head is without strain and wholly relaxed.

Don't look at the floor—just dangle! Next, bend the knees a bit more and begin rolling UP, keep head down until the body is parallel to the floor. Then thrust the pelvis forward and uncurl like a snake, little by little. Raise yourself up by using your back muscles only. Don't come up too quickly, or you may get dizzy.

And Now to Sleep

If you sometimes find it difficult to fall asleep, here are a few simple techniques that will help you relax at bedtime. Try any or all of these—they work!

1. Open the window even a tiny crack to allow fresh air in. It's a soporific.
2. Create a pleasant home for the night. A lightweight blanket or down quilt is best. Crisp, fresh sheets are a plus. (The lovely new permanent-press variety feel fresh from one bed changing to the next.)
3. Leave the world behind you. It's essential to change the pace and disassociate yourself from the hurly-burly of daytime life. Don't use pillow-time to rehash all your troubles. Swing your thoughts around to soft, happier ideas.
4. If you simply can't forget about it until tomorrow, write down a few of your gripes to get them out of your hair. Better yet, read an old-fashioned novel (Dickens, Jane Austen) that will transport, not stimulate, you. Geography, history, or even philosophy books are MOST effective, at least for me.
5. Music helps. Play favorite mood selections, a classic romantic Frank Sinatra, for example, or Debussy's CLAIR DE LUNE.
6. Find something to eat or drink at bedtime that "calms" your nerves. One famous actress sips a glass of champagne or dry white wine. A good standby is a cup of herb tea (mint and camomile are good) or some warm milk with honey.
7. A lovely soporific: a languid, tepid bath (regulated to body temperature via a bath thermometer). Add a little lemon scent or light, flowery perfume; relax for five minutes, then gently pat yourself dry (don't rub) before donning a fresh nightie.

Instant Sleep from Dr. Lauda

Lie down, fully stretched out on the floor or on your bed. Picture your right or left hand as becoming very heavy or very warm. Tell yourself, verbally, that your feet and thighs, too, are becoming very tired. As you repeat these incantations softly to yourself, your limbs will become heavy and warm, and you'll unconsciously eliminate all that's been keeping you from falling asleep. This exercise can be used for relaxation, too.

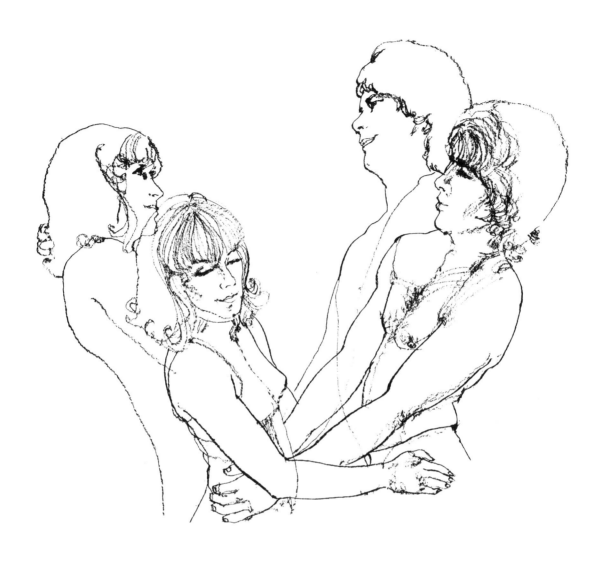

9
The
Wonder Weekend

Now I'm going to show you how to re-create an actual spa experience in forty-eight wonderful hours devoted to one goal: making you more beautiful all over.

Weekend for One

If you live alone, working out the preliminary arrangements for your Wonder Weekend is fairly simple. If you're part of a twosome, foursome, or anysome, you'll have to juggle some details, use a little cajolery, and arrange to have EVERYBODY out of the house for those precious two days. If you can manage my wonderful twenty-four-hour Water fast on Friday, your weekend will be twice as effective. See page 42.

If you have children, have your husband take them to Disneyland, New Hope, his sister's, his mother's—ANYWHERE for the forty-eight hours. If children aren't a problem, schedule your Wonder Weekend for a time when your husband has business out of town, has to see HIS children, or has tickets to the Super Bowl or the Indianapolis 500. AT LEAST THREE TIMES A YEAR, try to snag forty-eight hours just for you. Everyone you know will rave about the results. Promise.

With the house to yourself, you're ready to start your Spa Happening. Turn on some music, on your favorite station or pile on your favorite records. Have dinner early. Make it a light, but beautiful repast —broiled chicken breast and sliced tomato with basil; a glass or two of white wine; some fresh fruit for dessert. Arrange your servings attractively, colorfully, symmetrically. I want you to be aware of everything you do this weekend—colors, smells, textures, tastes, sounds.

After dinner, prepare your weekend's worth of Potassium Broth (page 41); and, as it simmers, stir up a batch of Wonder Water (page 42). Although this isn't a One-Day Water Fast regime, you will be enjoying some of the benefits of that fast in combination with a very spare spa eating program that will shave off at least five pounds by the end of the weekend.

I'm assuming that all the beauty supplies you need are in order. Now gather up the needlepoint you never have time to work on, the magazines that have been gathering dust, the book club selection you've been meaning to read, the thick soft towels you've been saving for guests (your crispest, prettiest sheets are already on the bed), and those delicate slippers and the great negligee your husband or boyfriend gave you. This is going to be an occasion.

With the Potassium Broth Wake-up Cup and Wonder Water in the refrigerator, turn down the telephone bell so it won't jangle you if there is an unexpected call. Slip off to bed with a nightcap of fragrant herb tea with honey and a thin slice of clove-spiked orange floating in it. Set the clock-radio for seven. (After all, we're trying to reproduce an authentic spa ambiance, and you can't dawdle in bed on BIG DAY NUMBER ONE.) Lay out a stack of your favorite records for your weekend—including exercise music. If you have no phonograph, find a good FM station. This is your chance to commune with YOURSELF, so keep TV viewing to a bare minimum or zero level. It's important to get a good night's sleep, for tomorrow is a busy day.

Saturday (or Day One)

8:00 Good morning!
      Wake-up Stretches (page 45)
      Rag Doll Shake (page 32)
      Wake-up Cup: ½ cup prune juice, ½ cup water, juice of ½ lemon, heated together until steaming and kept hot overnight in a thermos.

8:30 Hairbrushing
      Dental routine.
      Weigh in (record your weight).
      Jump rope or use exercycle or twist board for five minutes.

9:00 Breakfast: ½ cup fresh orange juice, ½ cup fresh grapefruit juice, and 1 tablespoon honey. Whip with 2 or 3 ice cubes in the blender, or beat together, without ice, with a wire whisk.

9:30 Relax or dance to your favorite music; dress.

10:00 Brisk walk outdoors.

10:30 Camomile face-steaming or sauna.
      A cleansing facial followed by iced witch hazel.
      Facial exercises (page 63).

11:15 Wonder Water: 1 cup hot Wonder Water. Sip it plain or steep a tea bag in it for instant lemon-honey tea.

11:30 Meditate or read romantic poetry you haven't looked at since your sophomore year in college.

12:00 Exercise routine: pick five new exercises from the suggestions in Chapter 14.

12:30 Steam up the bathroom, or use the sauna if you're lucky enough to have one, and follow this steaming with a cool-off shower.

1:00   Liquid Lunch: 1 cup hot tomato juice or V-8 Vegetable Cocktail with a squeeze of lemon juice, or best yet, fresh vegetable juice (tomato, carrot, celery, cucumber, green pepper, lemon); or half vegetable juice, half Potassium Broth.

1:30   Siesta.

2:00   Weed out lingerie and clothes closet.

2:30   Eyebrow shaping.

3:00   Cold Drink: 8 ounces or more of Wonder Water. Add ice if desired.

3:30   Make up experimentation session.

4:00   Abdominal exercise routines.

4:30   Tea: 1 cup hot Wonder Water (plain or tea).

5:00   Free Time: Plan a party, a picnic, or your next vacation. Dress for dinner in your prettiest robe or caftan.

6:00   Dinner: 1½ cups broth (Potassium Broth), plus ½ cup of the diced vegetables. Sprinkle with kelp or sea salt, if desired. 1 glass cold Wonder Water.
       If you like, follow your dinner with 1 cup of Wonder Water (or tea). You may have 1 piece of fresh fruit for dessert.

6:30   Tightening facial; rest in the Beauty Angle.

7:00   Use depilatory or shave legs and underarms.

7:30   Remove polish on finger and toenails (to air them).
       Beauty Bath: Choose one of the versions on page 22. Loofah-rub, pumice feet, soften, and rinse off under shower. While you're in the bath, sip an Herbal Tisane: 1 cup of Wonder Water plus 1 herbal tea bag or ¼ teaspoon very finely powdered mint leaves. Steep two to five minutes. Dry off, splash on after-bath cologne: use lotion on arms and legs; brush hair.

8:30   Prepare nightcap and Sunday's Wake-Up Cup. Nightcap: 8 ounces warm skim milk, 1 tablespoon honey. Sprinkle with pumpkin pie spice or cinnamon.
       Wake-up Cup for Next Morning: Same as Saturday's.

9:30   Apply favorite emollient; blot off after ten minutes.
       Evening dental routine.
       Cream hands and feet; wear bed socks and gloves so the treatment works overnight.

10:00 Sip Nightcap. Read a good book or

do a bit of knitting or macramé.
Lights out.
Countdown to sleep.
Pleasant dreams.

Sunday (or Day Two)

8:00   Good Morning!
       Wake-up stretches.
       Rag Doll Shake.
       Wake-up Cup.

8:30   Castor oil moisturizer, followed by ice toning (page 33).
       Brush hair.
       Morning dental routine.
       Weigh-in.
       Jump rope, exercycle, or twist board (5 minutes).

9:00   Breakfast: Stir 1 cup plain yogurt with 1 tablespoon honey, plus ½ cup fresh sliced strawberries or blueberries; or ½ diced ripe pear, apple, or orange. Plain tea or black coffee.

9:30   Wash hair; towel or blow dry; tie back until later.

10:30 Exercises.

11:00 Broth Break: 1 cup strained Potassium Broth, heated.

11:30 Dress and take a brisk walk.

12:00 Cat bath or quick shower.

12:15 Do-it-yourself foot massage.

12:30 Lunch: Banana milk shake: Blend 1 ripe banana in the blender with 1 cup skim milk and 1 teaspoon honey (optional: 2 drops rum flavoring). Or simply mash banana with a fork, stir in honey, and beat in milk.

1:00   Siesta.

1:30   Free time: Continue your nap, or write a letter or a poem.

2:00   Liquid Refreshment: 1 cup Wonder Water, hot or cold.

2:15   Exercises.

2:30   Super Rich mask (choose one from pages 34–35). Rest in the beauty angle for fifteen minutes. Remove mask.

3:45   Scented bath.

4:15   Dry off; apply lotion all over.

5:00   Manicure and pedicure.
       Do facial exercises while polish dries.
       Read or listen to music for the next hour.

6:00   Dampen and set hair. Dress for dinner. And REALLY dress. Tonight you're going to look wonderful. You haven't spent this spa weekend just for you; you did it because other people care how you look, too. If you're on your own, snag a friend to share dinner with; if you've shunted off kids and/or husband for the weekend, now's the time to prepare to welcome them back. So dress for the occasion.

7:30 Have a glass of white wine with your partner for the evening.

Bed-
time Try a late dessert of ½ cup plain yogurt mixed with 1 tablespoon honey or dark Barbados molasses and 1 tablespoon wheat germ . . .

or Have a nightcap of hot tea, herb tea, or Wonder Water with a slice of orange centered with a whole clove.

Weekend for Two

How's your love life? A little COMME CI, COMME ÇA? Haven't you noticed that it improves when you and your man are able to escape everyday life for a vacation, however brief?

The whole point of a weekend for two is to establish a "vacation" atmosphere with a plus: THIS weekend both of you will be working toward a new awareness of each other. This schedule doesn't resemble an ordinary holiday weekend. It has no built-in demands of dressing for dinner, or making that "must-attend" cocktail party. The main ingredients are two people who love each other, tranquility, aloneness (send the children to Grandma's), and a spa atmosphere.

This is not simply a twofold repeat of the Wonder Weekend for One. When a woman spends a weekend on her own, recreating a spa experience, it should be quite different from a weekend with her man. It would be unthinkable on this weekend to defuzz your legs or do your hair or give yourself a manicure.

Prior to your weekend, get yourself in the best condition—hair squeaky clean, body silky smooth, sexy lounging clothes at the ready, toes so adorable he can't resist kissing them, food that begs savoring, devilishly fatal perfume, music that takes him back, sheets that invite sliding into, and luxuriously thick bath towels you'll want to languish in.

Ideally, you will do things this weekend you've NEVER DONE BEFORE—even on vacation.

The Wonder Weekend for Two leaves you gobs of free time. I've sketched out a tentative schedule, but you should think about him and what he likes and —before embarking on your forty-eight-hour encounter—rearrange the schedule according to his preferences. Use your ingenuity to make this a really special adventure for the two of you.

Here is you sample weekend schedule. Fill in the details on diet, exercises, and massage from those that have been detailed earlier.

Friday Night

7:00 Cocktails: sherry or white wine, plus CRUDITÉS.

7:30 Dinner: Broiled lobster tails; baked potato shells; asparagus spears with lemon; sliced tomatoes with basil and oil dressing; carob mousse; coffee or tea.

8:30 Retire to your bedroom and slip into comfortable lounging clothes. This might be the time to present him with a thick terry robe, or a knit jump suit—something he can really relax in. Turn on music that's relaxing and romantic.

9:00 Time to massage his feet. I think the Maine Chance technique for making feet feel wonderful is the best. Using a pencil eraser, press gently over every square inch to discover any sensitive spots. Work out any soreness using your thumbs or the eraser. Then relax the feet by bending toes down and massaging the arch; massage sides of heel from the bottom all the way up past the ankle.

9:30 Time for him to massage YOUR feet.

10:00 Nightcap: Hot milk with honey and spices, plus a handful of raw cashews. Read him excerpts from an author you know he'll love. If he's not the type you read to, drag out your old photograph albums and high school scrapbook, and go over the good old days together.

11:00 Time to sleep.

Saturday

8:00 Wake him up gently, unless he wakes you up first.

9:00 Teach him how to stretch, really stretch awake—feet, legs, arms, shoulders, head, body. Hold hands and stretch together. Then, while he uses the bathroom you fetch a Wake-up Cup which you have cleverly prepared

BEFORE the weekend started. Un-Bloody Mary: tomato juice sparked with lemon juice and tarragon.

Now, you use the bathroom while he enjoys his Wake-up Cup and reads the morning paper. (While you're brushing your teeth and cleansing your face, remember to do your tummy tucks and one or two facial exercises.)

10:00 Breakfast: Wedge of melon; sourbread or French toast with honey (make the French toast beforehand and freeze; reheat in oven and serve with dollops of honey and butter; coffee or tea.

10:30 Dress. You go first while he reads the paper; and while he's dressing, spirit away the breakfast dishes and put them in the dishwasher. DON'T JUST STACK THEM; CLUTTER IS NOT PART OF THIS SCENE.

11:00 Go for an old-fashioned walk. And this time, instead of lagging behind, keep up with his longer strides. After you warm up, jog a little, and laugh when the people in your neighborhood (none of whom EVER walk) turn their heads.

11:30 Broth Break: Potassium Broth (page 41), sparked with tarragon.

12:00 Time for some active exercise before lunch. Get out the jump ropes and have a jumping match (to music) to see who can jump most rhythmically and gracefully. The cut off time is fifteen minutes. And you'll have to decide —since you may be in better shape—whether you want to out-class him or not.

12:15 HE takes a shower, while YOU get lunch squared away.

12:45 Cocktails: Bloody Mary; this time add 1 ounce of vodka, and spark up the drinks with some sweet basil.

1:15 Lunch: Quiche Lorraine, made with Swiss cheese, eggs, bacon bits, and green pepper; cole slaw; yogurt with blueberries for dessert.

1:45 You take a shower, while he gets lunch mess squared away.

2:00 Siesta or free time.

3:00 Rise and shine; fun time: each of you will enjoy a fruit-based facial. Choose avocado or strawberry or banana; let him apply your facial, and you do his; then both of you put your pillows under your feet—unless you are lucky enough to have TWO slant boards—and relax and talk for fifteen minutes, while you giggle over how silly you both look with all that goo slapped on your faces.

3:30 Rinse off facials and get ready for exercises.

Sitting Rock

Both of you sit down and face each other with legs apart. Grasp hands and let him pull you forward as he leans back as far as he can without toppling both of you; return to center and YOU pull him forward. Rock back and forth quickly, in rhythm to count of fifty.

Thigh Squeeze

Place two chairs twenty-four inches apart, facing each other. Each of you take a chair and scrunch forward on the chair until your knees are touching, his on the outside and yours inside. While he squeezes his knees together, you try to spread yours apart. Hold to the count of ten. Relax. Reverse positions so that his knees are inside and yours are outside. You press as hard as you can inward, while he tries to spread his knees apart. Then hold to the count of ten. Go slowly at first because you're using muscles that are rarely used in regular daily activities; eventually work up to count of twenty.

The Stomach Rock

Both of you lie down on your stomachs, locking legs, with knees bent. Working together try to raise your heads and your bodies as far as you can, with legs still locked in position; then return to head-down posture and repeat body-bending position. Work up a rhythm—first head down, rise up slowly as far as your back can arch, return to starting position. Try for ten back "rŏcks."

Although most exercise sessions that I've recommended have been limited to fifteen minutes or so, this time I've allowed an hour because you will have to practice new routines. There may even be some fun interruptions. (After all, playful grapplings are definitely permitted.)

4:30 He gets the bathroom to shower, shave, or whatever. You read a novel, do needlepoint, or just lie there, in your beautifully sheeted and scented bed and do nothing.

5:00 Dress for dinner.

5:30 Cocktails: Free choice of favorite cocktail. (Hopefully, you're truly happy with a glass of dry wine; let him have what he will.) Talk about art, talk about movies, talk about the economy, talk about anything BUT the children's grades, your mother, HIS mother, the weather, tomorrow. Keep it on an artistic and philosophical level.

6:30   Dinner: Rock cornish hen stuffed with rice and almonds; broccoli au gratin; lettuce and artichoke salad with oil/lemon dressing; fresh strawberries with (light) cream for dessert.

7:30   Relaxing time. Play Gershwin's "Rhapsody in Blue," Stravinsky's "Rite of Spring," a vintage Sinatra, or a current Streisand, while you enjoy your after-dinner TISANE: a pot of herbal tea, garnished with lemon slices centered with cloves.

8:30   Time to slip off to the bedroom and change into—nothing. It's time for a massage. You massage him first. If you've never had a massage, you've been missing out on a wonderful experience that can be tranquilizing or stimulating, an exercise substitute, a luxurious, sooth-

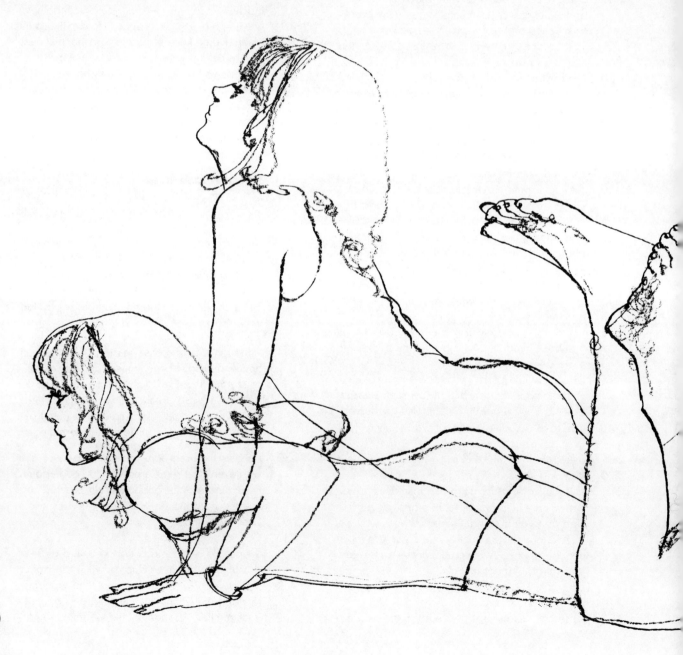

ing awareness of your entire body. For those who have enjoyed this delicious form of body pampering, no sales pitch is needed.

Massage Tips

During your weekend, you'll be on both the giving and receiving sides of the massage picture; if you've never played MASSEUSE, this is the opportune time to learn and to practice.

You'll want to select a special oil or cream. Unscented mineral oil is generally used for professional massages, but you'll want something a little more glamorous and sensual. Any favorite body or skin lotion is appropriate, and if your man prefers a non-creamy product, try plain old rubbing alcohol. Seek out herbs and spices such as musk, cinnamon, cloves,

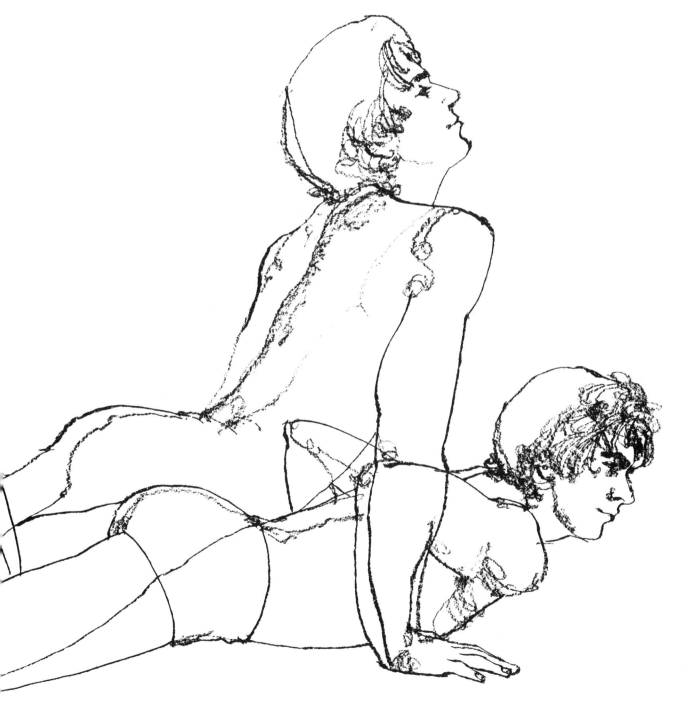

frangipani, myriad oils, waxes, honeys, and flower waters.

Although purists claim that mattresses are too soft to provide the foundation for a good massage, this weekend we think you should use your own bed.

Basically you'll be using the four techniques of Swedish massage: EFFLEURAGE (light strokes), FRICTION (for circulation building), PETRISSAGE (restful, calming kneading), and TAPOTEMENT (pummeling, slapping or tapping).

Start the massage with your man lying on his stomach, with his forehead resting on his hands.

Begin by massaging his NECK. Put a little oil or lotion on your hands and begin by stroking the neck very lightly. Use two fingers of each hand and work from the base of the head to the point where the shoulders begin. Be sure to work down. Then go over the neck area again, this time with small, circular movements, using your fingertips only.

Now apply the lotion to his entire back and SHOULDERS. First grab the shoulder muscle FIRMLY and knead the area while your thumbs stroke up along the backbone. This point applies to the entire massage: when your man responds with murmurs of appreciation or delight, keep on doing what you're doing a little longer; if you hear a displeased grunt or groan, modify your motions accordingly. After kneading, give the shoulders a few gentle friction strokes, using the palms of your hands.

Always massage the BACK from the BOTTOM to top. Starting at the base of the spine, work up, massaging in fairly firm strokes with your two middle fingers of each hand. This will cover the entire center back. Next, concentrate on the SIDES of the back. Do one side at a time, working with your hand perpendicular to his body, in circular strokes. Go over the area again, this time with fingers spread open to massage the muscles between the ribs. The final back area to be massaged is the LUMBAR REGION. Use light effleurage strokes again, circling and stroking up, up, up. Now, massage with smaller, firmer motions the muscles near the vertebrae.

It's time to turn over for arm and leg massage. Put a pillow under his head, and perhaps one under his knees. His arms should be outstretched while you massage his SHOULDER. First apply oil or lotion to one entire

arm from shoulder to fingertips. Then, using two hands, gently knead the shoulder area; work on the round part of the muscle, pressing hard.

For the upper arm, knead the biceps from bottom to top, one hand on the front and the other on the back muscles (triceps). Don't disturb the mood by touching the armpit. (This is NOT the time for tickling!)

Avoid the elbow area and apply light strokes (fairly firm) to the entire FOREARM, working up again from wrist to elbow. Finish the arm massage by a once-over light stroking all the way up from wrist to shoulder.

Massage the top of his HAND with your palms and follow by firmly massaging each individual finger, working from fingertip to hand. Apply lotion and repeat massage on other arm. Now you're ready for the legs. Apply lotion or oil to one entire leg, rubbing in lightly from hip socket to feet.

Use your fingers in a firm stroke to massage THIGH muscles. Then, working up from the knee, use entire hand in circular, pressured motions. As a third movement for the upper leg, start at the knee, and work up with a chopping movement, using the "flats" of your hands. This should be done rapidly several times.

In massaging the calf, first work up lightly from ankle to knee, using one hand after the other with light strokes. Have him bend his knee so you can work on the calf, beginning with slow strokes, and graduating to firmer ones. (Remember to work up and don't touch the under-knee area.)

Finally, repeat the earlier FOOT massage.

9:00	His turn to massage you. One good feel deserves another, right?
9:30	Bath-Time à Deux: You've prepared a deliciously relaxing herbal bath, plus bubbles, to be followed by lavish applications of body lotion or baby oil for both of you. This step may be skipped if the massage has induced you to better things.
10:00 or 10:30 11:00	Nightcap. Maybe tonight he'll read to you, or talk, or just cuddle. This is definitely super-relaxing, do-whatever-you-want-to-do-time.

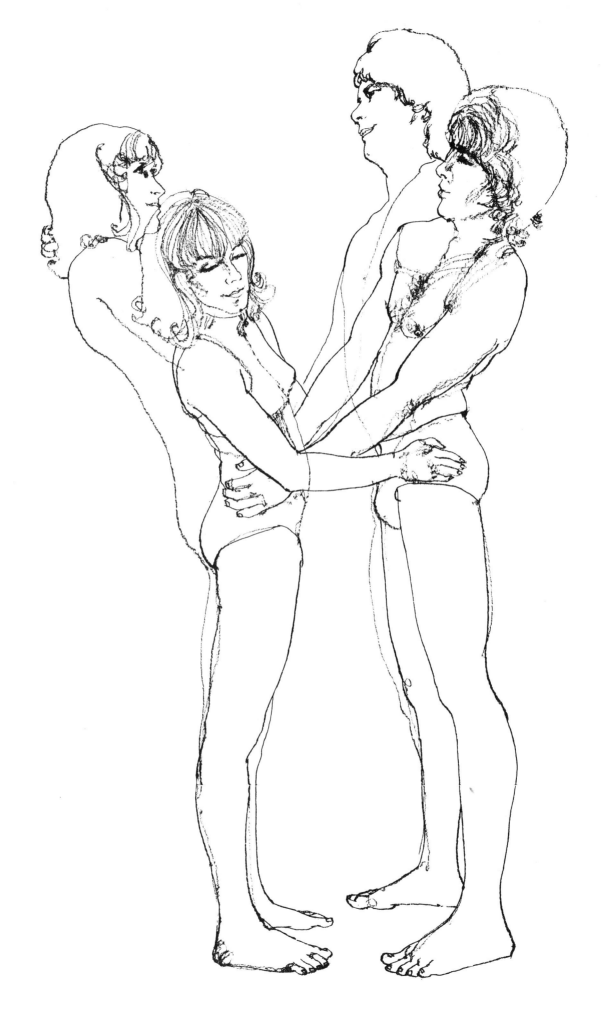

Sunday

9:00   Your turn to use the bathroom first while he fetches the Wake-up Cup: Fresh orange juice sweetened with honey and cinnamon.

9:30   While he's in the bathroom, you do your every-day exercises, on the mat or the slant board, with cream or oil on your face, or a tightening mask, which you'll remove before he emerges.

10:00   Breakfast.

10:30   Dress or free time, as the spirit moves you.

11:30   Go for a walk. Jog again. (Today you'll be much more organized and spirited than you were yesterday.)

12:00   Broth or Tea Break: Potassium broth in a mug, or herbal tea spiced with nutmeg.

12:30   Time to read the Sunday papers and share a footbath. Let him soak longer while you prepare lunch.

1:15   Lunch: Salmon salad; sliced tomatoes with tarragon, plus lemon and oil; cheese and fresh fruit for dessert.

1:45   While you clear away the dishes, he gets ready for a nap which you'll both enjoy, sans clothes.

2:30   Time to wake up . . . easily, no pressure; loll around another fifteen minutes or so.

3:00   Exercise Time.

Block Buster

Each of you needs a wooden block, or thick phone book or pillow. Sit on it with legs locked; fold arms, and each of you lean back as far as you can. Keep those legs locked. Then rise up to sitting position. Repeat twice.

Side Stretches

Both of you stand erect, about one foot apart so you can comfortably grasp each other around the waist. Then, while you bend your torso to the right eight or ten times, he bends his body to the left; then reverse directions.

3:30   Tea Break: Chinese tea with wedges of blue cheese and a fresh pear, sliced (half a pear each).

4:00   Shower Time: This is the ideal time for a shampoo. Prepare a double portion of the super hair-conditioning shampoo with eggs (page 38). In the shower, apply the egg rinse and emerge together (to be wrapped in the lovely, thick, extra size towels you bought just for this occasion) to towel-dry your hair and enjoy the lovely results.

4:30   Time for a massage. It's your turn to be massaged first. (If you don't get around to HIS turn, better luck next time.)

6:00   Time to dress for dinner. While he uses the bathroom, you rest on your slantboard wearing a firming mask (page 33).

6:30   Your time in the bathroom . . . and now you'll do your most glamorous makeup (lay on the eye shadow), plus a good dollop of perfume applied in strategic places, while he relaxes and prepares cocktails.

7:15   Cocktails: Your choice, plus raw peanuts (moderate amount) and yogurt, tarragon, garlic dip for selection of CRUDITÉS (including asparagus, brussels sprouts, carrots, celery, artichoke hearts, radishes, scallions, cherry tomatoes).

8:00   Let him take you out to dinner, where you'll concentrate on some aphrodisiac specialties to cap your love-in. Your eating-out choice might be seafood, or organ meats (sweetbreads, heart, liver, kidney), or fish amandine. Other selections could include anything with tomatoes, cabbage, broccoli, asparagus, or mushrooms; or desserts that include honey, yogurt, strawberries, or bananas.

10:00   If the family comes home now, lock the bedroom door and continue the love-spa mood by slipping into something sexy. Invite him back to the bedroom for a Sunday Night Special massage, taking up where you left off yesterday evening.

74

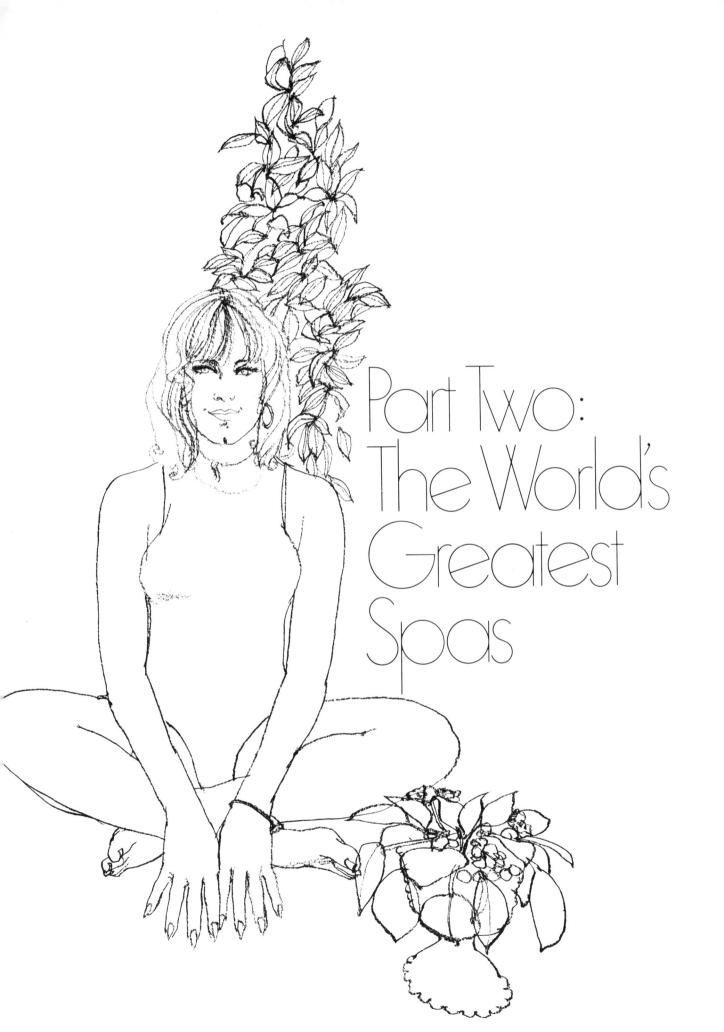

Part Two:
The World's
Greatest
Spas

10
Spas in the United States

Maine Chance Arizona

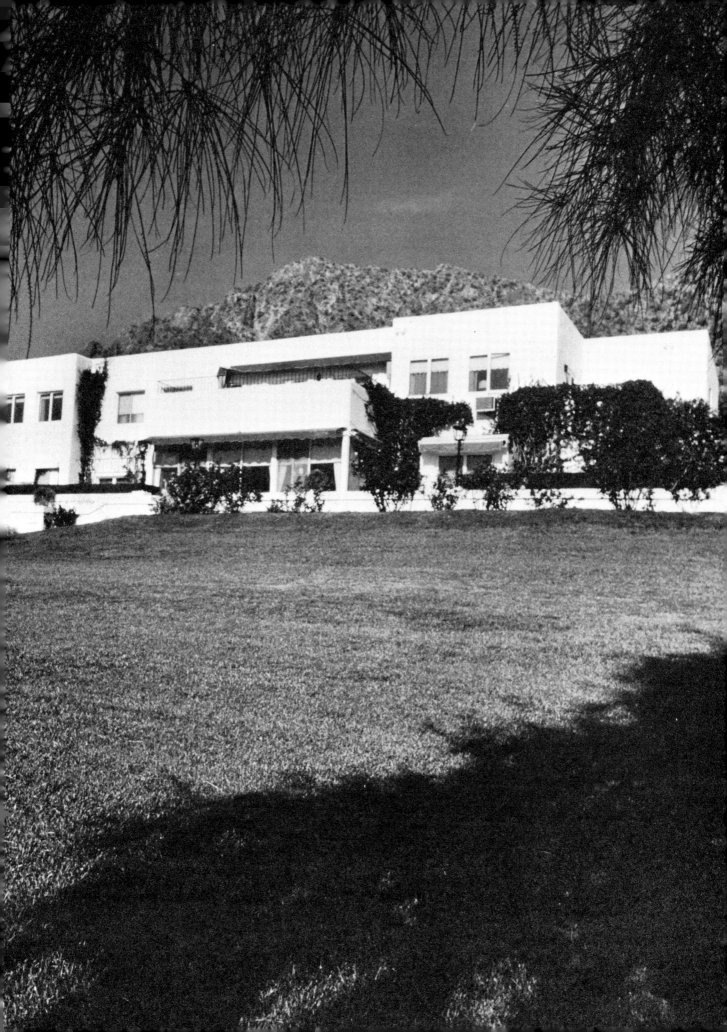

Maine Chance Arizona

In the Depression summer of 1934, with the whole world collapsing around her, Elizabeth Arden converted her North Woods vacation palace into a paying club for her friends and a few handpicked names from the Social Register.

At the suggestion of her beau, advertising executive Henry Sell, she called it Maine Chance. For the next forty years, the cream of American society came to her luxurious Waterville, Maine, estate to venerate this indomitable Canadian-born feminist and her pagan credendum that a woman could remain beautiful forever through particular rites of diet, exercise, and corporeal care.

Maine Chance was a reflection of the soul of this Canadian truck farmer's daughter, born Florence Nightingale Graham. It reflected her unquenchable ambition to erase the failures of her youth and to make the most of her multimillion-dollar cosmetics empire.

She used the 750 acres originally as a private weekend retreat, usually having on hand a gaggle of close friends, and several treatment and exercise girls from her salon to put the former through their paces. Following her divorce from Tom Lewis, who had helped her build the business from a six-thousand-dollar loan into a sixty-million-dollar-a-year enterprise, the idea of commercializing the retreat made sense. She also saw it as HER main chance to one-up the European spas she knew.

She put up two hundred thousand dollars to convert her estate into the first beauty spa in America worthy of the label. Everything reeked of class. It had loads of space, most of it in chalet-style housing. It was as luxurious as any Manhattan townhouse, replete with good paintings, fresh flowers, magnificent linens, silver, and crystalware. The staff-to-client ratio was never permitted to drop below two-to-one. The Maine Chance guest had it good.

The guest list, initially, was limited to twenty. (Later up to forty would be received.) The only males permitted on the grounds were servants and, for her special July 4 dinner, a Senator or two. It took her months to assemble a meticulous, minute-by-minute schedule of activity for her guests. Even today at Phoenix Maine Chance, that schedule varies hardly a jot from the original, beginning with a 7:30 A.M. breakfast in bed delivered by a personal maid and ending with a strict 10 o'clock bedtime.

Arden knew quality. She hired the best: Gaylord Hauser to fashion her meals; Ann Delafield to design the basic program and body exercises; Marjorie Craig to execute the program and incorporate into it one of the most effective exercises I've ever come across; and Maurice, her first fantastic chef, who drew up the healthy but gourmet menu.

She got into the nature fad early. She scorned chemical additives and put things like seaweed, orange blossoms, and natural oils into her products. Her Eight-Hour Cream is still one of the finest cosmetic creams you can buy. It smells bad, but works wonders on everything from horses' manes (Arden used it on the manes of her horses) to human scalps, faces, cuticles, lips, and feet.

Mainly, she used it to stimulate hair growth. Her scalp specialists used Eight-Hour Cream and two brushes to impart a lovely sheen to clients' hair. (See page 37.)

After two dreadful fires, the Maine spa was closed down in 1970. It signaled the end of Arden's GRANDE MODE style. Although the delicious routine of breakfast in bed, served by one's own maid still holds at the Phoenix Maine Chance (inaugurated in 1946)—to me it's, well, not QUITE the same.

Phoenix Maine Chance is more relaxed when it comes to its guest list. And, if you choose to spend a week there and leave all your cares behind, you have a great treat in store.

Much of the Arden personality remains in the Capo di Monte and English bone china, the monogrammed silver and linens, the paintings by Chagall, Magritte, and the Southwestern primitive Georgia O'Keefe, and in Arden's precious Peace rosebushes that adorn the grounds.

Phoenix Maine Chance is a sequined sandal buckled on the foot of Camelback Mountain, a 105-acre country estate with a white manor house and seven smaller houses. The eye feasts on acres and acres of rolling green lawns, such as one might see in Kent or Surrey, lush rose gardens creating a curious color chemistry with the indigenous citrus and palm trees and the imposing centuries-old saguaro cactuses.

The interiors are plainly Continental: marble statuary, travertine floors, crystal chandeliers, eighteenth- and nineteenth-century French antiques, bedroom four-posters, elaborate draperies, massive Italian armoires—all bathed in the almost palpable rosy glow of the flowers and the inevitable Arden pink.

The Phoenix spa, like the original one, seems to be a highly personal blend of country club, beauty sanctuary, European spa, summer camp, and boarding school. EVERYTHING is done for the client; all major decisions have been made well in advance—by the staff, not the client. They decide what you will eat, drink, play at, and have done to your face and body. Phoenix Maine Chance is a meticulously plotted escape from stress and frustration into a state of total pampering.

On a recent visit, as I alighted from the plane at Phoenix Airport, blinking in the blazing sunshine, I felt months removed from the mushy gray New York morning I'd left five hours before.

Despite the influx of NOUVEAUX RICHISSIMES, the old prejudice against what Miss Arden called "ordinary people" has left its mark. The women here are quieter, less ostentatious than at other spas.

Elizabeth Arden's greatest legacy to Maine Chance was, in a word, "CLASS." And THAT is why it remains a favorite retreat of Mary Lasker, Claire Boothe Luce, Bunny DuPont, Christina Ford, Mrs. Ogden Phipps, Greer Garson, Ava Gardner, et al.

Back to my Sunday arrival. As always, I was hot, tired, and thirsty. Did I head for the water fountain? I did not. Not HERE. A maid promptly fetched a cool glass of unsugared fresh lemonade.

"Plain water isn't good enough," she said solicitously.

I had the feeling I'd just been patted on the head. And that was a feeling that grew and grew with each passing day of my week there.

Maine Chance's culinary genius had prepared a superb cheese soufflé, served with lightly stewed tomatoes, a salad of dark greens with finely shredded beets, a dessert of fresh stewed fruit, and honeyed tea. Like most meals there, this one had a superlative FRESHNESS about it.

Let it be said that Maine Chance never stints on food in any way. It is always delicious, always first quality. I found myself trading the attractive junket desserts for fresh fruit. Otherwise, I approved of the menu.

Here is the terrific recipe for cheese soufflé, which every guest is treated to on her first day:

Cheese Soufflé à la Maine Chance

¼ cup butter or margarine	1 cup shredded cheddar cheese and ½ cup shredded Swiss cheese (about 4 oz.)
½ cup Gold Medal flour	
½ tsp. salt	
¼ tsp. dry mustard	4 eggs, separated
Dash cayenne red pepper	¼ tsp. cream of tartar
1 cup milk	

Melt butter in saucepan over low heat. Blend in flour and seasonings. Cook over low heat, stirring until mixture is smooth and bubbly. Remove from heat. Stir in milk. Heat to boiling, stirring constantly. Boil and stir 1 minute. Stir in cheese until melted. Remove from heat. Beat egg whites and cream of tartar until stiff but not dry; set aside. Beat egg yolks until very thick and lemon colored; stir into cheese mixture. Stir about ¼ of the egg whites into cheese mixture. Gently fold mixture into remaining egg whites. Carefully pour into soufflé dish. Bake 50 to 60 minutes or until knife inserted halfway between edge and center comes out clean. Serve immediately. (Serves 4.)

And here is that salad (my FAVORITE Maine Chance mixed salad):

Maine Chance Salad

Boston lettuce	Endive
Bibb lettuce	Shredded beets
Romaine lettuce	Water chestnuts

Vary the above in amounts to your liking.

And you MUST (well, try it ONCE, anyway) serve it with this dressing, which is good for any vegetable salad:

Maine Chance Dressing

1 bunch parsley, chopped fine (without the stems, please)	1 tsp. horseradish
	1 tsp. mustard
	1 tsp. Worcestershire sauce
1 bunch watercress, chopped fine (also de-stemmed)	⅓ cup tarragon vinegar
	½ cup Wesson oil
8 shallots, chopped fine optional	½ cup safflower oil

After lunch, I strolled around the gardens and took a dip in the Olympic-sized swimming pool from which one can gaze up at the bluest sky and the stark, arid majesty of Camelback Mountain.

The blue-green sparkling clean pool inspired me to swim several lengths. Swimming, by the way, is one of my favorite muscle-lengthening exercises.

While floating under a canopy of lofty orange trees, my toes jabbing at the sunshine, I felt the most marvelous sensation of letting go, of being utterly at peace with myself. I knew that life for the next few days would be simple and good.

At precisely 6:45—just fifteen minutes before dinner in the main house—the "Happy Hour" began. Leaving behind the ubiquitous tank suits and terry robes, we emerged from late-afternoon naps wearing caftans, long skirts and shirts, or evening pants and blouses. The undone hair was stashed under turbans, scarves, or washable wigs. Those with washable hair skinned it back into buns or topknots.

No one needed to worry a bit about overdoing the hors d'oeuvres. A double portion of the vegetable juice, cranberry juice, and raw vegetables couldn't have added a millimeter to the waistline. Black-uniformed maids circulated among the guests with tiny glasses of juice and exquisitely prepared crudités—carrot matchsticks, slivers of sweet pepper, wire-thin scallions, rounds of raw turnip, baby cherry tomatoes.

The dinner that night was broiled chicken, Swiss chard, cubed squash, with junket and honeyed tea for dessert.

A lot of the old despotism has vanished from the Phoenix Maine Chance. There's no more clandestine baggage-searching for liquor. The erstwhile prohibition on in-room phones has been lifted. ("Why court bad news from OUT THERE," Miss Arden used to say.) And Miss Ames ("Amesy"), the original beloved hostess, no longer monitors the dinner servings: more than two of the thin roast beef slices on a plate inevitably produced a stony scowl from Amesy. Now we were on the honor system, and guests were permitted to go back for seconds. The only penalty was a discreet, silent treatment from neighbors, who lashed the gourmande with raised eyebrows.

Entertainment at Maine Chance is of the do-it-yourself kind: bridge, conversation in the drawing room, television, reading (the library is excellent), some hopping off to Scottsdale, double-board bingo, and—a recent innovation—a once-weekly movie.

I retired early that first night to write letters and make a few calls to New York. I kept promising myself to get to the books and needlepoint I'd brought with me, but they lost out to the prospect of a good night's sleep in that big pink bed. After all, I was here to indulge myself!

My first full day began with a visit from the staff doctor and nurse, who checked my heart and general health condition and okayed the program of diet and exercise.

No woman should die before having one breakfast served in her pink boudoir by a Maine Chance maid. It's as close an approximation to Nirvana that I can imagine. After the doctor left at 7:30, my maid knocked at my door and brought in a tray covered with a crisp doily containing a bud vase with a single lovely rose, the morning paper, delicate Royal Adderley china in my favorite cornflower pattern (how did they KNOW?), and, almost incidentally, breakfast. Mine was a half of grapefruit, one coddled egg, whole-grain bread, a pat of sweet butter, and coffee. (I was not dieting severely. The usual is grapefruit and coffee.)

A reminder that the day will be a no-nonsense, busy one comes in the form of a red-white-and-blue appointment card—all filled in. Following the usual ritual, I tied it to my terrycloth robe, feeling a bit like a tot off to nursery school with her mittens pinned to her sleeves.

9:00	Exercise
9:30	Steam Cabinet
10:00	Massage
11:00	Exercise
11:30	Face Treatment
12:00	Hair & Nails
1:00	Luncheon
2:30	Make-Up Class
3:30	Exercise

At 9:00, I had an exercise class with none other than Marjorie Craig herself, followed by a face treatment from Miss Helen Wesley, using the classical Arden products and salon techniques. (For an example you can use at home, see page 33.)

I made it a point to request my facial after exercise and before lunch, knowing that I would—as always—fall asleep in the chair.

Water therapy came next. I chose the whirlpool in a delightful open-air area, to loosen the kinks and cricks I'd just acquired during my first exercise session.

By lunchtime, I'd felt as if I'd been through a full day's schedule. But I was hungry, and delved enthusiastically into the deviled eggs, cold shrimp, and salad. The salad was brushed with a delicious mustard-and-oil dressing, full of the dark vitamin-rich "heavy" greens Maine Chance is known for. There's a reason for those greens. When you cut carbohydrates so drastically, your elimination often suffers. Swiss chard, kale, raw spinach, and the like contain cellulose, which keeps traffic moving right along.

After-lunch repose comes in the form of a nail-and-hair treatment. This double treatment is more than an elementary prettifying exercise. Fingernails and toenails (on alternate days) are shaped, creamed, and buffed for twenty minutes; and the scalp is massaged and lubricated with Arden's standby, Eight-Hour Cream. Then the hair is brushed with the two-brush method. See page 37. Greased to a fare-thee-well, I headed for yet another exercise session.

The Arden exercise program, while vigorous, differs from most routines in one significant respect. We were encouraged to perform each movement accurately and completely. It's as vigorous as any high-school gym class, but, I think, far more rewarding—and less prone to strain a muscle or pull a ligament.

The yoga slant board is indicative of Miss Arden's fascination with and reverence for all kinds of Yogic routines. I remember a HARPER'S BAZAAR photograph long ago of her standing on her head, every hair in place, wearing white knickers. Her stretching, deep-breathing routines are in the yogic tradition.

There was no more than a three-minute interval between the exercise class and the unique Maine Chance paraffin bath. Long ago, Elizabeth Arden brought back a collection of large body-shaped baskets with stands from India. The baskets were lined with waxed paper.

I stripped, climbed into the basket and settled back into my crackling bed. Most people, out of a touch of claustrophobia, leave their arms hanging outside.

Then an attendant poured warm, melted paraffin over me, making sure to dab extra wax over the chubby spots. The number of dabs reminded me of how many chubby spots I had, and inspired me to considerable remorse. Then she wrapped me in waxed paper and a top cover to keep the warmth in. I lay there for what seemed an eternity, sweating out months of ill-considered desserts and APÉRITIFS. When I was "done," I was cracked and peeled like an Easter egg, helped to my feet, and asked how I felt.

I felt just great! Airy-fairy, light (in fact one pound lighter), limp, with each pore in my body purged of impurities. Still perspiring, I wafted to my 4:15 massage, where every remnant of tension was kneaded out of my body. Purring like a pussycat, tired, I curled up in my room for a pre-dinner siesta.

Dinner featured a thin but delicious four-ounce Kansas City-cut steak with cottage cheese (to raise the protein count), a few carrots and string beans (for vitamins), and fresh shredded pineapple topped with a juicy strawberry for dessert.

Then we retired to the drawing room for Sanka, congenial chatter, a round of bridge maybe, and then good night.

My day was typical of the Maine Chance routine. Concentrated sun-up activity, quiet evenings. Above all, there is time—time to collect and sort out your thoughts, time to remember or discover who you are, time to plot your future, time, if you wish, to do nothing at all but listen to the howling coyotes in the Arizona desert.

Maine Chance also gave me time to care for my feet even beyond the ritual pumicing and creaming every day. And what a luxury to be able to floss, brush, and Water-Pik my teeth properly!

Maine Chance's big bonus is the staff. They're accessible. (No disappearing acts when you need them.) They're wholly professional, and they share their expertise with you freely. My masseuse, for example, fed me nutritional advice as she unknotted my knots.

"Never drink water with meals," she said. "You should use your own saliva to break down food. A cup of bouillon or a glass of wine before dinner will stimulate your digestive juices. But the best DIGESTIF of all is time. Never bolt a meal. And never, never eat ANYTHING standing up."

A special staff member at Maine Chance during one of my stays was a wonder-woman who used acupressure (formerly known as zonal or reflexology therapy) to bring bliss, not only to the feet, but to the entire body.

The principle of acupressure is similar to that of acupuncture. She believed that there are nerve endings in the feet that affect every part of the body. And, although she did not pretend to diagnose illnesses medically, she insisted that one foot treatment would tell her a world about anybody's health problems.

After she had explored every spot on my feet, kneading, prodding, circling with her fingertips, palms, and knuckles, I emerged a limp, smiling rag-doll. In fact, I felt so CARNALLY good, it made me feel a bit guilty.

"If it feels good, DO it!" she said. "We Americans feel so self-conscious about anything that makes us feel good or relaxed or beautiful—as if it's wicked."

This woman, having traveled the world, touted a sensational Malaysian remedy for women who have no one to massage their feet. (See page 18.)

Rates vary according to accommodation, in the range of $1,850 to $2,350 single; $1,700 to $2,100 double per week, plus a 15% gratuity charge and applicable taxes.

SUMMARY: Maine Chance is class, and definitely first-class at that—prim and genteel. The top-notch talent that made Maine Chance—from Arden herself to Gaylord Hauser and Marjorie Craig, and as well as an unsung but super lower-level staff—spell quality, service, comfort and fulfillment for the guest. A lady's refuge in an unladylike world. Easily worth the tab if you've got it to spare.—E.W.

The Greenhouse Texas

Each spa leaves you with a distinctly different feeling upon departure. When I leave Maine Chance each time, I feel as if I've just celebrated my sixteenth birthday and once again said goodbye to childhood. The Greenhouse is another pampering Eden, but a grown-up one. After a week or two in Arlington, Texas, I feel that I am taking temporary leave of the world's most exclusive club.

The Greenhouse is loyal to its members (no casual preference is EVER forgotten), and its members return this loyalty by coming back year after year. In fact, four of every five women you'll see there are repeaters. But even on my first visit, I felt welcome. On the third visit, I felt as if I owned the place.

The Greenhouse is owned by The Great Southwest Corporation, and operated with the help of Neiman-Marcus and Charles of the Ritz. Stanley Marcus once said that the Greenhouse was meant to be a hothouse for wilted ladies. With proper care, feeding, and exercise, their bodies are brought back to life and their souls achieve a certain cultivation.

Fair enough. For $2,200 per week (plus 15 percent service charge in lieu of individual gratuities), the guest luxuriates in a great glass-covered Shangri-La, from which the sunlight streams down into a two-story glass-encased courtyard spoked with walkways leading to guests' suites. In all, there are some 52,500 square feet of white brick building in an exotic jungle landscape, scalloped into a series of interior gardens and patios. There is also an indoor heated pool that can be used in any season.

The living accommodations are as posh as one can imagine without being in any way garish. They come in single and double rooms, with or without private balconies facing the indoor pool. Suites enjoy private entry foyers, and some bedrooms connect to large sitting rooms with fireplaces. There is space galore, and each room is tastefully done in dulcet yellows, greens, beige, white, and gold.

The Greenhouse is a classic spa and the only major spa in the country open the year around for women exclusively.

It is unlike most spas in that it does not depend upon any natural attraction. The Greenhouse is a totally controlled environment—including controlled temperature, humidity, and light. It is able to sneer at the weather extremes that can torment that patch of Texas between Fort Worth and Dallas.

I cannot tell you how luxurious it feels to bounce on the mattress of your bed in your Greenhouse bedroom. The gadgets and indulgences surpass even Maine Chance. The bidet symbolizes the continental quality of the place. You also have your own air controls, sunken tub, lighted closets, makeup mirrors, separate bathroom and powder room, radio, and television.

While a woman could spend the entire week ensconced in these luxurious confines, those who long for the outdoors can enjoy it via an outdoor pool, hiking and jogging trails, tennis courts, and a full golf course adjacent to the property.

The nice thing about returning to the Greenhouse is that they remember every little preference from your last visit. My second time around was so pleasurable: they remembered to put my favorite flowers in my room, and they remembered that I like my daily facial before lunch and my massage late in the afternoon following exercise.

The schedule has discipline, but you're bound to it only insofar as you care to be. A staff of 125 cares for a capacity of 38 guests.

Breakfast was a delight (I was keeping to an 850-calorie-per-day regimen), served promptly in bed at 8:00 A.M. on a lucite tray with flowers. It consisted of egg baked in a cup, thin delicious toast (without butter), and tea with a tiny cup of honey. The day's schedule was carefully written out on a card.

I had always wondered how they got those pieces of toast so incredibly THIN. Last time I was there, I learned their secret. Here it is.

Paper-Thin Toast

Freeze an entire loaf of bread. Then use a slicing machine (if you have one) or a serrated knife, and cut the bread into 1/8-inch slices. Place the slices on a baking sheet greased with margarine or butter. Pop into the oven, or over a pilot light overnight, until it crisps. Best results with whole wheat, rye, or cinnamon swirls.

By 8:30, I was down by the pool doing the "wake-up-and-warm-up" exercises in a pretty blue exercise suit. (Yellow terrycloth cover-ups are worn to and from the treatment rooms. These, incidentally, are provided for each guest by the Greenhouse.) The exercises were meant to prime us for the rest of the day, and

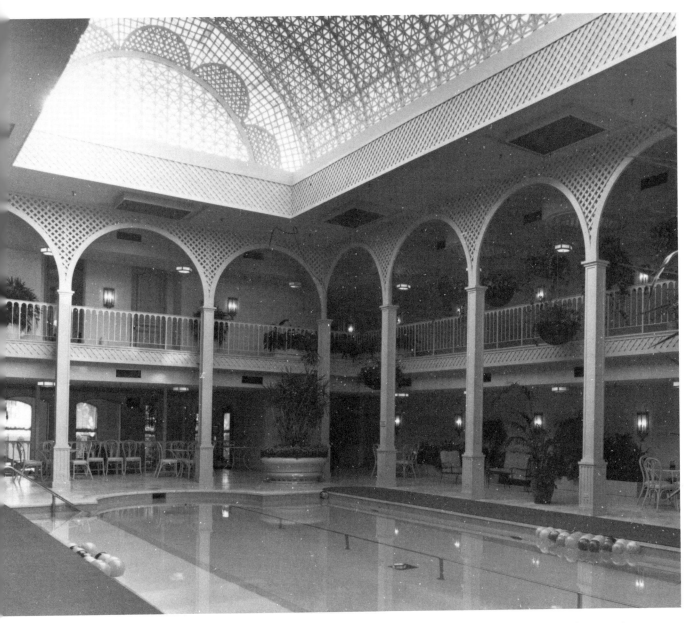

The Greenhouse Texas

involved mostly breathing and stretching movements. Veteran dancer Toni Beck developed the program along rhythmic, choreographic routines. She (like Marjorie Craig at Maine Chance) abjures fast, strenuous exercises. The entire period was built on dance principles, requiring minimal effort and tension, but yielding, in my opinion, excellent results.

Toni, now executive director, told me she feels the most troublesome areas for women over thirty-five are the abdomen and upper thighs, caused mainly by bad posture. There is, she said, a tendency for women approaching middle age to allow their shoulders to droop, causing a host of muscles to sag.

"You can recover a waistline," she said, "if you learn to keep your shoulders down and back, and your legs relaxed when you walk. Always hold your body with a 'lift'—and you'll find it working not only on your body but on your mood and attitudes as well."

Many youth-conscious women, she declared, make the mistake of mimicking their daughters, keeping themselves toothpick-thin. Every woman has a ten-pound differential on either side of her ideal

83

weight, within which she can be comfortable and look good. If weight rises or falls below those limits, then she ought to take action.

At 9:00 A.M. Toni started us on her "Swing and Sway" exercises to music from "Fame", Willie Nelson, Olivia Newton-John and a Ray Coniff album, "Turn Around, Look at Me", which I found superb for picking up my flagging spirits.

For one of Toni's best exercises, see page 45.

At 10:00 I had my manicure and pedicure, followed by water exercises in the warm pool, which makes exercise MOST relaxing. The pool is about four feet deep, and thus beautifully suited to working with balls and doing kicking exercises for a marvelous firming effect.

At noon, we were given makeup lessons, and I had the opportunity to have my scalp treatment. Many of us consider the Greenhouse our private beauty hotel. The products used are very special. Charles of the Ritz for face, Rene Guinot for skin care, Redken for hair—things you simply don't get from the average beauty salon without asking specifically for them and paying extra. The quality of care is such that you might get by combining the salons where you got your best massage, your very best facial, your best shampoo and set, and so forth.

Here are some of the Greenhouse beauty secrets I tucked away for you:

Greenhouse Home Beauty Secrets

Freshener should always be blotted with tissue. If it evaporates, it can dehydrate the skin.

A moistened sponge used as a big "eraser" will help you eliminate that matted, heavily made up look.

Cheek coloring should be applied to the cheekBONES. A touch on the chin and forehead will give you a nice, brightening look. But avoid getting too close to the eyes or nose, which pulls the face down.

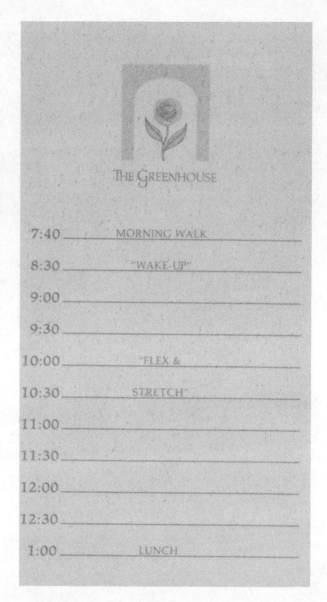

THE GREENHOUSE

7:40 _____ MORNING WALK _____
8:30 _____ "WAKE-UP" _____
9:00 _____
9:30 _____
10:00 _____ "FLEX &
10:30 _____ STRETCH"
11:00 _____
11:30 _____
12:00 _____
12:30 _____
1:00 _____ LUNCH _____

At 1:00 P.M. sharp, luncheon is served round the pool. My lunch consisted of one-half cold boiled lobster tail served on a bed of lettuce with lots of parsley (meant to be eaten), congealed gazpacho salad, coffee or tea and fresh fruit slices.

After lunch, more beauty treatments: nail massage, and curative pedicure. At 2:30, spot-reducing sessions. At 3:00, I was escorted to the sauna, which was followed by a needle shower, and massage.

At 4:30, I returned to my lovely room, where I napped and then dressed for dinner, which is preceded by a non-alcoholic "cocktail hour" featuring delicious juice concoctions and low-calorie dips. Dinner at 7:00

consisted of iced vegetable relishes, veal rack, zucchini fans, sauteed mushrooms, asparagus salad with mimosa dressing, coffee pots de creme and demi-tasse coffee.

Although many of the women there during my stay seemed to be going through either divorce or widowhood, the average age has dropped dramatically. The Greenhouse is a marvelous place to recuperate from the anxieties and traumas of separation. The one thing every woman who suddenly has to fend for herself ought to do is get into shape fast. Every challenge is easier if you look and feel your best. The Greenhouse has a blitz program—one that could take a very, very long time if you ran around trying to collect all the services they offer under one roof.

There are also many young girls at the Greenhouse these days. Some had no more than an eighth of an inch to work off before a wedding or a very special occasion. It seemed as if the girls with the twenty-four-inch waists were the most severe with themselves in adhering to the program.

This is the perfect place for a career girl who gets precious little exercise. The Greenhouse offers her a method of weaving self-care into the tapestry of her daily life. Health routines become automatic, once you've learned how to tuck your tummy in while brushing your teeth, to watch your diet, and to do a few yoga exercises in the course of your working day.

For many of the women with those plum-sized diamond rings and golden chokers and private planes parked outside, a visit to the Greenhouse was highlighted by the Tuesday evening fashion show. The Neiman-Marcus fashion coordinator arrived with exquisite clothes and models. Each woman was given a list of the fashions, including everything from basics to accessories, bags, shoes, and hats—with style numbers and prices. You simply checked whatever you wanted.

Then, on Thursday, after having your hair done and your facial, you could skip some classes and be driven to the store in a chauffeured car.

All these goodies could be charged to your Neiman-Marcus account. And anyone without a charge account could open one very quickly and painlessly.

A commercial touch, perhaps, but sweet, tasteful, and unobtrusive, like everything else at the Greenhouse. One remembers the little touches: the five-gallon dispensers of Mountain Valley Water all around the place, used not only for drinking, but in spray bottles, to set makeup or for use after facials; the unique fruit facials made of grapes and apricots; and the fresh leotard, tights, headband, toga, and robe that are distributed DAILY.

The food, by the way, is ALWAYS good. Here are some of the finest recipes from the Greenhouse that I've tried and loved:

Salade de Crudités
Use any vegetable cut into bite-sized pieces.

Sliced Brussels sprouts	Squash
Slivered asparagus	Cauliflower
Celery	Sliced carrots

Pour hot water over all to bring out color. Cool and add:

Cucumber	Belgian endive sliced
Green onion	Romaine lettuce in
Fresh mushrooms	small pieces
Cherry tomatoes	

Toss with clear, fresh dressing. Pour off dressing, sprinkle with chopped parsley, and serve.

Yogurt Dressing

1 cup plain yogurt	2 level Tbs. Dijon mustard, mild

Mix.

Ratatouille

1 eggplant, peeled and diced	1 onion, peeled and sliced thin
1 green pepper, de-seeded and sliced thin	1 Tbs. salad oil
1 tomato, peeled and sliced thin	1 tsp. lemon juice
	Salt substitute

Pile vegetables in casserole in layers. Pour oil and lemon juice over them. Bake at 300° until soft. Serve hot or cold.

Roast Veal au Citron

1 veal loin	Sauterne wine, dry
½ tsp. white pepper	Grated rind of ½ lemon
Pinch of cinnamon	Juice of 1 lemon
Pinch of Nutmeg	

Rub veal with seasonings. Place in 250° oven. Baste with dry Sauterne wine. Roast for 1½ hours. Add rind and juice of lemon and continue roasting for 1 hour or until veal is tender. Strain juices and serve as a sauce.

All these dishes come from the late Helen Corbitt, the original Neiman-Marcus and Greenhouse dietician. She stressed the importance of making all food ATTRACTIVE—visually as well as gustatorially. Once a week, she gave cooking lessons in the Greenhouse kitchen.

"For people who love good food," she said, "dieting must be a state of mind over matter. A new approach to a habit you enjoy, to lose weight and not find it again. Think thin, and you automatically say no-thank-you to the extra calories from breads and high-starch foods, to nibbling of sweets, to cocktails, to all the things you know add pounds."

In order to avoid falling off the diet once you're home again, she instructed us to avoid the stale, boring tomato-and-cottage-cheese routine. She felt that diet foods should be varied, NOT overcooked, and should be physically attractive. Each meal should have some fresh fruit and vegetables (she abhorred frozen varieties, but allowed them in a pinch). And these, she pointed out, should be prepared just prior to cooking.

I doubt if any woman ever spent a week at the Greenhouse without feeling years younger at the end of it. And that is the name of the game. I am reminded of that wonderful line in Robert Browning's "Fra Lippo Lippi":

> IF YOU GET SIMPLE BEAUTY AND NOUGHT ELSE,
> YOU GET ABOUT THE BEST THING GOD INVENTS.

SUMMARY: The Greenhouse is a Texas gusher of hospitality, good food, exquisite furnishings, and self-indulgence. While it's the only beauty spa I know of that places cigarettes on the dining table, or tells you that you can buy almost anything you see at the department store down the road, those are good indications of how deeply they've plumbed Milady's weaknesses. If it comes off as a mite materialistic, it's GENUINELY materialistic and not HYPOCRITICALLY materialistic. Their "Y'all come back soon!" goodbye is as much a real invitation as it is a farewell.—E.W.

The Spa at Palm-Aire Florida

"I would sell my bread for marmalade," said Théophile Gautier, in a variation on the give-me-luxuries-and-I'll-dispense-with-the-necessities credo.

It probably takes a French poet to understand some of the paradoxes of my life. I'm thinking particularly of the way I cheerfully pay $230 a day to stay at the new, posh Palm-Aire Spa—and then for the next six months boycott taxis, lunch on yogurts I keep in my purse, and recycle teabags.

When I walk into the lounge of the Palm-Aire spa and take in the mix of beige carpeting, off-white walls, and eye-reposing stretches of glass, shingles, and concrete, I get that serene, eager feeling that I'm entering a cornucopia where I won't have to forego any of life's delights.

And Palm-Aire itself IS a delight. For two million dollars it ought to be. The secret is not so much the money, but the brains that went into putting it all together. They hired creative experts from other Super Spas who were familiar with what was right and wrong in the old spas and who eliminated the nuisances (such as 5:00 A.M. reveille, spartan accommodations, one-hundred-miles-from-nowhere locations).

Palm-Aire is one of the few spas that cater to men as well as women, and even has duplicated all of the facilities and programs for them. But the two sexes normally do not meet in the course of the spa program unless they're getting facials in adjoining salons, enjoying the Olympic coed pool, a half-mile station fitness course, the coed gym and weight room, or the magnificent racquetball courts (four of them).

This gender segregation is, according to most of the men I've talked to, just fine. It turns their half of Palm-Aire into a kind of men's club.

"It's absolutely delightful to be without women's shrill, helpful voices for a few days," said a dashing young banker friend of mine. "Once you're all naked and in the pool, you begin to talk with the other men—seriously about serious things. They're mostly businessmen, lawyers, accountants, and bankers. You develop a genuine camaraderie as you perform exercises together, slam the medicine ball at each other's spare tires, play volleyball, do leg lifts, and so forth. With all the activity, even with the delightfully prepared and tasty food, I lost weight. I have only two minor reservations about Palm-Aire: the first is that there weren't enough sports, such as one has at La Costa, and the second is that the food was neither glorious nor adequate for the appetite you build up. But, let's face it, I lost-six-and-a-half pounds in the first two days. And THAT's why I was there."

I'd be astounded if anyone of either sex at Palm-Aire had any energy left over after a full day's program of open-air massages, exercises, herbal wraps, saunas, hot and cold dips, Turkish baths, facials, whirlpools, tennis, golf, and what have you. And beyond that, there are also bridge lessons, backgammon and volleyball, the racetrack and fronton, the theater, the cinema, and a complete series of health enhancement lectures and discussions, including luncheon lectures, cocktail hour discussions, and evening programs. After a day at the spa, I found that it was all I could do to lug an apple up to my room, glance at the paper, and fall asleep.

Incidentally, Palm-Aire boasts a most civilized touch. There is no crack-of-dawn splashdown up-and-at-'em torture. Absolutely nothing stirs or twitches before 8:30 A.M.!

The spa is part of a 1,500-acre condominium complex at Palm-Aire in Pompano Beach, Florida, located halfway between Palm Beach and Miami Beach. The spa guests stay at the luxurious Spa Hotel at Palm-Aire. Also on the property are five spectacular 18-hole golf courses, four championship and one executive, and thirty-seven tennis courts, many of which are lighted for night play. The clientele has a minimum of retired gentlefolk and a very high percentage of "doers."

At Palm-Aire, you'll bump into such exciting people as Jerry Lewis, Lee Elder, Lee Trevino, O. J. Simpson, Elizabeth Taylor, Goldie Hawn, Nancy Lopez, to name just a few.

Both sexes find a special serenity and discipline at Palm-Aire. Alcohol is a no-no; smoking and coffee drinking provoke frowns; and if you simply follow the leader, you can't help but lose weight.

The six-hundred-calorie diet need not spell gastronomic privation. Palm-Aire's dietetic staff tries to wean you away from high-fat foods and put you onto fish and fowl and fruit, away from coffee and tea and onto rose hips and herbal teas.

One dinner was so scrumptious, I asked the chef for the borscht, Palm-Aire dressing, shish kebab, and fruit torte recipes. The entire meal is well under 300 calories—but so GOOD!

Here is a typical menu, with each item's caloric value clearly marked.

Russian Borscht

Combine 2½ cups (No. 2 can) of shredded beets with the beet liquid and 4½ cups of bouillon. Simmer 10 minutes, then add 6 tablespoons of lemon juice and some pepper to season. Serve hot or cold and top with a teaspoon of low-calorie sour cream. (Serves 8, 40 calories per serving.)

Palm-Aire Salad Dressing

1 bunch parsley (stemless)	1 tsp. Worcestershire sauce
1 bunch watercress (stemless)	⅓ cup tarragon vinegar
8 shallots	¼ cup safflower oil
1 tsp. horseradish	3 egg yolks
1 tsp. mustard	1 tsp. Vege-Sal (seasoned salt)
	¾ cup water

Blend together. (15 calories per teaspoon.)

Shish Kebab

Place onto a skewer and broil:

2½ oz. raw tenderloin	3 cherry tomatoes or
3 mushrooms	3 tomato wedges
2 pieces of onion	3 pieces green pepper

(150 calories per serving.)

BREAKFAST
7:30 a.m. to 9:30 a.m.

135 CALORIES MAXIMUM

JUICE OR FRUIT
Choose One

☐ 4 oz. Orange Juice (40 Calories)   ☐ Fresh Melon Wedges (40 Calories)

☐ ½ Grapefruit (40 Calories)   ☐ Fresh Strawberries ½ cup (40 Calories)

☐ 4 oz. V-8 Juice (25 Calories)   ☐ 4 oz. Diet Cranberry Juice (30 Calories)

PROTEIN
Choose One

☐ One Medium Egg Cooked to Order (72 Calories)   ☐ Skim Milk 4 oz. (40 Calories)

☐ Low Fat Cottage Cheese ⅓ cup (67 Calories)   ☐ Double Egg-White Omelette with Parsley or Mushrooms (35 Calories)

STARCH
Choose One

☐ Bagel Thins (2) with Diet Jelly (25 Calories)   ☐ Bran Muffin (75 Calories)

☐ ½ Slice 7-Grain Toast (35 Calories)   ☐ ⅓ Cup 7-Grain Cereal (40 Calories)

☐ Cold Cereal ½ Cup (65 Calories)

Hot or cold cereal is not served with milk unless indicated under "PROTEIN" above.

BEVERAGES

☐ Rosehip Tea   OR   ☐ Decaffeinated Coffee

Any changes or alterations must meet with the approval of the Dietitian.

NAME   **ROOM NUMBER**

Fruit Torte

Drain an 8-ounce can of low-calorie fruit cocktail, saving the syrup and adding enough water to make one cup of the liquid. Bring to a boil, then dissolve contents of 1 envelope of lemon-flavored D-Zerta into the boiling liquid. Stir in a cup of ice and water. Continue stirring until the ice has melted. Chill until mixture thickens. Line the bottom of an 8-by-4-inch pan with split lady fingers. Whip gelatine until volume doubles. Now blend in a cup of prepared Dream Whip and the fruit cocktail. Spoon over the lady fingers and chill. When thoroughly chilled, slice into 12 servings. (45 calories per serving.)

MONDAY LUNCH

APPETIZER
Choose One

		PORTION SIZE	CALORIES
☐	Chicken Consommé	5 oz.	20
	or		
☐	Romaine Salad Lemon Dressing	1 Cup	20

ENTREE
Choose One

☐	Cottage Cheese Fruit Plate with Cinnamon Yogurt Dip	1 Cup Fruit	160
	or		
☐	Spanish Omelette with Green Beans	1½ Eggs ½ Cup	160

DESSERT
Choose One

☐	Fruit Torte	2½	50
	or		
☐	Fresh Seasonal Fruit	½ Cup	45

BEVERAGES

☐ Rosehip Tea OR ☐ Decaffeinated Coffee

Any changes or alterations must meet with the approval of the Dietitian.

_____   _____
NAME   ROOM NUMBER

MONDAY DINNER

APPETIZER
Choose One

		PORTION SIZE	CALORIES
☐	Spinach Soup	6 oz.	20
	or		
☐	Tossed Salad Italian Dressing	1 Cup	20

ENTREE
Choose One

☐	Flounder Marinara with Tomatoes, Oregano and Garlic	4 oz.	150
	or		
☐	Broiled Lamb Chops	3 oz.	150

VEGETABLE

☐	Steamed Artichoke		20

DESSERT
Choose One

☐	Vanilla Tart with Blackberry Sauce	2½ oz.	40
	or		
☐	Fresh Fruit	½ Cup	40

BEVERAGE

☐ Rosehip Tea OR ☐ Decaffeinated Coffee

Any changes or alterations must meet with the approval of the Dietitian.

_____   _____
NAME   ROOM NUMBER

I mention the food first to put you at ease. Palm-Aire's diet-conscious gastronomic ingenuity really takes the martyrdom out of spa-ing.

The water programs are also fun. They are designed so that anyone with two left feet can perform them effortlessly. Never mind if you've got a bad back, partial paralysis, arthritis—the directors use the water's buoyancy to make the exercises easier and more efficient.

Palm-Aire's well-rounded approach to fitness includes classes that will help you lose pounds as well as inches. With over 15 classes, all designed with a level of difficulty, guests receive the maximum in individualized exercise prescriptions and receive the utmost of benefits both physically and psychologically.

You begin the day in one of three modern locker rooms, in which you're given a yellow robe, leotard, sweat shirt, sweat pants and slippers. There's also a supply of plastic, disposable shower caps and a complete array of toiletries from tanning lotions to razor blades.

Water EVERYWHERE. There is a luxurious outdoor whirlpool with eight jets spurting warm water at you from all directions. It is so relaxing and refreshing just

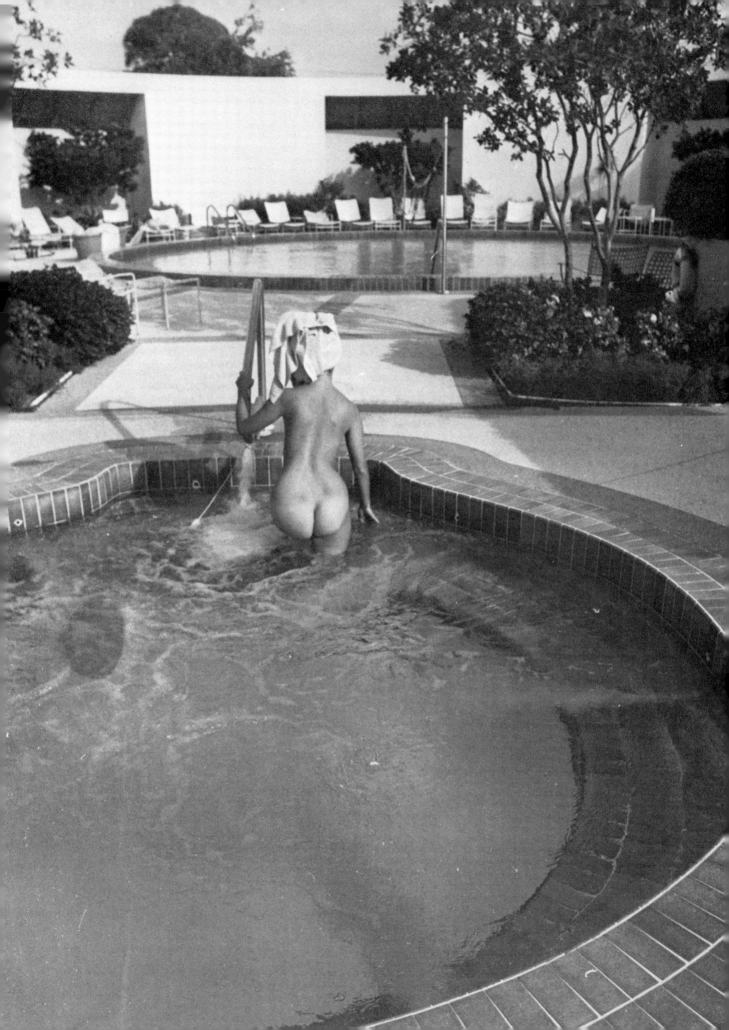

to chat in the Jacuzzi bath under the blue skies and baking Florida sunshine.

Just beyond the Jacuzzi is a large circular blue-tiled swimming pool, surrounded by scads of yellow and blue reclining chairs and lush palm trees, bushes, and other greenery. The total effect is one of unbroken gaiety. Also, there's an outdoor secluded, massage area and a solarium in both the men's and ladies' sections for nude sunbathing. In another area out in back of the spa there is the Olympic coed pool and a half-mile, nine-station fitness course. All areas have piped-in, soothing music.

The SPECIALITÉS DE LA MAISON are the loofah and Salt Glow treatments. Usually the Salt Glow is given first. The attendant rubs the avocado oil blend with medium-grained salt into the body to remove dead, scaly skin and to improve the circulation. Then the salt-oil is hosed off and an Ivory-soaped loofah is scrubbed all over the body. This creates a vibrant tingling that gives an extraordinary sense of well-being, of glowing and softness.

Palm-Aire has assembled a well-organized program of diet and exercise. It is closely supervised, with no loose ends, in superb indoor and outdoor facilities. There is also a physician who won't let you lift a barbell without a physical exam. The philosophy underlying the program is to give the clientele self-discipline and self-knowledge. These qualities inspire the confidence and pride that are the cornerstone of beauty.

From long experience, I can say that they're on the right track. They know how transient the spa experience can be. A sincere commitment is made to help motivate, stimulate and educate all guests. Take-home exercise programs, as well as a splendid array of health enhancement lectures and tapes are given to all guests so that they may get more involved in the process of lifestyle management and behavior modification. Palm-Aire is well ahead of its time with innovations and maintaining quality in all that it does. Genuine care and concern are shown to all guests with individual attention and expert professionals on hand at all times.

The usual schedule runs something like this:

8:40	Walk
9:00	Spa special
9:40	Water class
10:20	Whirlpool
11:00	Herbal wrap
11:40	Aerobics
12:20	Yoga
1:00	Lunch
2:00	Water class
2:40	Conditioning
3:20	Steam sauna and Roman bath
4:00	Stretch
4:40	Facial
5:20	Massage

No spa can keep the kind of clientele Palm-Aire has without appealing to their aesthetic sensibilities. And I found most becoming the citrus green and yellow color scheme and the impressionistic paintings that adorned the walls, as well as the immaculate cleanliness.

The bright green gym is filled with the finest Nautilus equipment, bicycles, rowing machines, rollers, belts, weights, poles, volley and medicine balls, jogging machines, walking machines, exercise benches, strap-on weights, ankle weights, and wrist weights.

Their slant board was a joy to me. It had a slope to hug the backs of your knees and was pitched high. Your feet are strapped across the bottom for anchorage while you do your sit-ups.

Palm-Aire has added a tea bar to the gym, where you can help yourself to fresh herbal teas. There is also a large Eagle drinking water dispenser, which you're encouraged to tap as your thirst rises from the exercises.

I explored the sauna and steam room. An attendant is there to assist you in and out and offer you wet washcloths wrapped around ice. When put on your face or body, you maintain your comfort while sweating off the excess water in your body. Following this, you can take a shower in one of the eleven new stalls and help yourself to Eurobath soap and shampoo, razors, combs and body lotion.

The Siesta Room is a kind of siesta lounge, very soporific with its pebble-mosaic California-style paintings and carpets of chartreuse, pale, and deep forest greens. There are three bunk beds with stretched white sheets and green, fluffy blankets.

Then there are the 14 massage rooms with very efficient masseuses and the 12 spaces devoted to facials.

The beauty salon at Palm-Aire is fully equipped and staffed with a highly skilled group of professionals.

Some of the valuable tips for day-to-day living, that I remember and practice which Palm-Aire offers its guests include:

1. Exercise at least three times a week for 30 minutes at a time.
2. Become more physically active by doing things

yourself instead of relying on machines and gadgets.

3. Protect your back by keeping a pelvic tilt, knees bent.
4. Eat well-balanced meals. Avoid too much meat, fats, and sugars.
5. Get adequate sleep.
6. Modify your behavior so that you eliminate bad habits such as overeating, lack of exercise, and smoking, and try to avoid stress.

SUMMARY: Palm-Aire is a conscientious blend of sophistication, seasoned expertise, and a rigorously commonsense program that works. It has irresistible appeal to schizoids like me who yearn for escape but can't survive without civilized diversions.—E.W.

La Costa California

When you first lay eyes on La Costa's seven thousand rolling green acres near the California coastline, I promise you will be smitten, just as I was.

You will feel as if you'd finally discovered the last word in luxurious spa-dom, a made-in-the-U.S.A. potpourri of Shangri-La and El Dorado.

Located thirty miles from San Diego, La Costa has become many things to its denizens and visitors. It is a weekend love nest for Hollywoodians and others. It is a veritable sports palace with inviting swimming pools, assorted gushing waters, tennis courts, new jogging path, and his-and-her gyms. It is also a magnet for the flamboyantly dissolute who choose to flee the sun and the greenery and the beaches and just sit in the bar and get uproariously sloshed.

It is also an American Super Spa with precious little debt to any other in décor, belligerently breaking all the old rules and erecting new ones.

It is also good eating—for dieters and non-dieters. The eating is perhaps too good, and frequently destructive of the best intentions. La Costa immediately evokes memories of crispy and delicious rolls, marvelous black bread, country-fresh butter, superb roast beef, imaginative desserts, and the best of wines, all served low-key to those lucky guests who did not come to diet.

The spa is only one part of the La Costa resort community. There are guest lodges, two hotels (one reserved for spa guests), glass-fronted chalets for spa guests, a racquet club, a saddle club, a beach club, cinemas, ballrooms, and boutiques. You can buy an ultra-modern condominium, townhouse, or a plot of land on which to build your dream house in this eternally sunny land. If you do, you will find yourself bathing in a sea of celebrities, mostly TV and movie people—many owners rent out their châteaux or houses while they're away.

Careful, though. If you have the notion that La Costa can provide you with a quiet retreat, forget it. This is one of the few spas on earth where you have hard-core glamor along with your saunas and exercise classes. Unspoiled it is not.

The spa facilities are excellent. But the program works only if you avoid the temptations of high living. If you can, forget about bringing fancy daytime clothes, because you'll be spending all your day hours in leotards, bathing suits, bathrobes, or birthday suit.

The spa celebrity register is long. It includes Valerie Perrine, Cindy Williams, Penny Marshall, Carrie Fisher, Stephanie Powers, Carol Burnett, Albert Finney, Gore Vidal, Louis Nizer, Sidney Sheldon, Bette Davis, Burt Bacharach, Carol Bayer Sager, Edie Gorme, and Steve Lawrence, to name a few.

Figure upwards of $275 per day single; $405 per day double plus 15% gratuity charge and 6% tax. Minimum stay on the Spa Plan is four days.

The plus on the side of spa-ing at La Costa is that it is a spa-oriented resort for both men and women. Each can do his or her own thing and still not be separated, except for the time spent in the spa program itself. Daytime attractions include golf (there is a 27-hole golf course) and tennis (there are 25 courts), and it is a rare guest who does not incorporate these into the spa program—both are included in the price. A couple may dine together, incidentally, with one person sticking to the spa diet and the other not restricted to it.

Every evening there is some special "activity" all spa guests can enjoy. An effort is made to involve the guests in bingo, backgammon, duplicate bridge, and lectures. And there is a special spa cocktail party to help the social side get going.

Let the staff know your arrival time at San Diego airport and a limousine will be sent to meet your plane. It's only a half-hour's drive. And if you're winging in on your own Lockheed or Cessna, you can touch down at Palomar Airport, only three miles away.

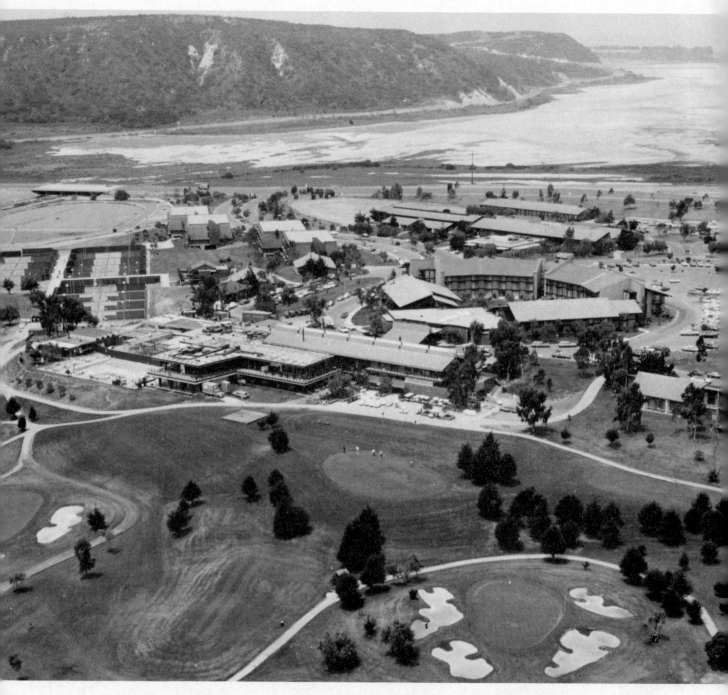

La Costa California

You're here to unwind, so tote along all those patience-demanding doodads you haven't yet had time to tackle.

If you stay at the regular hotel instead and qualify as a "regular" guest, the spa facilities are yours to use for an extra charge. Those on the special spa program stay at the comfortable spa building and have un-

limited use of all the health and beauty equipment. But be sure to book your appointments ahead of time.

You must begin your program with a consultation with Dr. R. Phillip Smith, the medical director. Then you are interviewed by the dieticians to help set your daily caloric intake and any special dietary course you might require. Their kitchen, which provides meals for nine thousand guests per month, has created tempting dishes for diabetics, ulcer victims, and clients on low-salt, low-residue, and low-purine diets.

Programs are individually tailored, but a typical spa day for a female guest might go like this:

LA COSTA

8:00 Breakfast: strawberries, small filet mignon, coffee.
9:00 Two consecutive exercise classes of your choice, followed by a Roman or whirlpool bath. Afterwards, the sauna or steam room and a Swiss shower (seventeen different hot and cold jets).
11:00 Makeup class.
11:40 Pool exercises.
12:40 Facial massage.
1:00 Lunch: consommé, fruit platter, turkey breast, vanilla custard.
2:40 Exercise class and herbal wrap.
4:00 Indoor or outdoor massage.
4:40 Shampoo, set, manicure.
6:00 Makeup session.
7:00 Dinner: Purée of tomato soup, salad, chicken amandine, toasted potato shell sprinkled with Parmesan cheese, caraway seeds, and chives, green beans, fresh pineapple.
Bedtime: one small apple.

Among La Costa's specials are the Ion Bath, the Luffa Massage, the Sunbrella Suntanning Program, and a daily herbal wrap. My espionage capability failed me here; I could not identify the twenty-one herbs infused into the mummy-style linen wraps that envelop you while you're being steamed. Most prominent, according to my nostrils, were eucalyptus, wintergreen oil, and mint. The wraps are soaked in the herbal solution and carted in steaming hot.

The attendant then sets you down on this hot sheet, which is placed over a plastic sheet on the cot, and wraps you in it. After the wrapping, several blankets are added for insulation. A cold compress is placed on your head, and you can nap, read, or daydream. Benefits: total release and relaxation. You may also find, if you've been exercising hard, that your muscles are less stiff after an herbal wrap.

The open-air Roman pools are very stimulating. Pulsating jets of water pounding all over your body can be extremely erotic. There are, in fact, so many different swirling, whirling, bubbling hoses and nozzles and faucets and tubs that I have trouble telling one from the other.

The gyms are not for lolling about in, and they are unlike anything you've ever seen before—lavishly mirrored, with a totally co-ordinated color scheme, right down to the carpeting, exercise bikes, rollers, slant boards, and bust-development machines. After too many sessions with the Costa Curves, Costa Capers, Isotonics, Isometrics, yoga, self-defense, water exercises, Swedish exercises, and stretches of one kind and another, you are liable—if you are both ambitious and out of condition—to turn the same shade as your surroundings.

Most of the exercise seems geared to improvement of respiration. And many guests take two classes consecutively, followed by a whirlpool bath and a half-hour in one of the siesta rooms.

Action Central at La Costa is the dining rooms. It is here that your spa tale acquires either a happy (pounds less) or tragic (pounds more) ending. You'll find your neighbors in the dining room counting calories with maniacal precision. And the only dietary slip-ups are intended, since each course is listed with its specific calorie content. So, whether you're aiming for a one-thousand- or eight-hundred- or six-hundred-calorie day, your only obstacle to success should be your arithmetic.

On an eight-hundred-calorie diet, for instance, you can lunch on fresh asparagus soup, sole a la Jardin, baked squash, cole slaw, cinnamon custard, and coffee. The quality is midpoint between haute cuisine and home cooking. One thing is sure, it is never dreary or tasteless.

Here is another luncheon I found most appetizing—and one you can re-create at home for a nice change of pace: cold blueberry soup, spring chicken cacciatore, salad with French dressing, and pineapple yogurt.

Cold Blueberry Soup

1 qt. apple juice	Very thin lemon slices
4 cups fresh blueberries or frozen berries without sugar	Whole cloves, if desired
	1 tsp. unflavored yogurt as garnish

Blend apple juice and blueberries until fairly smooth. Refrigerate at least 1 hour to mix the flavors. Strain, allow to settle, and skim to clear liquid. Serve in chilled

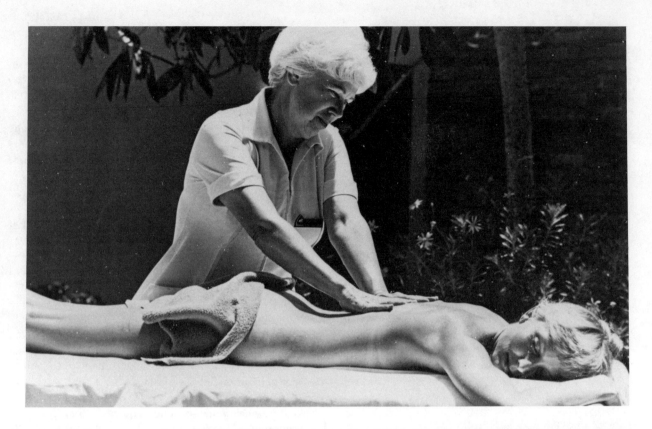

La Costa California

bouillon cups, garnished with 1 very thin slice of lemon, centered with a little dab of plain yogurt and 1 clove. (Serves 4.)

Spring Chicken Cacciatore

5 chicken breasts	½ tsp. mixed herbs—
½ cup each of chopped	rosemary, oregano,
green onion tops	sweet basil,
and green pepper	black pepper
1 cup diced, peeled	5 oz. unsalted tomato
fresh tomatoes	juice
½ tsp. chopped garlic	

Brown chicken on all sides in a hot dry pan. Add chopped vegetables, herbs, diced tomatoes, garlic, and tomato juice. Cover and allow to simmer until the chicken is tender. Remove lid and reduce the sauce if too thin. (Serves 4.)

La Costa French Dressing

2 rounded tsp. vegetable	1 level tsp. dry
gum (available in	mustard
pharmacies)	1 pinch ground
4 oz. white vinegar	celery seed

½ lemon, juiced	1½ cups pure pine-
and strained	apple juice
3 tsp. paprika	1 pinch sugar
⅛ tsp. white pepper.	

Dissolve vegetable gum in small amount of vinegar. Mix remainder of vinegar, lemon juice, paprika, pepper, mustard, celery seed, pineapple juice, sugar, and vegetable gum mixture. Blend lightly with wire wisk. Store in refrigerator until served.

Pineapple Yogurt

Just add 1 cup of coarsely chopped fresh pineapple to 2 cups of plain yogurt. Chill. (Serves 4.)

Dinner menus include Roast Duck Normandie, New York sirloin steak, and even chocolate mousse. The question that must occur to you, as it did to me, is by what magic does the chef pare down the calories of such fattening fare?

There are essentially two tricks.

The first consists of serving puny portions. After a day or two, your stomach suddenly realizes that two thin slices of Turkey Marco Polo are enough. What's more, they don't produce a bulky and bloated Thanksgiving Evening Syndrome. And a 3-ounce filet mignon (2 ounces in the broiling) makes a fabulous nonfattening and self-indulgent breakfast.

Bagel Thins are a terrific calorie cheater at La Costa. Regular bagels (horrendous plumping agents) are frozen firm and sliced with a meat slicer into 16 paper-thin "flying saucers." Then they are toasted. Only two are allowed at breakfast. These are delicious and satisfying and guaranteed not to bring you into the clutches of Jean Nidetch—IF you don't stray and wolf them down like potato chips. (But the temptation IS almost overwhelming!)

La Costa's kitchen also works wonders with low-fat meat cuts, dairy products, poultry, and fresh fish.

The second La Costa dieto-culinary trick, however, is one that I am obliged to label "unfair." It consists of using substitutes, like saccharine (which you'll find on the table), in the confections and preserves, and in the cooking. Their mousse turns out to be diet chocolate pudding whipped up with water, ice,

air, and egg white. Calorie-poor, to be sure. And ANYTHING but mousse.

This is not to say you can't eat decently and lose weight at La Costa. You certainly can. One solution is to tell the dietician you want only fresh food—with no make-believe sugar or salt. Another method I have used is to have these customized meals sent directly to your room so that it doesn't make your friends jealous, and does keep you far from the non-diet wood-paneled dining room (with its gluttonous, aromatic temptations) and the bar—both of which you must cross in order to get to the spa dining room.

While dieters may be tempted by the excellent choices on the non-diet menu, La Costa advises guests that they can cheat on their diets if they want to, just as they can at home, but if they can't deal with temptation at La Costa, they can't expect to be able to deal with it at home.

La Costa offers a new vitamin and mineral regimen as an important supplement for daily nutrition. They call it pre-planned meals to go. Conveniently packaged in foil packs each containing a day's supply, it

La Costa California

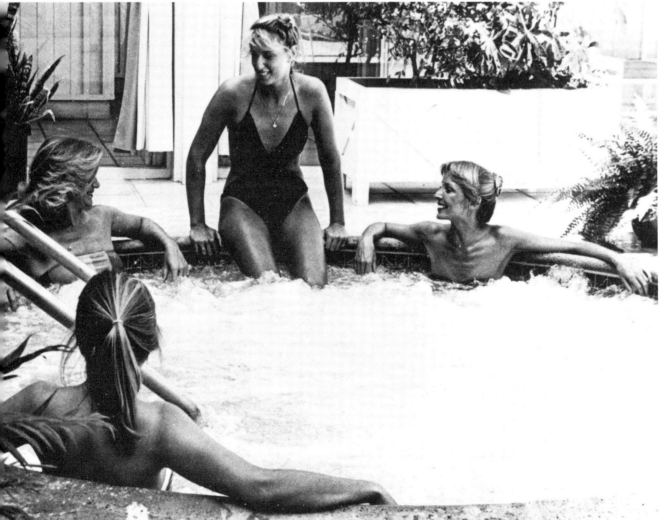

95

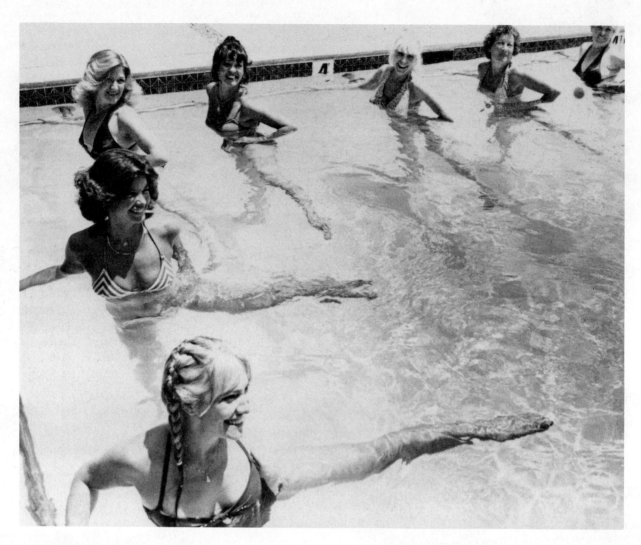

La Costa California

is available on the tables at La Costa, as well as to take home to help you continue the La Costa look of health and beauty.

While La Costa has an excellent exercise program, a lot of emphasis is placed on walking. The only acceptable way to get around is by foot or golf cart. There ARE cars, if you insist, but the unwritten rules of the game require you to walk everywhere. And there's no better way of firming your figure. (So keep it in mind, it's the cheapest transportation around.)

Speaking of exercise, many devotees find the headstand a most rewarding pose, good for the mind, good for the figure, circulation-enhancing, relaxing and—take note, dieters—stimulating for the thyroid, which assists you in weight reduction. Many people, however, find the classical headstand too demanding of their non-acrobatic bodies.

One must item for La Costa: a wig. With all the water sports and roughhousing, your hair is bound to suffer—yet, with all the nocturnal activity, you will want to look your best.

While few things can truly "condition" your hair in the sense of increasing its body or reducing its spongy and porous nature, you CAN improve its LOOK and FEEL with some trickery. For home use, see the La Costa strategy on page 38.

SUMMARY: La Costa is a sleek, fat microcosm of the good and bad in American life generally. It is highly permissive—endowing only the fittest and most disciplined with a healthier, slimmer look. While it's long on comfort and options and gadgets, it's short on soul and the feisty, nagging, idealistic guiding spirit that makes some other spas so dynamic and vivid an experience. It is in the process of evolving a creative identity all its own.—E.W.

Safety Harbor Florida

For nearly forty years, Safety Harbor Spa has had one goal—to send each guest home feeling as finely tuned as a Stradivarius.

During a stay, discordant notes are eased into sweet physical harmony via a program that combines sensible diet and exercise-to-taste with lots of POP (POP stands for Plenty of Pampering). Could one ask more?

The spa is in a perfect setting—on the site of the Espiritu Santo Mineral Springs. If you remember your history, you may recall that in 1539 Spanish explorer Hernando De Soto and his men restored their strength by sipping from the five mineral springs, which have been a source of refreshment ever since.

De Soto would be surprised to see the setting today. The springs are now surrounded by a lush com-

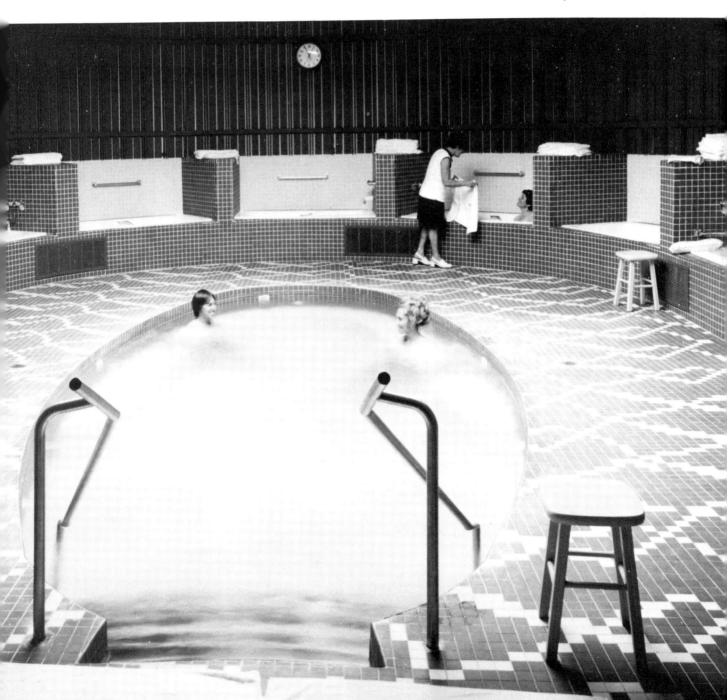

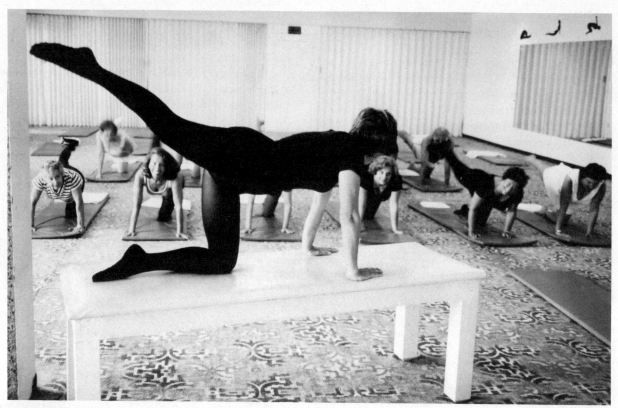

Safety Harbor Florida

plex of elegant pavilions with luxurious facilities, including pools, saunas, solaria, gymnasium, physical therapy rooms, medical offices, health and beauty salons—all this plus 11 tennis courts and an executive golf course. Safety Harbor is an oasis of tropical landscaping so extensive you can take a two-mile walk without ever leaving the grounds.

The big plus at this spa: An atmosphere as elegant as that of the great resorts of yesteryear as a background for personal beautification. Healthful diet and exercise programs—plus a good 101 ways to pamper body and spirit—are prescribed in an environment that's just heavenly. It's the little things that count—gracious service, friendly staff (guests are addressed by name), and lots of fresh flowers. It's nice to find your bed turned down each night so all you have to do is slip between lovely sheets and reap the reward of the healthful life—superbly sound sleep.

A stay at the spa begins with a medical examination by a staff, which is headed by a noted cardiologist. The objective: to determine the level of exercise and diet best suited to individual needs.

Some guests are not concerned about counting calories. Others come to lose weight, which the Spa helps them do in a most pleasant fashion. The rate of weight loss averages a little over a pound a day per person. Dieters find it difficult to feel deprived because the spa's master chef has mastered the fine art of making one thousand gourmet calories per day taste like ten thousand.

You have lots of delightful choices to make at this spa. You can create your own program, using such facilities as swirling heated mineral pools, saunas, massage sessions, and men's and women's solaria. There are classes in yoga, body-building exercises, and dance.

For athletes or would-bes, clinics and lessons in tennis are available from a resident pro. It's easy to get a game going when there are 11 courts. For those with drive, a four-hole, par three course, a 300-yard driving range and an 18-hole putting course spell G-O-L-F. Spa guests also have privileges at a nearby championship golf course.

Part of the tune-up program includes expert cosmetologists who prescribe for men as well as women. They teach such valuable how-tos as smoothing out tension and worry lines. They also provide professional advice on skin and beauty care. Hair styling, manicures, and pedicures are available.

The spa cuisine emphasizes natural foods—the

tropical fruit is superb. Meals build around low-fat and salt-free choices. Menus are appetizing but do not include: butter, iced drinks, beverages with meals, or liquor.

To make it easy for guests to think thin, Safety Harbor has an "Eight S" rule of diet. The eight S's are all no-nos for calorie counters: snacks, starches, sweets, second helpings, slippery (greasy) foods, soft drinks, spirits, and salt.

When it comes to exercise that really stretches out the kinks, I cherish a series of morning stretches which the late Dr. Salem Baranoff, founder of Safety Harbor Spa, once prescribed for me. They should be done very deliberately and slowly every morning, and every day. (See page 47.)

Dr. Baranoff's wife's recipes are just as delicious and right for slimming down as her husband's favorite exercises. I couldn't resist jotting them down, especially for you. All can be prepared easily in your own kitchen:

Safety Harbor Birthday Surprise
Make 3 packages of diet gelatin dessert, adding 1 tablespoon of unflavored gelatin.
    Add fresh fruit and pour into a mold.
    Let chill in refrigerator until firm. Unmold on cake stand.
    Decorate as a cake with low-calorie whipped cream, and add strawberries or cherries as a trim.
    Pop a sparkler on top and sing!

Safety Harbor "Natural" Laxative
1 cup prunes   ½ cup senna powder
1 cup figs   ½ cup blackstrap
1 cup raisins   molasses

Soak the prunes in hot water and remove pits. Put all fruit in grinder. Mix in senna powder and molasses. Use tablespoonful at bedtime. Keep stored in refrigerator.

Vegetable Patties
1 cooked potato   1 chopped onion
  (mashed)   1 stalk of chopped
1 beaten egg   celery
2 cups of cooked   ½ Tbs. unsaturated oil
  vegetables—cauli-   Seasoning to taste
  flower, carrots, peas,
  asparagus, mushrooms

Saute onion and celery in oil to brown. Add mashed potato and beaten egg to vegetables. Form patties, brush with a bit of melted margarine or oil, and bake on baking sheet in 350° oven till brown—approximately 40 minutes.

Costs including all meals and spa treatments are $140-205 per day for single occupancy and $90-130 per day per person for double occupancy.

SUMMARY: There are other pluses. Safety Harbor Spa endorses 101 ways to pamper the body and rejuvenate the spirit. Its founders and management have spent years in researching and developing ways to make the entire body function more efficiently.—E.W.

Harbor Island Florida

On the shores of Biscayne Bay in Miami Beach is an eight-acre tropical island. Owner Larry Paskow recently installed a new nine-story tower of lavish apartment accommodations with complete hotel service, which, together with the beautiful old accommodations (the poolside lanai suites are so convenient), constitute a heavy challenger in the sunny spa sweepstakes.

It's quite plush, with Roman marbelized tubs, whirlpool baths, steam rooms, solaria for sunlight massages, day and night tennis, Olympic saltwater pool, herbal wraps, men's and women's gyms, free massages daily, sauna, exercise and yoga classes, beauty and facial salons, and diverse sports and entertainment.

Basic Mousse Recipe
Sprinkle an envelope of unflavored gelatin over ¼ cup cold water. Now add ¼ cup of boiling water and artificial sweetener. Remove from heat and stir in ¾ cup skim milk and ¾ cup fruit concentrate. Chill until the mixture has a jello-like consistency, then fold in 2 well-beaten egg whites and chill.
(You can make your own fruit concentrate by mixing equal parts of fruit and fruit juice in a high-speed blender.)

Prune, Apricot, Pineapple, and Strawberry Variations

Add 2 tablespoons of fresh lemon juice and ½ teaspoon of grated lemon rind plus fruit concentrate. (Add ½ teaspoon cinnamon to Prune Whip only.)

Mousse au Chocolat

Increase skim milk to 1½ cups. Omit fruit concentrate and add 2 or 3 tablespoons of low-calorie chocolate syrup. Fold in ¼ cup low-calorie whipped cream.

Mousse au Mocha

Substitute 1 tablespoon instant coffee for flavoring and proceed as for chocolate mousse, but use one less tablespoon of chocolate syrup.

Many gentiles have the suspicion that kosher food is not terribly palatable. This is simply not true. Harbor Island's kosher food is as delicious as their regular menu, a sample of which is included on page 101.

This spa bears the imprint of one man: Larry Paskow. He began his career with no more than the desire to create a spa that would please HIM and a generous friend's $400,000. But with that going for him, he created a spa where I feel tremendously comfortable and relaxed and pampered. I even lose weight there.

Here are excerpts of Larry's own story, as he told it to me:

"In 1955, as a partner of the Vitamin Corporation of America, I weighed 280 pounds. I'd lose thirty pounds in a month at a spa, and then put them right back. I never learned a thing about proper eating habits because the spa food, salt-free, was tasteless.

"Then, in 1956, I had a chance to buy a hotel on a bad place called Harbor Island—monumentally unsuccessful. I wanted to create a place I would enjoy. I told my friend, 'How could you put up all this money to create a spa and let ME run it? I know nothing about the hotel business.'

"He said, 'Don't worry. The first guest that checks in will teach you the hotel business.'

"That's the secret. Here we've done everything for the guests. They don't have to think. We think, we plan for them.

"Our consulting nutritionist, Dr. Norman Jaloff of New York, believed in a balanced diet: protein, carbohydrates, and fat. One diet won't fit everybody. Diets should vary according to the individual's weight, age, height, activity. He warned us that we must prepare TASTY quality foods and find a chef who could substitute herbs for the salt we would omit.

"The real secret is moderation. You can eat almost anything you want—in moderation. Eat when you're hungry, not when they tell you to eat. If we feed you properly, every three or four hours, you should not be hungry.

"You're used to something sweet after a meal. Okay. We make a sweet dessert with fifty calories instead of five hundred. A rich dessert satisfies for maybe five minutes—but its toll is taken over days and days afterwards.

"We call our waitresses 'jailers' because they can't be bribed. If by chance they are bribed, we fire them. They simply will not give you anything not on the menu.

"Our exercise girl is the best. She knows, for instance, that you can't give the same exercise to a supple woman of twenty that you give to a woman of fifty. You don't treat an overweight person the same as you do one who isn't.

"Unfortunately, God didn't charge us for our bodies. Maybe we'd take better care of them if they had a price tag. Most people abuse their bodies.

"We put vitamins on the table. Every two weeks we invite doctors to talk to our guests about nutrition, proper diets, diets as prophylaxis against disease. We won't serve cold drinks with meals.

"In the morning, you should have a hot drink to start your body metabolism working properly.

"Most people with indigestion don't see a doctor. They take an antacid pill. Our food is low-fat, salt-free, and is either boiled, broiled, or baked. There's no aftertaste, and you just don't get indigestion. With no water or cold drinks during meals, the body will digest food properly.

"We don't give severe massages unless they're asked for. We discourage them. We don't put the whirlpool on a particular muscle: it's for general circulation. We don't call people to the phone during a meal unless it's an emergency.

"Ours is a personal business. We know our guests by name and idiosyncrasy. When our guests check in, we find out if they prefer soft or hard pillows, where they like to sit in the dining room, which waitresses they like. We know each and every idiosyncrasy. We treat every bed and pillow to ultraviolet radiation before giving it to a new customer.

"Of our 170 employees, 135 have been here more than ten years. We are good to our help. We know their families, their children—and treat them all as our own family. If an employee doesn't work out, one of

LARRY PASKOW'S HARBOR ISLAND SPA
Good Afternoon

TABLE NO. _____ NAME _____
DIET _____ WAITER _____

SUNDAY

CHOICE OF

HOT CHICKEN BROTH
COLD BORSCHT
CHILLED APRICOT NECTAR

CHOICE OF

BERMUDA ONION OMELET
*WHOLE WHEAT SPAGHETTI, POLONAISE –
    PRITIKIN SUGGESTION
DIET PEARS WITH COTTAGE CHEESE
SALAD BOWL WITH JULIENNE MEATS
NOVA COMBINATION PLATTER, CREAM CHEESE,
    ONION AND BAGEL
BROILED FILET OF FRESH RED SNAPPER,
    PROVENCALE

CHOICE OF

SECTION SALAD
BRAISED SPINACH

CHOICE OF

FRESH STEWED RHUBARB   DIET JELLO
REGULAR JELLO   BAKED APPLE
ICED MELON   PISTACHIO MOUSSE

YOU EAT OUT AT YOUR OWN RISK

PLEASE CIRCLE DESIRED ITEMS
COFFEE • TEA • DECAFFEINATED COFFEE
AND TEA, SALT FREE MARGARINE AND
BUTTER BUDS 5 CALORIES PER OZ.
AVAILABLE AT ALL TIMES

AN ADDITIONAL CHARGE FOR ITEMS NOT ON MENU, AND
SECOND MAIN COURSES.
15% GRATUITY WILL BE ADDED TO CHECK
FOR INVITED GUESTS.
THANK YOU
PURIFIED WATER USED IN ALL COOKING

LARRY PASKOW'S HARBOR ISLAND SPA
Good Evening

TABLE NO. _____ NAME _____
DIET _____ WAITER _____

SUNDAY

CHOICE OF

BISQUE OF CHICKEN, DE VOLAILLE
CHILLED APPLE JUICE
HOT CHICKEN BROTH
FRESH FLORIDA FRUIT CUP

CHOICE OF

BAKED SPRING CHICKEN, CACCIATORE
ROAST SLICED SIRLOIN OF BEEF, AU JUS
BROILED KOSHER KNOCKWURST, SAUERKRAUT
BROILED FILET OF FRESH BOSTON SCROD
* EGG WHITE OMELET WITH MUSHROOMS–
    PRITIKIN SUGGESTION

CHOICE OF

FRESH GARDEN BEANS BAKED IDAHO POTATO
SQUASH GRECQUE
BAKED SWEET POTATO

CHOICE OF

HEARTS OF LETTUCE
COMBINATION SALAD

CHOICE OF

BAKED APPLE   PISTACHIO MOUSSE
ICED MELON   DIET JELLO
REGULAR JELLO   DIET JELLO CAKE
FRESH STEWED RHUBARB

YOU EAT OUT AT YOUR OWN RISK

PLEASE CIRCLE DESIRED ITEMS
COFFEE • TEA • DECAFFEINATED COFFEE
AND TEA, SALT FREE MARGARINE AND
BUTTER BUDS 5 CALORIES PER OZ.
AVAILABLE AT ALL TIMES
ALL BROILED OR SPECIAL ORDERS
APPROXIMATELY 30 MINUTES.

AN ADDITIONAL CHARGE FOR ITEMS NOT ON MENU, AND
SECOND MAIN COURSES.
15% GRATUITY WILL BE ADDED TO CHECK
FOR INVITED GUESTS.
THANK YOU
PURIFIED WATER USED IN ALL COOKING

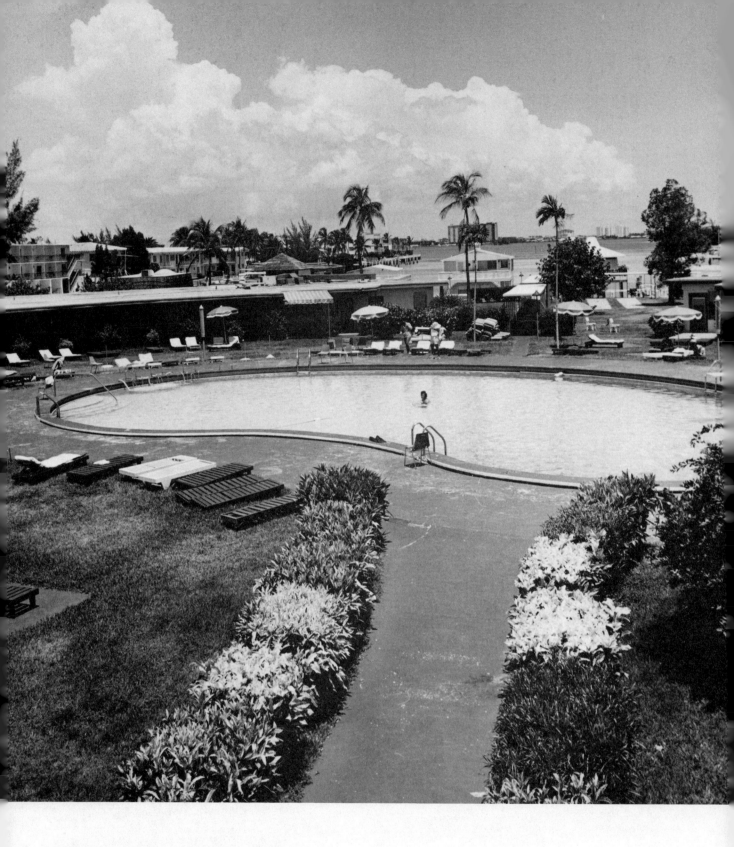

Harbor Island Florida

our other employees will generally come and tell us to dismiss him."

SUMMARY: A diet resort with good food, camara-derie, good accommodations, and Larry Paskow himself at the piano. As for the kosher cooking: try it, you'll like it.

11
Deborah's Places

Memory, they say, is the power to gather roses in winter. For many a winter I thrived on the memory of beautiful spells at Maine Chance, beginning with my first fairy-tale visit in 1946.

The war had been over for a year, and we wanted to forget it had happened. The days of rationing were past, and we celebrated their passing with indulgences. Maine Chance was, for me, a supreme self-indulgence.

I can still taste that first festive Fourth of July salmon dinner with Elizabeth Arden's favorite lemon meringue pie dessert. I can still see before me each of the fourteen exquisite, different settings of china and silver we would use during our two weeks there. I can still feel the cold, infinitesimally moist freshness of Elizabeth Arden's monogrammed sheets as I slipped between them at night. I can still see the famous quality Arden preparations piled high on my crystal-and-mirror dressing table. And, perhaps the greatest luxury of all, stepping into those irridescent, velvet bubbles churned into my bath—a bath lovingly drawn by my very own private night maid.

When the Maine spa burned down, those memories sustained me. They made humdrum and hectic days endurable. They were at the time, I confess, the best part of my life. They were a solace and a crutch.

It was foolish, I suppose, to live in the past so heavily. And so it was with great relief that a stunning reality superimposed itself upon my daydreams. That reality was a new spa called the Golden Door.

The Golden Door was pruned from Deborah Szekely's Rancho la Puerta. The Ranch, as we call it, was the Mexican proving ground for the elements that went into the American Golden Door.

For thirty-five years, Deborah had used the Ranch to try out every technique, product, exercise, recipe, and décor that she thought might enhance the beauty, health, and tranquility of her guests. The things that won big were imported to the Door in Escondido, California.

Deborah Szekely and Elizabeth Arden were both women with dreams they themselves would work to make come true. But the resemblance stops there.

Arden's spas were basically retreats for close friends, a sporadic diversion for herself and her class. She was to her toenails a lady. The spa was only incidentally a business. Her real business was her hugely successful cosmetics empire. The spa was an extension of her private life.

For Deborah, on the other hand, the Ranch and the Door are her whole world—commercial and private. No woman I know has ever welded the two together more successfully.

Arden was an ingenious and tasteful borrower, mostly from the European spas. Deborah is, too, but far more innovative, more rugged, and more daring. Most of the American spas have copied her ways and hired their key personnel from the ranks of her instructors and attendants. In many ways, Deborah Szekely could be called the Mother of the American Spas.

Deborah has, for the decades I've known her, always cared deeply about people and ideas. She listens to and registers indelibly every word you say. She smiles irrepressibly, talks positively, and is curiously at ease with her great responsibilities. I recall her once leaving an important meeting to assist a guest who had just sprained her ankle.

But she's a super executive and a hard-nosed administrator. (However, her staff seem genuinely to like and respect her.) If you ever ask her to do something, it is taken care of immediately. It is NEVER forgotten.

Both of her spas are nearly full year round—and she does not begrudge surrendering the overflow to her copiers elsewhere.

"More places," she says, "will make more people healthier, and we'll have a better world for that. You need vitality to be able to surmount all obstacles and problems with fun and delight. After all, each of us has only so long a lifespan. Whatever we can do to increase our energy will let us achieve twice or three times as many things.

Deborah, whose San Diego home is blessed with a marvelous warm, dry climate, begins each morning at 7:30 with a walk-jog in the park. If she's been traveling, she'll walk more than jog. If she's been home, she'll jog more.

"But it is ALWAYS a full hour. And everybody knows not to call me before a quarter to nine. Because I just won't be home. You HAVE to make a daily investment in health—making deposits, if you want to make withdrawals. So I not only make an absolute issue of the morning schedule, but no less than four times a week I swim after my day's work. I have to—because I've just turned sixty and I intend to be very energetic in my seventies and eighties and nineties."

Deborah believes that women have never had it better. She espouses Sartre's view of freedom as the opportunity to choose. Accordingly, women are freer because they can do more varied things today than ever before.

"Women," she says, "are no longer worried about what other people are going to think. They realize that what REALLY counts is what THEY think. And they are beginning to take responsibility—not blaming their ills and misfortunes on husbands or in-laws. At the Golden Door and Rancho la Puerta, we teach that no one else can take care of your health or enjoy it but you. After all, the hand you hold the longest is your own. We work on giving you your own strength."

Vital Statistics of Deborah's Spas

	Golden Door	Rancho la Puerta
BIRTHDATE	1959	1940
LOCATION	Escondido, CA	Tecate, Baja California, Mexico
MAXIMUM CLIENTELE	34	110
STAFF	110 private instructors and attendants, extremely attentive	Varies seasonally, but usually 1:1 based on clientele, up to 110. Casual, but good service.
COST	$2,500 per week per person	$600 to $1,750 depending on occupancy.
FOOD AND DIET	Continental gourmet, non-vegetarian, low-calorie with high proportion of natural, organic foods grown at the Golden Door	Vegetarian with proportion of natural, organic foods. Honey produced nearby. Fish twice a week.
CLASS LIMITATION	5 per class	None

GENDER RESTRICTIONS	Year round for women only, except for first two weeks of March, June, September, and December, which are reserved for men. No small children. Couples week the last two weeks of March, June, September, and third week of December.	None. Children welcome, but no babysitters and no children's programs available. Men's week in December. Couple's week in October.
TELEVISION AND RADIO	Yes	Bring your own radio. No television.
COST OF PHYSICAL PLANT	$3,500,000	Approximately the same
AMBIANCE	Restful, Japanese Honjin inn	Mexican hacienda-ranch, ruggedly restful
AREA	150 acres	Somewhat over 500 acres, of which 190 are developed
SPECIAL FACILITIES	3 gyms, 3 pools, tennis, steam, sauna, Scotch hoses, biofeedback	9 gyms, 3 pools, tennis, Fitness Parcours (2½ mile jogging track with 20 special exercise stations), 3 saunas, 3 jacuzzis
SPECIAL PROGRAMS	da Vinci exercises Jazzex Water exercises Water volleyball Tennis Hatha Yoga Hiking Jogging Special diets Herbal Wraps All beauty treatments with Golden Door cosmetic and skin care products Varied entertainment and evening programs Golden Door cosmetic skin care workshops	Over 30 classes a day to choose from (same as Golden Door) Varied Entertainment and evening programs Golden Door cosmetic lectures and workshops on skin care All beauty treatments with Golden Door cosmetic products

Rancho La Puerta Tecate, Baja California, Mexico

When fulminating spavelitis has me champing at the bit and my bank balance will not permit super pampering, I often opt for a week or two at Rancho La Puerta, about one hour's drive from San Diego and some thirty miles east of Tijuana, Baja California, Mexico. The Ranch just happens to be the best bargain in American spas, considering the low rates (from $100 per day, per person, including all meals and fitness activities).

There is something uniquely memorable about those acres of Mexican scrub carpeting the Baja California Coast Range foothills. The climate is dry and hot. The fresh mountain air scampers down the hills through the olive trees and vineyards, carrying sage- and succulent-scented breezes to the Ranch. The magnificent natural setting alone has a way of quickly reviving my sense of humor, refreshing my lungs and purging the grimy feeling of city living.

The Ranch is famous for letting you do your thing. I go there to write, read, relax, and chat with Deborah on her weekly visits, as well as to drop a pound or two.

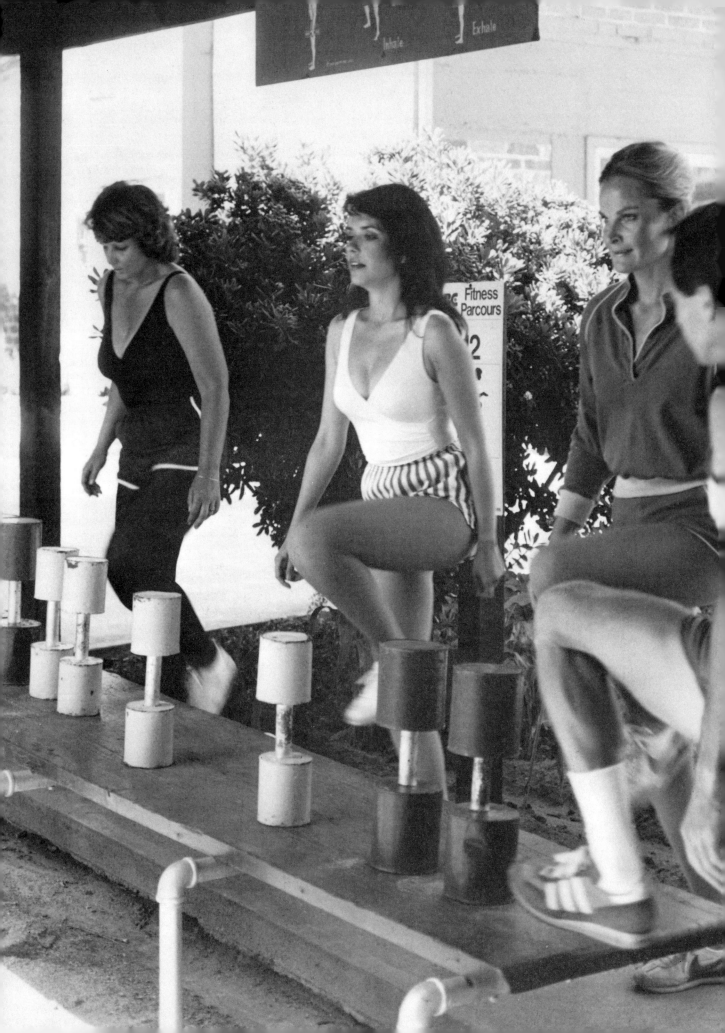

For Herschel Bernardi, the Ranch was "the one place where I once had found peace. I went there for three months, just staring at the rugged dusty hills, living in an adobe house, and not communicating with anyone."

For Michael Murphy, the Ranch was the inspiration for his famous Esalen Institute at Big Sur. For Aldous Huxley, it was the ideal ambiance for a weekend encounter marathon that first defined the Human Potential movement.

And it's just a vegetarian refuge for a lot of the famous: Joan Kennedy, Catherine Bach, William F. Buckley, Jr., Milton and Rose Friedman, Erica Jong, Burt Lancaster, and hundreds more.

There are just under 100 buildings on the 190 acres—mostly low, brick buildings flanked by vineyards and jacaranda trees. The whole area is beautifully landscaped and constitutes a cosmopolitan oasis in the midst of brush plains and craggy, purple mountains.

The senses can feast at the Ranch. The ears gourmandize on the rich dollops of silence, broken only by the splashing of water, the snapping of twigs, the buzzing of bees, the chirping of birds and crickets, the crackling of a hearth fire, and good dinner talk.

The nose is glutted with a hundred new perfumes emitted from unfamiliar blossoms and leaves and herbs and roots and soils.

The eyes probably have the most sumptuous treat as they savor the Ranch's gallery of element-buffed gray boulders on the slopes, the year-round yucca, manzanita, sage, broom, and buckwheat bushes, the seasonal peonies, rosemary, violets, moss roses, daisies, geraniums, oleanders, daffodils, and clumps of lush grapes.

The palate is tickled, too, by the wildflower honey produced in apiaries nearby, the tangy acidophilus (a cross between Bulgarian buttermilk and yogurt), the new sensations of the herbal teas, the creatively seasoned vegetable recipes, and, most especially, the magnificent multi-whole-grain bread served in the cheerful, spaciously windowed dining room.

In fact, the whole body seems to ripple in gratitude as you awaken muscle after muscle, even if you do no more than trek around the grounds getting from one place to another.

The spa was started from scratch by Deborah and her then philosopher-biochemist husband, Edmond Bordeaux Szekely. As a bride of seventeen in 1940, she wept when her groom carried her across the threshold of their honeymoon cottage. It was an adobe stable, with no amenities and a dirt floor.

Deborah was a Brooklyn girl, and her late husband was a cosmopolitan Hungarian dreamer, who,

she once said, had never earned a penny until he met her. But it was she who knew how to realize his dreams and commercialize them so that others might savor them. They tried everything and anything, at least once.

"I always tell my guests that it has been a matter of trial and error. But you don't see our errors anymore, they're so far away behind."

The successes have been borrowed by almost every other major spa in the western hemisphere. It doesn't bother her a whit that others have ridden to small fortunes on her adaptations, such as the English organic gardens, the French grape cure, the Swiss sunbathing bins, the Sumerian sun-and-water baths, and the Aztec herbal baths.

The Ranch diet has always been vegetarian, and very light on sodium, cholesterol, and calories—with one thousand the maximum for the dedicated dieter. Of course, one is always free to walk or drive to nearby Tecate for a Mexican meal, but those who do, abandon all hope of winning the weekly maximum weight-loss first prize.

Actually, you can diet any way you please at the Ranch. The strict dieter, for instance, would breakfast on an orange or grapefruit, black coffee or tea, and a single slice of that marvelous Tecate bread with a dab of honey or a little bowl of granola.

I remember the last lunch I had at the Ranch. Walking down the buffet salad bar, one sees each dish listed on a sign with the exact caloric value and a sample plate is displayed to guide your portions. One is free to take whatever one wishes, and go back for seconds.

There were, to begin with, little glasses of that marvelous acidophilus (I usually take two); a large bowl of escarole, fresh as could be; string beans with toasted, sliced almonds; diced broccoli spears; cauliflower, cucumbers, fresh pimiento, and green and red peppers in a marinated salad; then a hot vegetable salad on cold greens. At the end of the line there is always coffee and tea; parsley, mint, or alfalfa tea; and a dessert, such as a pudding. There is always ripe fruit, too.

Here are a couple of the Ranch's best recipes:

Tecate Bread
(Whole-wheat bread)

½ ounce	dry active yeast (2 packets)
4 cups	water, lukewarm
¼ cup	corn oil
¼ cup	honey
10–10½ cups	whole-wheat flour
1 heaping cup	miller's bran, unprocessed
1 teaspoon	sea salt

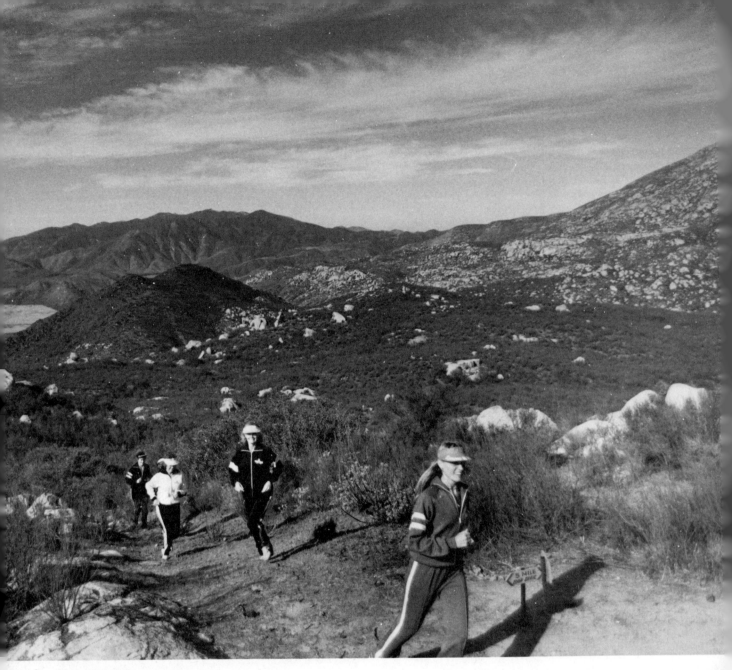

Rancho La Puerta Mexico

Place yeast in large bowl. To dissolve, gradually add lukewarm water. Stir in oil and honey. Add flour, bran, and salt. Blend together with your hands. Knead till dough no longer is sticky or adhering to your hands. It should feel tough and elastic. (Add more flour if necessary.)

Lightly coat dough with oil, top and bottom. Place in bowl, and cover with towel not touching dough. Let rise in warm, draft-free area till doubled in size (about 1–2 hours).

Punch dough down. Placing on lightly greased board, knead about 1 minute. Divide into 3 equal parts, and throw dough against board 3 times. Generously oil three 8½" × 4¼" × 2½" loaf pans (preferably clay); line bottoms with wax or parchment paper. With a little oil on your hands, shape dough into loaf shapes; place into pans, pressing gently. Run knife tip down center of each loaf. Cover again with towel, and let sit 30 minutes.

Preheat oven to 350°.

Bake 1 hour and 15 minutes, till well browned. Remove from oven, unmold by running knife around edges. Wrap in towels and plastic bags till cool. Rewrap in plastic, and refrigerate or freeze.

This bread is most enjoyable when toasted before serving.

Calories per loaf: 1,657
Calories per slice (16 slices per loaf): 104
Preparation time: 2 hours
Baking Time: 1 hour 15 minutes

Huevos Rancheros

2 tablespoons	sesame-seed or safflower oil
3	onions, medium size, sliced
1	bell pepper (optional), chopped
1 tablespoon	dried whole oregano
1 tablespoon	dried sweet basil
1 teaspoon	vegetable seasoning
1 28-ounce can	whole tomatoes, chopped, or 4 large fresh tomatoes, peeled and chopped coarsely
½ teaspoon	black pepper, freshly ground
4	eggs
8 tablespoons	Monterey jack cheese, freshly grated, or 4 thin mozzarella cheese slices

In heavy pan, heat oil. Gently saute onions over low fire till light golden brown; stir with wooden spatula. Add bell pepper, and season with oregano, basil, and vegetable seasoning. Cook 2-3 minutes. Add tomatoes and pepper. Simmer 10-15 minutes, till sauce is somewhat thick.

With spoon, make 4 pockets in mixture, and drop in eggs. Cover eggs with cheese. Cook covered, 10 minutes for soft eggs, 15 minutes for eggs more done. Serve immediately.

Serves: 4
Calories per serving: 244
Preparation time: 30-35 minutes.

Tecate Tostadas

4	corn tortillas
8 ounces	homemade refried beans
½ head	iceberg lettuce, shredded tomato, medium size, chopped fine
1	
4	radishes, sliced thin
4 ounces	Monterey jack cheese, grated
4	avocado slices

Preheat oven to 375°.
Heat tortillas 5-10 minutes, till crisp.
Spread each tortilla with beans; top with lettuce, tomato, radish slices, cheese, and an avocado slice.
Just before serving, warm in oven.

Serves: 4
Calories per serving: 258
Preparation time: 30 minutes

The routine at the Ranch is so vigorous that I understand why Deborah's diet includes more carbohydrates than most dietetic spas. You need them for energy. Or at least that's my suspicion.

If you want to follow a program, the spa offers two to choose from. One is the "moderate" program, the other is a "vigorous" program. If you're in anything but good shape, I suggest you keep to the moderate pro-

Rancho La Puerta Mexico

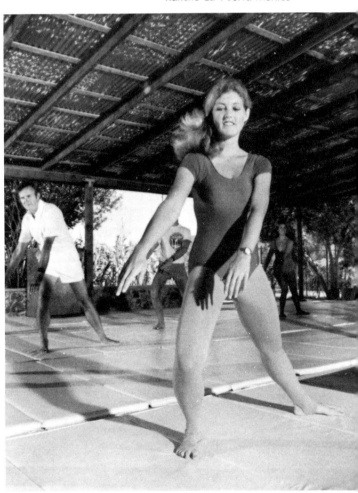

gram, which is vigorous enough for the likes of me. You can also register between the programs. Deborah suggests alternating active with less active classes.

Remember, these are only suggestions. You—or the staff—can prepare any kind of schedule that pleases you. If you opt for the whole Tecate enchilada, in addition to your daily exercise schedule, you'll also opt for herbal wraps, massages, facials, and pedicures (using Golden Door cosmetic skin care products), all available for a minimal fee. Plus, there are skin care workshops and private consultations to take advantage of.

There is also a reconstruction of the ancient Mexican Toltec Ball Game on a specially built court. It's not as easy as it looks. The game combines aspects of football, golf, croquet, soccer, and basketball.

It you're Cathy Rigby or Burt Lancaster—or want to develop builds like either of them—you might choose the new two-and-a-half-mile Fitness Parcours, or Circuit Training, adapted from the Marine Corps training program. The Parcours is an exercise track with twenty stops at which you perform special calisthenics. This has proven very popular with the more athletically inclined visitors.

La Puerta also offers folk dances, movies, bingo, bridge, chess, pocket billiards, ping-pong, and topical lectures.

But my most blissful moments are spent in the herbal wrap, which almost everyone who tries it has described as a quasi-mystical experience, some even claiming that their souls leave their bodies and soar.

The Ranch's "happy feet" treatment is another delight you can duplicate CHEZ VOUS. It not only stimulates your feet, it relaxes your entire body. (See page 17).

Two other Ranch specialties—from the food department—are well worth taking home. I pass on the recipes to you.

La Puerta Do-It-Yourself Salad
Prepare individual bowls of sliced beets, shredded red cabbage, large sprouts, radishes, sliced tomatoes, green peppers, shredded carrots, cucumber, diced celery, whole chicory, Romaine lettuce. Then place alongside these bowls small dishes of sesame seeds, shelled Indian nuts, crushed black peppercorns. Add cruets of wine vinegar, olive oil, and sesame oil.

La Puerta Do-It-Yourself Fruit Platter
Set out plates with pieces of banana, melon, papaya, orange, grapefruit, apple, pear, grapes, and strawberries. Serve plain yogurt, grated coconut, and sunflower seeds as toppings.

The truly beautiful thing about Rancho La Puerta to me is its do-it-yourself spirit. Nobody's conned, compelled, or cornered into any activity. Somehow Deborah Szekely has discovered the secret of inspiring her guests to make the most of their opportunities at the Ranch—and feel totally, exhilaratingly FREE!

As a reporter for the CLEVELAND PLAIN DEALER recalled a visit to the Ranch:

"Morning mists rise over the Western mountains, and I picked rosemary in bloom, and sage, and I was glad I was born. Every night I walked back to my cabin . . . and the stars were so close that I knew I could touch them if only I could stand tiptoe."

SUMMARY: Savage country, manicured ranchscape, wizardly dietetics and exercises, sports galore, and a very hearty welcome for the whole family make this venerable and sprawling Mexican spa a Wilkens Best Bet for the budget-minded spa-nik. Whether you live in the Manhattan jungle or the Iowa flatlands or some coastal enclave, Rancho La Puerta is guaranteed to give you a healthy, rugged change of pace you won't regret.—E.W.

The Golden Door Escondido, California

Whether Deborah Szekely got the name Golden Door from the legend on the Statue of Liberty I don't know, but her Super Spa certainly represents an emancipation from oppressions. The difference is the exclusivity of her guest list, which is rather more elite than the Immigration and Naturalization Service's. With some rubberizing of the analogy, one might consider her crowd occasionally "tired" and even "huddled"—but scarcely "poor" or "wretched." Not at two thousand five hundred dollars per week.

The Golden Door in Escondido, California, has been the smallest, most distinguished Super Spa in the United States. Take the trumps of her Mexican Ranch program, carefully preserve the Good Life, enforce a rigid exercise schedule and special diets, and sprinkle with all kinds of pampering such as breakfast in bed,

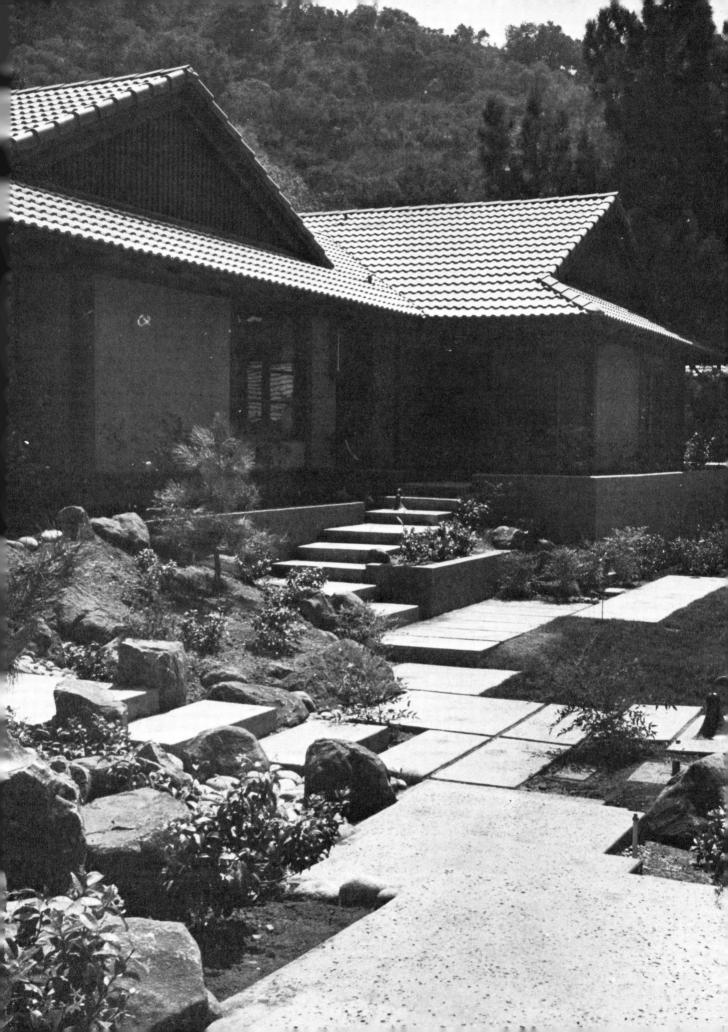

and three staff members to serve every guest, turn everybody on to some sophisticated head-tripping from time to time, sort the women from the men—and you have the Golden Door.

On July 20, 1975, Deborah relocated her original Golden Door a mile or so down Deer Springs Road to a brand-new location, adapted a Japanese Honjin inn style of architecture, and spent three-and-a-half million dollars on the new facility. The schedule remains basically the same, alternating active and passive 60-minute and 30-minute periods. It goes without saying that the famous East-Indian golden door itself still graces the new entrance.

The Door towers above its competition mostly by virtue of its staff's empathy and expertise. They are continually being schooled in sensitivity and new techniques to relieve guests of their natural anxiety and vulnerability. Thanks to this atmosphere, visitors tend to develop close and lasting friendships.

Although the Door and the Ranch have almost identical health and beauty courses, the former operates like the Monterey Army Language School and the latter, a set of Berlitz records. You emerge from a week at the Door absolutely fluent in the neologisms of self-discipline and self-care. When you're back home, the leap from bed to full-length mirror for ten minutes of stretch exercises is practically a conditioned response.

When Deborah announced the new Door would have a Japanese motif, many of her regular clients worried that the old charm might get swallowed up in the wake of an interesting but unrewarding experiment. Judging from their enthusiastic reactions to the new Door, however, this fear was unfounded.

Hers was the first health and beauty spa to use biofeedback machines, which she has experimented with over the past five years. The director of the Golden Door is a biofeedback and stress-management specialist and teaches the guests how to influence their emotions and physical well-being by regulating their own brain waves, temperature, heart-rate, etc.

"Our hope," Deborah told me, "is that our guests will then be able to go home with the added conviction that they REALLY ARE the masters of their own destiny. This should help their resolve to continue the good habits they've acquired at the Door. They'll have an extra delight, an extra dimension to their self-knowledge. They'll be able to increase the intensity of their own thinking processes."

The biofeedback courses are used in conjunction with individual stress-management sessions where guests learn to identify and eliminate the unnecessary stresses in their lives. They learn practical ways to incorporate the time and space for introspection and play in their daily lives. This "balanced" approach to stress management has provided many guests with the means to completely eliminate stress-related illness from their lives.

The water-therapy building (equidistant from the four clusters of buildings) has a Japanese vibrating communal tub, which will hold nine people "chum-mily." The tub is a kind of reward before bedtime to insure total relaxation for sleep. Around the tub are low beds, where a Japanese-style massage completes the ritual.

"You can't help lying there limp as a washrag," says Deborah. "My problem then is to get you into your bed."

She has exploited beautifully her exquisite natural setting. Guests cross a Japanese footbridge and, at the gatehouse, exchange street shoes for slippers, and are handed a hot wash-cloth and a cup of green Japanese tea.

The interior colors of the buildings reflect the garden flowers—largely irises and wisteria—and have a weathered wood trim. The buildings seem to be floating in a sea of gardens and courtyards. There will even be a traditional flowered shrine, a Japanese carp pond, as well as side-by-side hot and cool pools and a new warming room.

My first visit to the old Door in 1966 was a disappointment. I knew that this was Deborah's new baby, her pride and joy. Perhaps I'd been over-coddled by Maine Chance and the Greenhouse and was looking for the wrong things. I found the Door overbearing and dull. When I told Deborah this, she told me:

"Please, Emily, do me a favor. Be my guest and go back. We have a new program. See if you don't enjoy it this time."

I did—I fell in love with it. The program was just as rugged, just as strenuous. But this time the staff made all the exercise classes enjoyable and, above all, meaningful. They seemed to care about me as a person. The director glanced at me and knew immediately what was wrong and what to do about it. Sitting together the first day, we discussed every conceivable physical and dietary need. Then I received a movement assessment with a physical therapist who analyzed every joint in my body for flexibility and range of motion. Finally I emerged for my first morning class adorned with a flurry of brightly colored ribbons that alerted the staff to my special physical strengths and weaknesses. The staff continued to take me aside and brief me as if I were their sole concern. And when they did that, I stopped floating. I felt I belonged.

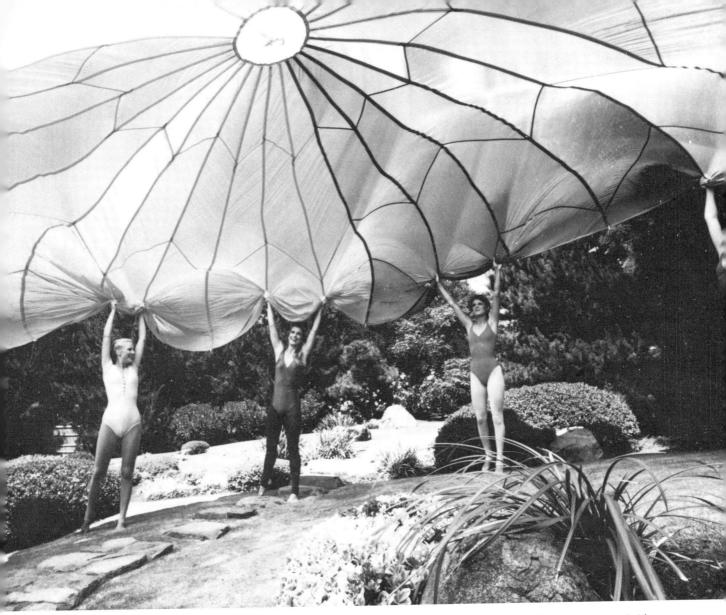

The Golden Door California

What's an average day at the Door like?

It is more flexible than the rules might indicate. If you really have a preference for beauty treatments instead of the massage before lunch, it can be arranged. Just speak up. I found it miraculous that the staff worked so smoothly with the tastes and preferences of thirty-four women.

The day begins with a 6:30 A.M. hike (6:00 for men), followed by breakfast and wake-up and stretch exercises; then "da Vinci" exercises (extremely tough movements with towels, volleyballs, hoops, Indian clubs, and sticks).

Then comes individual spot reducing. A special program is prepared just for you and your inimitable lumps and bulges. By the end of your week, you will be sure to have made significant inroads on them. You are assigned to spot-reducing classes, grouped according to Fitness Level and taught by your own personal Fitness Guide who watches your progress and determines when you are ready for more challenges.

As you can tell, those exercises are terrifyingly businesslike and rigorous. They are topped off by an herbal wrap, steam or fragrant dry-heat sauna, and eventually a massage in your room.

Lunch is at 1:00 P.M. Although most of the women eat lunch together, I prefer to eat alone. The midday hour is the best time for me to catch up on my writing.

Incidentally, the chef, Michel Stroot, is marvelously proficient. His food is tasty and light on the calories. Here (from *The Golden Door Cookbook*, which Deborah has published privately) are two of his luncheon recipes that I fell in love with:

113

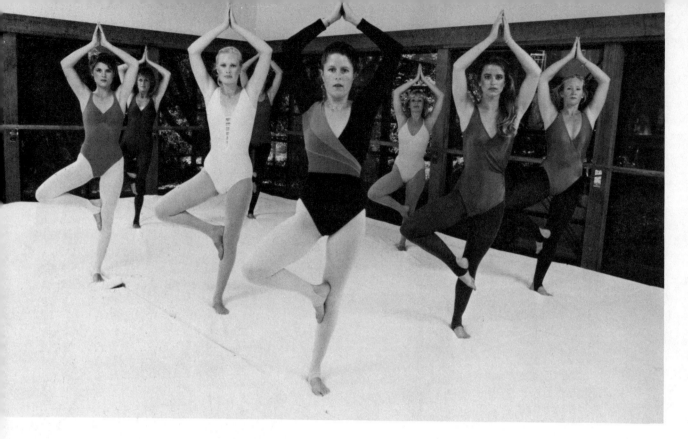

Golden Door California

Mushroom Salad a la Greque

1½ tablespoons
    Sun-dried white
    raisins
1 tablespoon shallots or
    scallions, minced
1 teaspoon garlic, minced
2 tablespoons olive oil
1 pound fresh
    mushrooms, trimmed,
    washed, and dried
1 teaspoon dried whole
    thyme, or ½ teaspoon
    fresh thyme

1 teaspoon vegetable
    seasoning
½ teaspoon black
    pepper, freshly ground
¼ cup dry white wine
1 cup tomato, peeled,
    seeded, and diced
1 tablespoon fresh lemon
    juice
¼ cup fresh parsley,
    chopped
garnish: lettuce leaves or
    watercress

Pre-soak raisins in warm water to cover, till plump. In heavy skillet, gently saute shallots and garlic in 1 tablespoon olive oil till they start to soften. Add mushrooms, thyme, vegetable seasoning, and pepper; stir with wooden spatula. Quickly add wine, tomato, raisins (drained), and lemon juice. Remove from fire as soon as mixture comes to a boil.

    Sprinkle with parsley and remainder of olive oil. Garnish and serve, warm or cold.

Serves: 4
Calories per serving: 127
Preparation time: 15 minutes

Honeydew and Crab Meat Bali

4 grapefruit halves,
    large, hollowed (drain
    insides, and reserve ½
    cup juice)
2 teaspoons olive oil
1 tablespoon shallots,
    minced (or white parts
    of scallions)
2 teaspoons curry powder

2 cups king crab meat
3 cups honeydew melon
    balls (and their own
    juice)
4 tablespoons coconut,
    grated, freshly toasted
2 tablespoons scallions,
    chopped
garnish: 4 strawberries

In heavy skillet, heat oil and shallots. Add curry powder. With wooden spatula, mix to make paste. Add crab meat. Mix together quickly. Cook, covered, over very low fire for 5 minutes.

    In separate, preheated pan, quickly saute melon balls in their own juice, just enough to warm melon. Add ½ of toasted coconut.

    Add mixture to crab meat. Mix well over fire.

    Add grapefruit juice. Sprinkle with scallions or chives. Fill grapefruit halves, and top with remaining coconut. Garnish and serve.

Serves: 4
Calories per serving: 226
Preparation time: 25 minutes

After lunch there is Aquatic Aerobics (a sort of "da Vinci" in the pool) and possibly a water volleyball game. This is followed by Shape-Up which combines spot reducing with "da Vinci." Then a Yoga, or Stretch and Relax class, and finally a facial or skin treatment.

At 6:00, it's bath time, and the women dress for cocktails at 6:30 (low-calorie hors d'oeuvres and non-alcoholic beverages). Evening programs vary from day to day and include lectures on nutrition, stress management, posture, and orthopedic health. Another evening, after dinner, there is a low-calorie, gourmet cooking class conducted by Michel.

During the week, there is a lecture by Deborah herself on how to make the benefits of your Golden Door exercises last.

What to wear?

Each guest is provided with a warm-up suit, T-shirts and briefs. Bring your own sneakers. The Japanese slippers and attractive kimonos are supplied by the house. Although some women dress up in caftans for dinner the first night, usually by the second or third day, post-exercise fatigue impels everyone toward increasing casualness.

Deborah's thinking on diet differs from most authorities. For one thing, she thinks in terms of "unfatness." For another, she likes to talk about "good eating" for enjoyment, creativity, health, and looks.

What's interesting about Deborah's theory is that she is fully aware of the tensions that burst forth the instant one contemplates a "diet."

"You say: 'I'm going on a diet,' and you create another tension that sends you right to the refrigerator. The more you think about dieting, the hungrier you get."

Since we were children, she points out, food has been a kind of reward. But heavy rewards inevitably make us unlovable adults. And diets are punishments.

The focus, she declares, must be a balanced lifestyle—taking the four or five hours daily that belong to us and ORGANIZING THEM TO DO WHAT WE REALLY WANT TO DO. This implies forethought and planning. It also implies taking stock of the long-buried wishes we anxiously repress—and REALIZING THEM!

Deborah, for instance, jots down in a notebook exactly six things that she'd like to do more than anything else that month. She continually surprises herself as to how greatly she surpasses her goals, once she's declared them.

Probably to inspire the guests, Deborah encourages her attractive exercise instructors to dress in leotards and tights that show off their trim forms to best advantage.

Deborah places far more emphasis on exercise than on diet, contrary to much popular philosophy on the matter of good looks. She makes exercise more palatable by breaking her at-home sessions into ten-minute segments scattered throughout the workday.

You've achieved the essential of any exercise, she says, at the point of "huffy-puffy." The simplest way of reaching "huffy-puffy" is with a jumprope (she has one in her car, one in each office, one in her purse, and one in her bedroom). She recommends the solid sporting-goods store jumprope rather than the toy variety. When you get to a fifty-skips-per-minute rate, you're up there with the pros and doing just fine.

Cycling machines, swimming, running (in place or around the block), and walking are splendid huffy-puffy generators, she says, and are done best before mealtimes. NOT before bedtime, because you may have trouble sleeping.

Guests leave the Golden Door with personalized cassette exercise tapes. Soon individualized video tapes will be available for guests to use at home.

Here are the best Golden Door take-home exercises. They are simple to do, effective, and can be done during five- or ten-minute breaks.

Golden Door Stretches

Stand straight with feet wide apart, knees relaxed, toes pointing forward. Arms straight up with palms facing forward. Begin reaching for the sky. Reach up with the right hand, then with the left, feeling the stretch start at the waist and go all the way to the fingertips. Breathe deeply with head at a slight angle upward. Repeat 6 times.

Pause with arms straight up and next to ears, knees still relaxed, lean first to the left side, then come up through the center and then lean to the right side. Exhale as you lean, inhale as you come up to center. Repeat 6 times.

Bring hands down to sides and with knees still slightly bent begin exhaling as you curl the upper body down one vertebra at a time until you are hanging rag-doll fashion with neck completely relaxed. Slowly inhale as you curl the body back up, vertebra by vertebra. Repeat 5 times.

Cross one leg behind the other, sink down to a sitting position, then roll down flat on your back with both knees well bent. Bring knees to chest and clasp behind the knees with both hands, straighten arms and legs upward as straight as possible. Flex the feet to stretch your calves. Now begin a slow exhale as you lift the upper body and head toward the knees, elbows bending out to the sides. This will stretch the upper back and warm up the abdominals. Inhale as you re-

REGULAR EXERCISES FOR TONING

START 10 x's INCREASE 5 x's DAILY TO 30

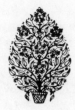

1. ARMS: Stand with legs apart, toes straight ahead, buttocks tight. Using a 3-lb. weight, lift right arm straight up overhead—elbow next to ear. Holding elbow stationary, slowly lower the weight toward the right shoulder and back. Then lift straight up—slowly—Exhale while lifting weight up, inhale while lowering weight. (Repeat on left side.)

2. WAIST: Stand with legs apart, toes turned in, tighten buttock muscles. Slowly slide right arm down your right side; right hand reaching for ankle, while your left elbow bends and the left hand touches rib cage. Straighten up and repeat on the left side. Use a 3-lb. weight. May be increased to 5 lbs.

3. HIPS & THIGHS: Down on the floor on hands and knees—keep eyes focused on the floor between hands. Lift right knee perpendicular to the floor, holding the calf at right angle to the thigh. Then lower the knee to the original position. Exhale on each lift of the leg. Keep the back flat and the shoulders still. (Repeat on the left side.)

4. HIPS: Down on the floor on hands and knees—keep eyes focused on the floor between hands—neck relaxed. Lift the right knee straight behind you, upper right leg parallel to body with knee bent and foot toward ceiling. Keeping the back flat, lift the knee up about 8"—then back to parallel. (Repeat on left side.)

5. WAIST & HIPS: Down on the floor, back flat. Separate your legs and bend your knees. Keep your shoulders down, and bring your knees down to the right, kneecaps touching floor, and then bring knees down to the left side. Be sure your legs are far apart, and that you work with resistance in legs.

6. STOMACH: Down on the floor, back flat, with arms and hands tucked under your lower back and buttocks. Put your legs together and bend your knees. Bring knees to chest, then straighten legs and extend them over head. Bend knees back to chest and touch toes to the floor.

7. HIPS, THIGHS & WAIST: Lie on the floor, legs straight, arms outstretched. Bring your right leg up, keeping it straight, lift it up and down to the floor, right side, flexing your foot. Repeat with left leg.

turn the upper body to the floor and bring the knees to the chest. Wrap your arms around your knees and draw the knees tightly to the chest. Lift the head to the knees to stretch the lower back. Repeat 3 times.

Curl upper body to an upright position, sitting with one leg extended forward, one knee bent on floor. Inhale first and then exhale as you sink your body forward over the extended leg, head dropping toward the knee. Use hands on the leg, knee may be slightly bent if needed. Breathe deeply, and slowly sink into the stretch. Hold, then inhale as you come up to a sitting position and change legs. Repeat six times, three times on each leg.

Come up to rest on your hands and knees for the cat stretch. Head is up, back is flat and abdominals relaxed. Inhale in this position, then a slow exhale as you sink the chin toward the chest, pull your stomach in toward your back, lifting back toward ceiling, tuck the hips under and hold with a full exhale. Inhale coming back up—the head comes up, back is flat and abdominals relaxed. Repeat three times.

Come up to rest on your knees, arms at your sides. Bring right foot forward. Place hands on upper right thigh and push yourself up to a standing position. With feet shoulder width apart, knees bent, reach arms straight overhead as you inhale, exhale as you slowly swing upper body down reaching arms between legs near the floor, then inhale and swing your body back up with arms overhead. Repeat five times.

Nine weeks are set aside for men: the first two weeks of March and June, three weeks in September, and two in December. Plus, there are seven weeks for couples: the last two weeks of March, last two weeks of June, last two weeks of September, and the middle week of December.

The men require less pampering than women and rarely ask for special services. For them the breakfast-in-bed option is not even offered. But they do enjoy the typical female indulgences of facials, manicures, and pedicures. The difference between the way the men and women play water volleyball is quite dramatic. Often the women look as if they are swatting flies. The men churn the water to a froth as if they were getting six-figure pro salaries.

"Captains of industry" is the phrase the Door publicist uses to describe the male guests. Besides U.S. chairmen of the board and company presidents and Hollywood luminaries, there are international personalities like Alex Papamarkou, who recently bought out a whole week for himself and titled and nontitled friends from both sides of the Atlantic. ("Isn't that going to be very expensive?" Deborah asked him. "My dear," he said, "have you ever rented a yacht?")

Designer Bill Blass' regard for the Golden Door is typical. He sees it as a semi-annual retooling or "kick-off" ritual for the next six months—making it easier for him to perform his exercises and stick to his thousand-calorie diet.

Golden Door fans include Cher, model Christina Ferrari, Phyllis George Brown, Olivia Newton John, and other public faces like TV's Barbara Walters.

At last count, I've been to the Golden Door seven times. And, with the exception of my first visit, I've been enthralled each time. One of my biggest pleasures has been exploring the very beautiful Honjin Inn.

SUMMARY: True to past performance, the Golden Door once again leads its elite passenger list luxuriously to tauter muscles, decompressed pouches, zingier complexions, and shameless narcissism.—E.W.

ADDENDUM: Long before the jet age, the wealthy went abroad for spa visits. Now they're going "aboard" because Deborah Szekely's Golden Door Spa At Sea has just opened the first Spa at Sea on the sixth and seventh deck of the Queen Elizabeth 2 for those who want to cruise their way to fitness.

It's a bargain buy because cruise and spa combined cost less than a stay at the Golden Door in California. Bonus: Bracing fresh air (the kind you can only get at sea these days) and a program that guarantees to work off any calories that accrue because sea breezes whet your appetite. (Those who want to go Spartan all the way can dine on Golden Door calorie-trimmed meals in the QE2 dining salon.)

The spa program aboard offers such pleasing programs as ballet barre exercises, whirlpool baths, in-pool exercising, aerobics, dance exercise, parcours on deck, jogging, swimming, and yoga. The active routines alternate with classes in relaxation techniques, biofeedback, stress-management, and nutrition. Help yourself to as much spa self-improvement as you like, then supplement with shipboard activities such as arts, crafts, bridge, backgammon, or classes in speed reading or languages.

Prices for QE2 cruises and trans-Atlantic crossings, including The Golden Door program, begin at $1,185. What a way to go!

The Phoenix at the Houstonian Texas

Within the last three years, a new world in spa-dom has been created in Houston, Texas. It's called The Phoenix located at The Houstonian, an unprecedented $100 million healthful living complex on 21 lush acres—right in the heart of the city.

Once the "impossible dream" of founder and chairman Tom J. Fatjo, Jr., (also renowned founder of Browning-Ferris Industries, world's largest waste management firm), The Houstonian has clearly materialized into an incomparable health and fitness facility.

Sharing its heavily-wooded acreage (the grounds of three former estates), are the elegant Phoenix Spa, an elaborate 126,000 sq. ft. Health & Fitness Center, the highly-respected Houstonian Living Well Medical Center, the 300-room Houstonian Hotel, a conference center with 29 major meeting rooms, a private club, the 28-story Houstonian Estates luxury condominiums, along with superb sports and recreation facilities of the finest resort. The Houstonian is also national headquarters for the American Leadership Forum, the American Productivity Center, Living Well, The Houstonian Foundation, and the National Fitness Classic (annually co-sponsored by The Houstonian and The President's Council on Physical Fitness and Sports).

It's obviously a do-everything place, expanding upon the "total fitness" philosophy I so greatly admired at the Dallas Aerobics Center back in 1973. That's how I met Houstonian's current president of membership, and exceptional fitness motivator, Russell A. Harris. He had helped Dr. Kenneth Cooper found the Aerobics Center in 1971, and in 1976 joined Tom Fatjo to found The Houstonian.

Today, thanks to Russ Harris and the other outstanding professionals on Tom Fatjo's team, you can enjoy spa weeks at The Phoenix, spa weekends and Living Well lifestyle changes programs at The Houstonian Hotel; refresh and renew daily as a member of the exclusive Houstonian Club; even embrace the entire Houstonian lifestyle by actually living on the property at The Houstonian Estates.

My first contact with The Phoenix came some four years ago when it was a mere gleam in The Houstonian's eye. Since then co-founders Frances Baxter and Judith Fatjo (wife of Tom Fatjo), along with spa director Chris Silkwood, have put The Phoenix on women's annual calendars across the country and in many foreign cities.

Like its famed namesake from Greek mythology, The Phoenix represents a unique capability for a virtual rebirth and continuous renewal. Unlike traditional spas, this contemporary health resort emphasizes education, "take-home fitness" and total beauty of body, mind, and spirit.

Each week-long session features programs on healthful eating, beauty, fashion, exercise, personal growth, individual fitness evaluations, and sufficiently pampered rejuvenation programs.

The complete and varied exercise program was developed and is supervised by spa director Chris Silkwood, well known fitness authority, formerly of the Golden Door in California. It emphasizes cardiovascular activity while integrating toning and stretching, brisk walking, aerobic dance, and water exercise.

Beauty care includes daily massages, individual make-up and skin consultations, hair styling and treatments, manicure, pedicure, and facials.

Evening activities and special events run the gamut: wok cooking classes, wardrobe planning demonstrations, country and western dance lessons, investment seminars, open forums with staff psychotherapist, healthful eating while dining out sessions as well as quiet personal time for the proper balance of rest and activity.

A typical day at The Phoenix looks something like this:

6:30 Wakeup call and juice served—to help pick up the blood sugar level before the brisk walk.

7:00 Walk-Jog—to stimulate the heart early in the day and enhance overall circulation.

7:30 Breakfast—usually a high fiber breakfast.

8:15 Extender—½ hour of static, comfortable stretches to prepare the body for the day's activities.

8:30 Toner—45-minute class working on specific body parts for tone, strength, and overall definition.

9:30 The Beat—45-minute class of dance exercise to strengthen the heart and burn up calories.

10:15 Juice Break—to keep the body in balance.

10:30 Circuit Training—45-minute class combining the weight machines with walking for a toning and aerobic effect.

11:30 Beauty-treatments include three facials, manicure, pedicure, makeup, hair treatment, and styling.

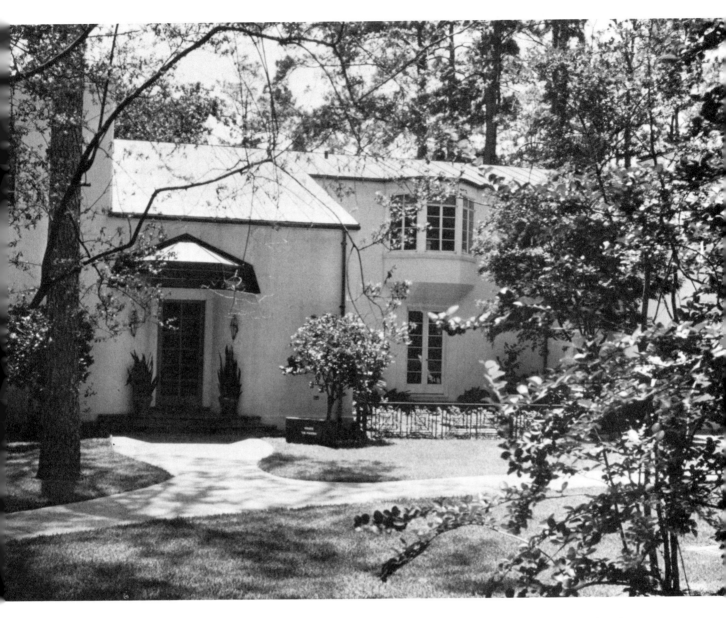

The Phoenix Texas

12:30 Lunch.
 1:30 The Revivor—relaxed toning exercises in warm water.
 2:30 Massage.
 3:15 Juice Break—pick up blood sugar and energy level.
 3:30 The Phoenix—fun dance classes and aerobic activities.
 4:30 Your Time—brisk walks, tennis, racquetball, lap swimming, or relaxation.
 5:30 The Roundup—summing up the exercise day with a stretching and relaxation session to pre- pare for a relaxed evening.
 6:30 Non-alcoholic cocktail hour.
 6:45 Dinner.
 7:30 Program.

Phoenix guests enjoy private accommodations in the lovely Phoenix Wing of The Houstonian Hotel— just a pleasant stroll across a charming wooden foot bridge from The Phoenix main house. The atmosphere and suggested dress is decidedly casual and relaxed. Apparel provided are T-shirts, shorts, warm-ups, terry robes, and caftans.

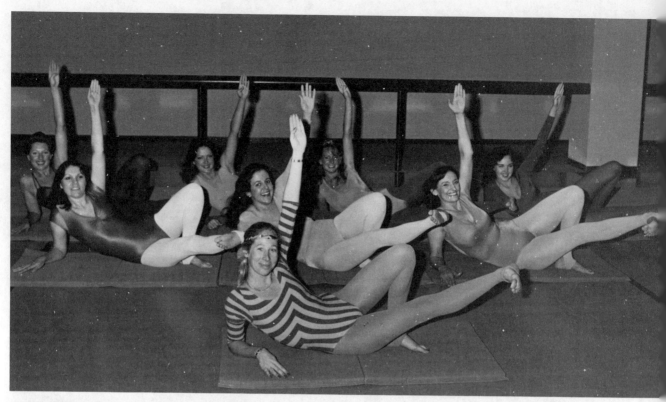

The Phoenix Texas

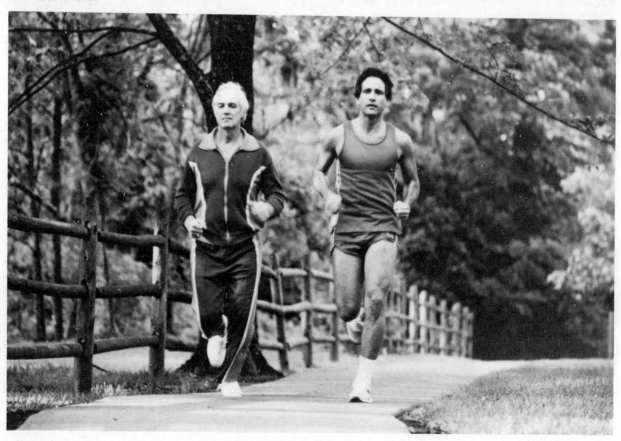

The Phoenix Texas

Cost for the week of total renewal is $1850 which includes all meals (breakfast in your room, if you wish), lodging and detailed handbooks containing Phoenix menus, recipes, caloric information as well as tips on skin care, fitness, nutrition, massage, and individual style and beauty. Also available are videotape cassettes of varied exercise routines by Chris Silkwood for home study, as well as other fitness literature and post accessories in The Phoenix Boutique.

For an additional $495, guests may receive a complete physical exam next door at the Houstonian Living Well Medical Center.

The smallest private spa in the country, The Phoenix accepts only up to 13 guests each week. Staff members outnumber guests approximately two to one, insuring a high level of service and especially serene surroundings.

Particularly distinct is the feeling you're visiting someone's wonderful estate home. Because in fact, you are. The Phoenix is housed in an Art Deco landmark mansion exquisitely renovated to accommodate complete exercise, beauty, dining, and lecture facilities.

Also, Phoenix guests have access to all The Houstonian's elaborate health and fitness amenities. These feature two swimming pools (besides The Phoenix' own pool), eight racquetball/handball courts, five tennis courts, a scenic 1-mile outdoor track, a gymnasium, a vast exercise room complete with weight training equipment, and a banked indoor track with pacing lights, plus spas with whirlpool, sauna, and steam.

The Phoenix, as a progressive health and beauty facility, provides its guests—on land or sea—with the opportunity to greatly enhance the quality of their lives. Each Phoenix department creates a stimulating environment for learning, productivity, and a total grasp of individual human potential.

Here health and fitness is not for the fainthearted. Exercise is fun but vigorous. Beauty is self-acceptance—assessing and developing the best you, primarily through immaculate grooming, and expression of individualism and personal style.

As Chris Silkwood continually stresses: "Too often, people come to health facilities with the intention of undoing in a single week all the wrong they have done to their bodies over a period of years. We do not under any circumstances promote quick weight loss, starvation diets nor extreme heat treatments for the purpose of losing weight."

SUMMARY: A visit to The Phoenix should be more than a physical experience. Guests are urged to spend reflective time on all aspects of their lives—intellectual, emotional, physical, and spiritual—and ways to permanently improve them. The Phoenix suggests you approach your stay as a rebirth. You'll leave with a fresh start for a more vital, productive life—a new beginning that will improve and strengthen through your own self-discipline.—E.W.

The Phoenix Texas

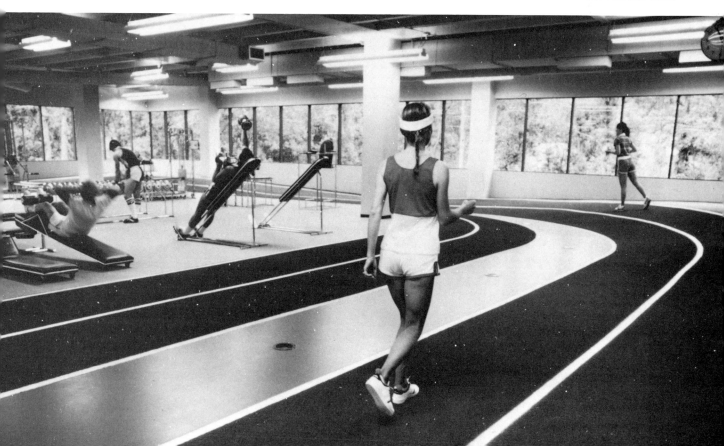

The Bonaventure Inter-Continental Hotel and Spa
Florida

The beautiful people have found a new hideaway, The Bonaventure Inter-Continental Hotel and Spa in Fort Lauderdale. Its spa facilities are part of a $50 million complex that includes a 600-room hotel, condominiums, private homes, golf courses (two), swimming pools (three), and tennis courts (two).

The spa itself is a veritable Tower of Babel. You can shut your eyes, tune in to conversations in French, Spanish, Greek, Japanese, and English (both the American and clipped British versions). It's the nearest thing to a European spa experience.

Whatever their nationality, spa guests are out to banish all signs of the sins of the social season. The spa directress tends to this matter with a strict program of body beautifying. She keeps guests busy with a vigorous program of exercise designed to diminish measurements and puts guests on a diet of 900 calories a day guaranteed to make pounds disappear. Nobody complains because vigorous and Spartan (synonyms for

exercise and diet) also mean physically fit and healthy. It's what everyone wants to be.

A plus for the program: It banishes stress and strain and sends guests home feeling relaxed, revitalized, and super refreshed.

They don't do a spa diet per se. They think in terms of complete nutrition. Their 900 calories a day are concentrated on fresh fruit and vegetables, whole grain products, fish, and poultry. Their goal is to establish sound eating habits that will last a lifetime.

They recommend that their guests do a lot of drinking—not cocktails but water. Mountain Valley, from Hot Springs, Arkansas, is the very special aqua pura favored. Six to eight eight-ounce glasses a day are recommended. You can usually find guests sipping away just prior to meals (a good way to take the edge off the appetite).

Diet soft drinks and alcoholic beverages aren't served. The aim here is to instill the tenets of healthful

The Bonaventure Florida

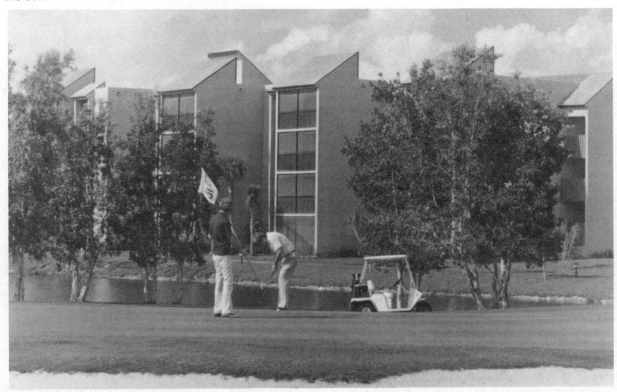

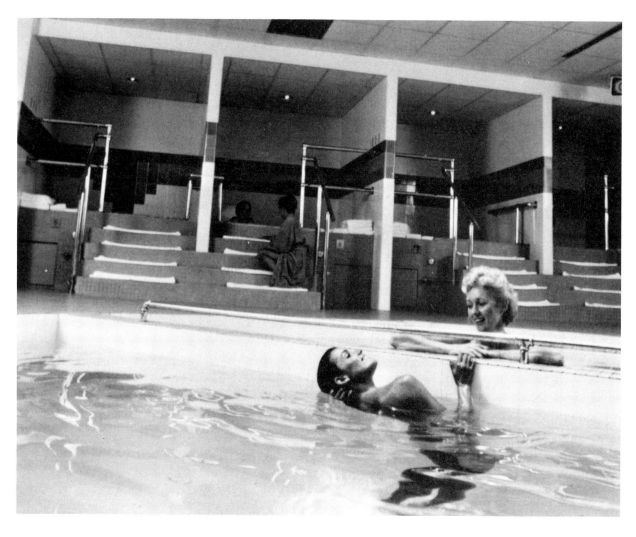

The Bonaventure Florida

eating and drinking. Nor will you find salt shakers on the dining table. Instead seasoning medleys of herbs and spices minus salt are available at the spa—and at your nearest health food store.

To sweeten the menu, the spa chef uses fructose, honey, or blackstrap molasses.

In the dairy department, acidophilus milk (which is low-fat and aids digestion) and yogurt are stressed.

Brewer's yeast (three tablespoons a day for energy and clear skin), fresh wheat germ (sprinkled on cereal to give you a vitamin fix), and natural bran or miller's bran (one to three tablespoons on breakfast cereal for roughage) appear on the daily menus.

The spa program includes Swedish massage, Shiatsu, hydrotherapy, Swiss needle showers, Finnish saunas, classic Turkish bath or steam rooms. For men, a salt glow loofah scrub with avocado oil and salt is fabulous. For women, a less vigorous treatment in-volves creams, cleansing gels and loofah sponging, with a fine mist of oils for the grand finale.

Bonaventure's soundproof gymnasiums are deco-rated most attractively with spectacularly soothing colors, with beautiful music piped in. An in-between room for both sexes encourages togetherness with all sorts of body building apparatus, under expert super-vision. You just might meet the man of your dreams on one of the strectching machines. Be sure to be dressed appropriately.

Depending on the season, prices for a four-day spa stay can range from $640 to $760 for a single; $520 to $620 per person in a double room. A seven-day deluxe fitness stay is $1,768 to $1,833 single; $1,543 to $1,575 per person double occupancy. An 18 percent service charge is tacked onto the bill.

SUMMARY: A new addition to the Spa World, beau-tifully equipped.—E.W.

New Age Health Farm New York

Back in the Golden Age, those glorious Greeks pioneered the principle of a sound mind in a healthy body. They believed in the intrinsic power of the spirit too. They were taking a holistic approach to life, an idea that is very much at the heart of the program at New Age Health Farm in Neversink, New York.

Much as the Greeks built their temples on scenic sites that encouraged man's spirit to soar, Elza and Graeme Graydon's farm is set on 152 acres of lush land, virgin ground untrampled by civilization and remote from the smoke, soot, and smog of urbanization. It's a two-hour 125-mile drive from Manhattan by car, bus, or taxi service.

When I visited, I discovered a program, unique for its emphasis on inner strength, that can lead to external improvement. The Farm is famed for its fasting regimens but they involve a great deal more than a diet of juices.

While weight loss is the goal, the Graydons help guests to achieve it not only with diet but by directing them to the deeper, often hidden causes that lead to overeating. The twofold focus is on HOW to lose weight and WHY it's a problem. You've got to get to the underlying cause before you can stay slim forever.

The Graydons are an interesting, complementary couple. He's a New Zealander—dairy farmer, archeologist, sailor, herbalist, pilot, student of homeopathic medicine. She's a bouncy blonde Austrian formally trained in music, yoga, psychology, astrology, cosmetology, and holistic therapies. Guests tend to be young—though all ages come—and the atmosphere is appealingly informal and fun.

Graeme Graydon's philosophy is simple. "All we are trying to do," he told me in his quiet, low-key way, "is create a relaxing situation in a very beautiful environment. We use nutritional programs of simple but therapeutic value and we give our guests tools in the form of advice, ideas, and experiences so they can return to their everyday lives better equipped to handle whatever is out there. We set a stage that they can use to make their own discoveries. They have to work for it, however, because we won't do it for them."

While the majority of the guests hope to head home slimmer, there are some, particularly the working professionals, men and women, who head for New Age to unwind and escape stress. "I had to get away," is a phrase I heard more than once.

Evening workshops and lectures are a popular feature. Presented by Graeme or Elza with some assistance from other staff members, these programs provide New Age's very special learning experience. Nutrition and healthful living are prime topics. Graeme has a knack of keeping abreast of new developments, sifting out the "discoveries" that turn out to be nothing more than flash-in-the-pan fads. He zeroes in on what makes sense for a balanced approach to healthy living, guiding his guests through the shoals of both entrenched orthodoxy and the wild excesses of the new health industry.

Elza's psychological workshops and guided programs of meditation offer guests opportunities to experience new feelings, gain new insights into old problems, and discover inner serenity.

The farm offers an excellent skin care salon but the emphasis is more on the values of health that stem from discipline and self-improvement. I found the guests interesting and cerebral, inclined to introspection and ready to make changes in lifestyle to attain their weight goals. I didn't encounter even one get-thin-quick-no-matter-the-cost-to-health type.

The program is tightly structured but I found it sound. The approach to diet and nutrition was not fanatical. "Put your energy into becoming a real person and your eating habits will improve automatically" is the Graydon's approach.

The day begins at 8 A.M., when the scales are set in the weigh-in-room. If you think you can't function without food, you'll be pleasantly surprised to discover how invigorating a 30-minute walk before breakfast can be. There's something about taking to the forest trail and spying on nature while the morn's still young that's positively bracing. At 9 it's back for the first liquid food-fix of the day, then on to a really fine exercise class followed by sauna and whirlpool before lunch at 1 P.M.

At 2, it's an hour-long hike or, in winter, the fun of stepping out in snow shoes or on cross country skis. The Farm has a number of scenic trails.

Afternoons set you up for an excellent yoga class, more sauna, and whirlpool. Dinner is served at 6 in a colonial dining room with a wonderful view of the countryside that sometimes includes grazing deer. The atmosphere is cozy in winter, cool and delightful in summer.

Evening lectures start around 8 when guests gather around the fireplace or assemble in the main lounge. At 9:30, it's a night cap of herbal tea or hot

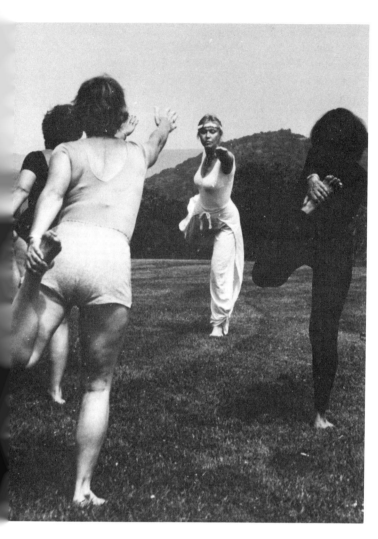

That almost instantaneous feeling of slenderness is the big reward.

The juice fast has advantages over a water fast. For one, it makes it easier to return to normal eating patterns with far less likelihood of binging off on a wild eating spree. I go on the juice fast any time I need to shed a fast few pounds or have been over-indulging in rich foods.

As guests check in, the program is explained and questions about fasting are handled in an orientation session. Guests also are briefed on the detox process. It includes enemas which, the Graydons believe, reduce all adverse effects of fasting, making it safe and more comfortable.

Surprisingly, no one seems to feel weak or light-headed on the juice fast. Instead, everyone seemed

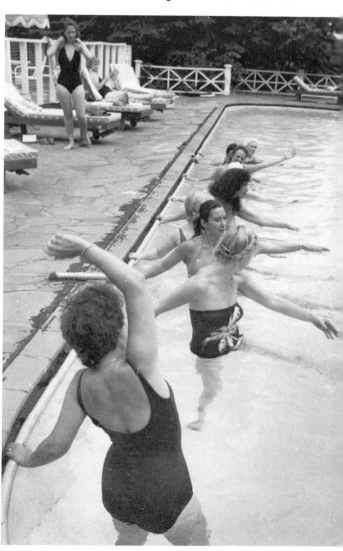

water sparked with lemon that tastes positively delicious. By 10, you're pleasantly done in and ready to retreat to your room in one of the surrounding houses.

Most guests follow a juice diet that serves up an imaginative and tasteful menu of fruit or vegetable blends during the day. It's fruit juice for breakfast, fruit or "veggie" juice for lunch, and vegetable juice plus broth at night. Herbal teas are an extra choice at each meal.

A water fast is an option for those who have their doctor's approval.

Diets limited to from 600 to 1000 calories are a possible choice. Also available is a vegetarian regimen which includes some chicken or fish.

I tried the juice diet, which is the preferred choice for weight loss, general cleansing, and relief from stress, and felt wonderfully full of energy throughout.

buoyed up. It could be the average weight loss—a pound a day—kept spirits high. Men often lose more than that. The big plus: inches disappear as new self-esteem surfaces.

Most guests stay a week. Some weekend or sign up for the popular mini-week, Monday to Friday. Arrivals and departures are daily occurrences that make for interesting new mixes.

The spa also offers massage, Quick Slim body wraps, and a full range of salon services—all at an extra charge. Private consultations with the Graydons are included in rates that range from $260 to $500 per week, depending on single or double occupancy and the room selected in one of five surrounding houses.

Accommodations range from large motel-type rooms with full baths to bungalow rooms that have showers but no tubs. Wherever you rest your head at night, the program and services are the same.

SUMMARY: The rolling, forested hills of the Catskills are a super setting for a super beauty farm. Since the program here caters to body and soul, the wonderful walking trails, secluded outdoor pool, garden, orchards, and greenhouse supply the perfect background for communing with nature—and your inner self. The Graydons enhance a stay by alternately playing teachers and warm, friendly hosts. Most guests return again and again which says something about the holistic experience—E.W.

Gurney's International Health and Beauty Spa
New York

Right at the very tip of Long Island, New York's Montauk Point juts into the mighty Atlantic. It is one of the world's most scenic spots. As far as the eye can see, the ocean rolls in, wave after wave, each breaker a seascape of its own, hypnotizing the eye with movement, lulling the spirit with soothing sound.

This is the magnificent setting for Gurney's International Health and Beauty Spa, chosen because owner Nick Monte believes the sea is good for what ails you.

"If people spent more time at the shore," he is fond of telling guests, "they'd never need a psychiatrist."

And there's no doubt that Gurney's is a relaxing place to stay, for the sea is ever-present. In summer, there's a resort-like atmosphere, for this is an inn as well as a spa. The main building is terraced down to the beach, so that each guest enjoys the happy illusion of a private ocean view. The sound of the surf is a surefire prescription for insomnia as is the bracing air.

Gurney's is open 365 days a year—366 in Leap Year from 8 A.M. to midnite. Many prefer winter and the quiet that remains when summer crowds head back to New York City.

Five years ago when I first met Nick Monte, we discovered we shared an enthusiasm for the great European spas. "It can happen here," he insisted, and shortly thereafter Gurney's was "born." It's no coincidence that the spa's symbol is a sculpture reminiscent of Botticelli's *Birth of Venus*. It depicts Youth as a shapely woman and symbolizes the sea giving birth to life, beauty, and health.

When I visited Gurney's I discovered that the "treatment" starts almost instantly. The air is invigorating. Just going on one of the spa's aerobic beach walks helps you breathe in new life. Negative ions in the air (inhale deeply), no pollution, no congestion, one of the nation's lowest pollen counts (a boon for hay fever sufferers) are all unique assets.

Clean sea water is used in hydro-therapies at the spa, including the renowned thalasso underwater massage. Water is pumped into the sensuous Roman baths and, needless to say, makes a swim in the king-size indoor pool refreshing. The pool is heated to the same temperature as the controlled air in the pool area. All the indoor comforts plus, through a window wall, a breathtaking view of the ever-changing blue sea!

The menu of sea-related treatments at Gurney's is extensive. For example: sea water plus Dead Sea salt combine for a scrub that leaves the body glowing. Seaweed cell fluid, which is imported from Brittany, plays a most important part in the spa's new cellulite control program. This corresponds to the most effective treatment techniques at the most famous European thalasso therapy centers.

You can choose from a menu of massage therapies: Swedish, Shiatsu (facial), tissue, polarity, reflexology. Try one, try all, or at least several. For something

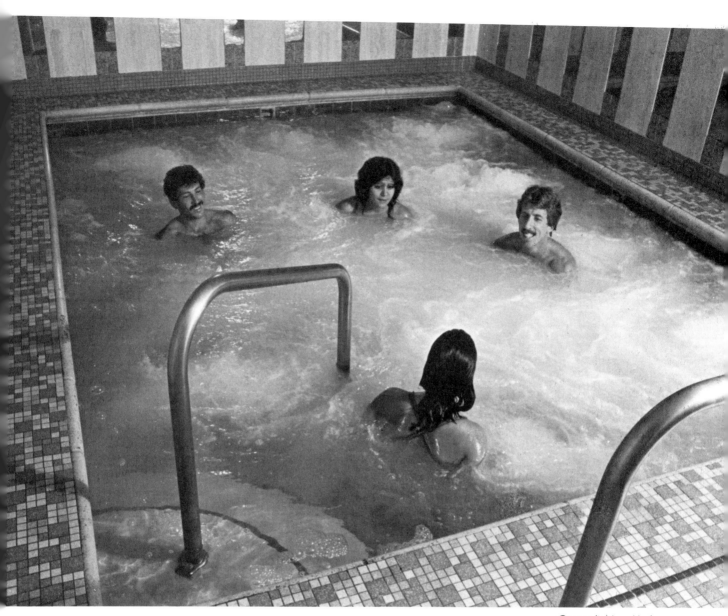

Gurney's New York

different, there's a unique massage developed by the well-known Hawaiian physician, Dr. Milton Trager. It's special.

Before Nick Monte brought European Spa techniques to our shores, a fango treatment was something you could only enjoy abroad. Now this deep-heat mud pack is a popular treatment at Gurney's. The beneficial mud is imported from Battaglia, Italy, then mixed with paraffin to give it heat retention. I oozed with what the ads so fondly refer to as "immediate relief" as it worked its soothing magic on tense shoulders and aching muscles. Aches evaporated and I could feel myself thinking "mmmmmmmmm" as each foot was gently, (oh, so gently) massaged.

Relaxation is a treat and a treatment at this spa. Seminars zero in on escape routes from the stress that's synonymous with modern living. Special techniques can help you summon up Nirvana and feel serene and peaceful once you master them.

To put matter over mind, you can enjoy a session in a thalasso tub, imported from Germany, that's somewhat akin to returning to the womb. You float in body temperature sea water on a cushion of air bubbles (luscious thought, isn't it!) while a trained nurse guides you with gentle imagery and soft music to a Never-Never-Land of profound peace and weightlessness. Is this how the astronauts felt, cushioned and weightless, as they conquered space?

A super spa for all seasons and reasons, Gurney's caters to men as well as women, allotting private treatment pavilions to each. You can choose to stay for a day, a weekend, or a week. Some spa facilities are open to guests at the inn.

The Executive Fitness Program is a new lure for

127

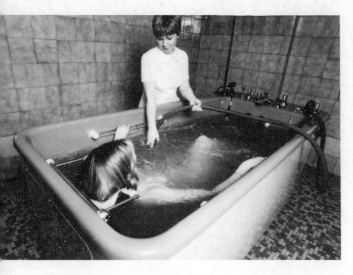

Gurney's New York

New York career women who escape the stress of skyscraper city to relax, reduce, exercise, and learn how to deal with the stress that seems to go hand-in-hand with success. At the end of a program, the executive Ms. heads home with a personalized file that provides a customized Rx for beauty of body and peace of mind.

Gurney's New York

Dining is a mixed bag at Gurneys—the haves and should-not-haves share the same dining room. That's a bit of a drawback for someone whose will-power wavers at the first whiff of a delicious aroma.

Still, the dietwise choices for those on the spa program were excellent during my last visit. Nutritionally well-balanced meals were high in fiber, low in fat, cholesterol, salt, sugar, and refined carbohydrates. Spa guests have their calories counted for them. The choices were good including the fresh catch of local fishermen.

As you slim down, tone up, and get ready to ship out for home, a stop at the L'Institut de Beaute, the spa salon, could be a perfect finishing touch. Wow the folks waiting for your return, not only with your new svelte shape, but dazzling beauty. It's a full-service operation offering everything from hair cutting, coloring, conditioning, and styling through manicure, to facials.

SUMMARY: Gurney's is the best of everything—old-world magic in treatments, new-world informality in an atmosphere that's casual. The staff was skilled and amiably ready to serve. The keepers of the inn, Joyce and Nick Monte, exude a friendly warmth that makes you feel you're a VIP guest in their super spa beach home.—E.W.

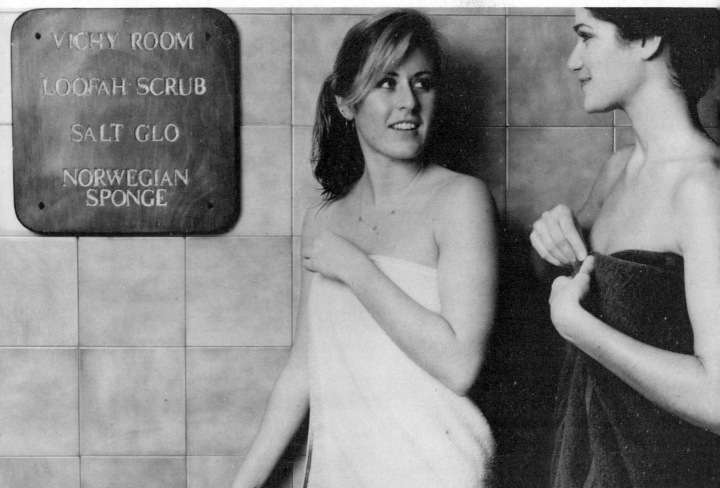

12
European
Spas

Getting There

The thousands of miles I've logged flying off to the world's most famous spas have taught me a lesson. With rare exception, B.Y.O. (Bring Your Own) is a wise rule for the diet-conscious when you fly. I've tasted too many starchy, dreary dishes aloft to fall into the "I'll try it one more time," trap again. This time I made an exception. I'd been hearing happy rumors that a spa visit to Germany begins aboard a Lufthansa flight with healthful gourmet meals that merit high marks. Bonus: I was told about an in-flight exercise program. I was intrigued with both notions. What better recommendation for good food than word of mouth.

I was not disappointed.

The food was appetizing from the moment I was handed the first class menu with its full-color cover photograph of garden vegetables. Reading it was a gastronomic thrill. The best was yet to come: A meal worthy of the finest restaurant.

The hors d'oeuvre choices included several var-

ieties of fish, including smoked salmon with dill. It was superb and not at all salty. My seat partner dipped into luscious caviar with all the trimmings. Alaskan king crab with kiwi, and crayfish with a flavorful dressing were other choices. Everything was beautifully presented. The bread basket was filled with crispy rolls, delicious dark and whole grain bread, making for a pleasurable choice. I noticed that most of the men were hearty bread eaters; the women settled for a little taste of each.

The salad—so crisp you could almost hear it crackle—was followed by sorbet and then the main course. What a presentation! When there's nothing else to do, as is sometimes the case when one flies, food assumes major importance. One could almost hear oohs and ahhs of appreciation as the *piece de resistance* was served. I selected roast breast of chicken garnished with tomato and seasoned with fresh basil. It looked as delicious as it tasted. My seat partner was digging into roast beef that really was prime, accompanied by fresh garden vegetables, and wild rice. For the spa-minded, there was fresh fruit for dessert; and for those who weren't keeping count of calories such delights as pistachio ice cream with hot raspberries, or morello cherries with vanilla sauce.

I checked out the breakfast menu and found good light choices, including fresh fruit and yogurt as well as the usual eggs and cereals.

Lunch offered light salads as well as heartier fare.

The food aloft was hot, well-prepared, and downright delicious. I liked the young, robust, superb German wines.

Before take-off, I'd wisely picked up a copy of Lufthansa's "Fitness in the Chair" booklet for executives so I could get a headstart on exercise and begin my spa program before landing in Germany. It is must reading for jet-setters because its mini workouts (10 minutes whenever muscles feel cramped) improves your circulation and keeps the blood zipping around.

I'd been airborne for more than an hour when I tried the Muscle-Toning Technique: With one-third of your strength, systematically tighten first your left thigh, then right; right buttocks, then left; back, then shoulders. Relax.

Next, I startled my neighbor slightly by doing the Stomach Press: Stomach pulled in, place palms against it and tense stomach muscles, using two-thirds of your strength. Hold for a count of seven before relaxing.

I also followed the booklet's instructions and moved around. I waited until the aisles were clear (a good reason to reserve an aisle seat) before getting up to stretch. Then I strolled around the plane, striking up some interesting conversations en route.

The end result: The light, satisfying diet of fresh food plus the mini exercise plan left me feeling vital and ready to go when I reached journey's end.

Wiesbaden Germany

We landed at Frankfurt, half an hour from my first stop, Wiesbaden on the Rhine, the spa city where kings once left their calling cards. My destination was the Nassauer Hof (managed by the charming and elegant Karl Nuesser), a world-class luxury hotel. Its beautifully baroque, columned facade was a preview of the many splendors inside. I was ushered into a spacious bedroom containing sleek contemporary furniture and with windows overlooking the most charming old-world view. I felt like a queen. After all, it was royalty that made taking the waters at Wiesbaden fashionable in the first place.

The Nassauer Hof is "the" place to stay. It's a happening all by itself.

You can dine informally in its brasserie "Die Pfanne" (The Pan) which is rustic and cozy. Or you can celebrity-watch as you enjoy a leisurely three-hour dinner in "Die Ente" (The Duck) where the fabulous food created by Peter Wodarz is simply delicious and as famous as such celebrated diners as Andy Warhol, Bianca Jagger and Charlton Heston.

Directly opposite the hotel is the "Kurhaus," a recreational center with a theater, opera, a gambling casino, and galleries. So entertainment and some interesting sightseeing are readily at hand.

What lures travelers to Wiesbaden, just as it lured the crowned heads of Europe, is mineral waters from springs which are famed for easing rheumatism, arthritis, and other aches and pains.

Water therapies vary. The most unforgettable—the Roman-Celtic Bath at the Kaiser Friedrich Bad which, three days a week, caters to a mixed male-female crowd. When in Wiesbaden do as the Wiesbadians do—so I shed my modesty along with all my clothes and followed the regimen. I don't think I've ever looked so many men straight in the eye. It managed to be exhilarating and exhausting at the same time plus great to pep up circulation and metabolism. Although designed to treat rheumatism, bronchitis, sinus, and circulatory disorders, the routine is strenuous and not advised for those who suffer heart trouble or circulatory disorders.

You're alternately hot and cold as you follow the attendant into a hot air room and a steam room, then shower and settle into a hot water pool. Next comes a dip in a cold, cold thermal pool, followed by a fantastic massage that completely loosens every tight muscle. Finally, it was heaven to stretch out in the relaxation room and marvel at the limp state of my body. The whole procedure takes three hours. It left me in a state of languor and positively purring.

There's a wide choice of revitalizing treatments at the Friedrich Bad. You can drink the healthful waters. You can bathe in them. Modesty prevails when you step into the biggest pool I've ever seen. It's grandeur puts the ancient Roman baths to shame. This is a fun

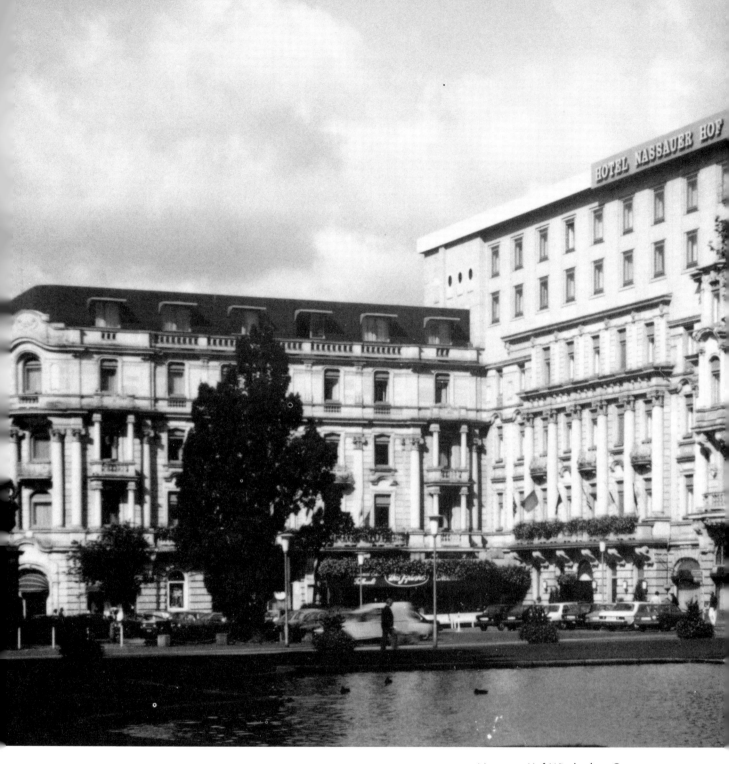

Nassauer Hof Wiesbaden, Germany

and social dip in mixed company and, yes, bathing suits are de rigeur.

Small pools of varying temperatures from steaming hot to arctic cold offer various therapeutic treatments, including under-water massage. Special mud packs soothe aches, pains, and the symptoms of ad-vancing age as do physical exercise therapies involving thermal waters.

Wiesbaden's reputation as a revitalization center is due in part to Professor Dr. Med. Klaus Miehlke, who operates two clinics that specialize in arthritis and rheumatism treatment and research. A tall, handsome man, totally dedicated to his work, he spoke of rheumatism as not one disease but many. His clinics are famous for treating the most severe forms, as well as for being a clearing house for worldwide research. Happily, he offers both help and hope for those who are threatened, prescribing special medication to help arrest the ravages of this painful condition. Annually a prize is given for the best research. The coveted award, which carries world-wide honor and prestige, has been won in the U.S. by researchers in Birmingham, Alabama, and Houston, Texas.

When your water therapy is over, there are pleasant walks in Wiesbaden that take you past charming outdoor restaurants, posh little shops, beautiful fountains and ornate buildings dating from the 17th century, each with a historic or romantic story to tell. It's a pleasant drive to the Taunus Mountain where, from the restaurant at Keller's Kopf, you have a cineramic view of the countryside. Or you can travel up the Rhine past castles, vineyards that produce great German wines, and breathtakingly beautiful gardens. Some prefer to spend idle hours at the magnificent casino where your passport and a good supply of cash are your ticket of entry. I kept my passport but left my money behind.

If you can visit Wiesbaden in May, you'll luck into a month of festivals that bring opera and theatre companies from the world over.

All this plus a revitalization boost recharges your batteries.

A week at the Nassauer Hof should cost $650–950, therapies extra.

Book reservations through Hotel Representatives, Inc. 770 Lexington Avenue, New York, N.Y. 10022.

Baden-Baden Germany

I slipped into Baden-Baden, that queen of spas, without the kind of pomp and circumstances that once heralded the arrival of the Kaiser or, before him, Napoleon III. But I felt like royalty traveling incognito. It's that kind of city—bejeweled, dressy, posh, stunning —and it's set in a bower of copper beeches, birches, maples, oaks, willows, chestnut trees, and stately pines.

Everywhere you look there's the kind of pre-World War I elegance that's dazzling. For example, no other casino in the world uses, on special occasion, gold and silver chips. The town orchestra and theatrical company are excellent and the National Art Gallery is a treasure trove of paintings that seem familiar because they're so famous.

Everyone who's visited Baden-Baden offers the same advice: Stay at Brenner's Park. Not for nought does this elegant hotel rate among the world's very finest. Heel-clicking service is everywhere at hand. Porter's appear magically. An attendant quickly spun the revolving door for me. The concierge was a welcoming committee of one who made me feel my arrival had made his day complete. I had barely crossed the lobby before I knew this was a stay I'd long remember. One gets accustomed to old-world charm in a thrice— even quicker when weary after a journey.

My "cure" began with a walk to my room along the lush, deep indigo carpets that led through endless marble corridors studded with exquisite furniture and delightful etchings and engravings.

In my room there were fresh flowers and fruit, champagne and chocolates, Persian rugs, furniture styled two centuries ago, a crystal chandelier, and heavy draperies. Whether the good old days were gentler, I can't say. All I know is that I felt as if I'd strolled into history's womb—utterly safe, protected from round-the-clock headlines, commercials, and the mindless clatter of civilization.

I could have spent the entire stay contently in my room—but there was too much to see and do. Brenner's Park has added a Lancaster Beauty Farm and a hairdressing salon to its many other attractions.

I didn't sign up for the entire cure, which ideally lasts from three to four weeks but I planned to put myself on the spa diet for a day or two to try it.

My host, the managing director of Brenner's Park-Hotel, Richard Schmitz, took me through the formal dining room into a delightful hunting-lodge room, the Schwarzwald Grill. The menu was excellent—and good for my figure. My first dinner began with an appetizing salad of cucumbers, tomatoes, carrots, and lettuce—each morsel crisp as a fresh fall day. The dressing was marvelous, and I pass it on to you:

Brenner's Park-Hotel Franka Dressing

Mix 2 egg yolks with salt, wine, vinegar, pepper, Worchestershire sauce, and English mustard to taste. While stirring, add slowly a pint of peanut oil. Dilute this mixture with as much heavy cream as you like—careful not to thin it unduly. Then, according to your palate, add tomato ketchup and chopped herbs, such as parsley, chives, tarragon, and basil.

Just a teaspoon or two of this magical mixture will give salad an out-of-this-world flavor without adding too many extra calories.

Richard Schmitz, a devastatingly attractive young man who has done a fabulous job at Brenner's Park-Hotel, ordered a very enjoyable white wine for me, Staufenberger Schlossberg.

The entree he suggested was excellent—a small steak and delicious fluffy rice. For dessert, I had fresh raspberries and champagne sorbet.

After dinner, I let myself get swallowed up in the down pillows and comforter for a sleep so sweet I'll never forget it.

The floor-to-ceiling French windows opened onto a little balcony, from which I surveyed the leafy Lichentaler Allee and the scenic Oos River.

As a delicious breeze wafted in through the windows, I thought of the Swiss governess I'd had as a child. She always took us children for walks among the pine trees.

"The pines, the pines," she used to say, "nothing heals like the air from the pines."

Breakfast next morning was carried in and placed on a gleaming white tablecloth. The bio-yogurt (dietetic) was good, as was the coffee. I managed to exert willpower and extracted from a huge basket of rolls only the Knackenbrot (a kind of Rye-Krisp) and a small rye roll.

Then I was ready to visit the raison d'etre for Baden-Baden: its baths.

Although no one is certain of the origin of the waters themselves, the springs that furnish the water have been analyzed with German precision. The large salt deposits in the Schwarzwald probably explain the slightly briny taste.

In times past, a Baden-Baden sojourn meant outrageous gourmandism, tumultuous promiscuity, and round-the-clock gossiping—after all there were all kinds of goings-on to talk about. In the 16th Century, there were 399 communal baths that would put any of today's swinger's colonies to shame. Men and women used to sit for six or seven hours straight in the baths—eating, drinking, doing EVERYTHING and ANYTHING you can think of together. The Reformation put

an end to that and on St. Bartholomew's Day in 1689 Louis XIV put the torch to the Baden-Baden margrave's residence and other buildings. It took the spa one hundred years to make a comeback. Life is much tamer these days, for most people come on a serious search for revitalization.

At Baden-Baden, as at any other spa with a vigorous program, watch out for what's known as the "spa reaction." It strikes after one or two weeks of the program. It's a "blah" syndrome that leaves you unable to sleep, not hungry (that's a blessing), somewhat pessimistic, and worn out. Give it a day or two and you'll be yourself—in fact better!

Baden-Baden ought to be of special interest to women who have chronic gynecological complaints—some of which, doctors say, may be of psychosomatic origin. Dr. Nobakht an outstanding Baden-Baden gynecologist, has an edge: medical expertise plus first hand knowledge of the benefits of the thermal waters for a variety of ills. Whatever the origin, the water routine seems to help one over the roughest spots. A lack of true relaxation, escape from routine—and what an escape Baden-Baden is—helps. When you add the water therapies, exercises, fresh food, fresh impressions, fun and games, you can cast the whole baggage of psychosomatic ailments overboard.

If you stay for a week or more, you'll spend some time daily at the baths. Both Augustabad and Friedrichsbad have full therapeutic treatments. Before you plunge in, be sure to have a local doctor check you. While the baths are "cures" for some, they're not for all. Good personal health is a key consideration.

I decided to try the fango (a mud and thermal water treatment) at Augustabad. What is there about mud that attracts adults? Is it a throwback to childhood and the don't-get-dirty warnings that were never-ending?

Anyway, I was rewarded. The fango, which eases aches and pains, especially those caused by arthritis, proved penetrating and invigorating. I was glad not to be on Candid Camera as I sat on a bench, my hands or my feet, immersed in pails of hot mud. Your doctor prescribes muddying-up time, which varies from person to person. You take another part of this treatment lying down—a nice glunky mud pack that felt strangely pleasant. Next came a marvelous massage.

One of the specialties at the nearby Friedrichsbad is the Roman Irish Baths and, indeed, its more invigorating qualities are evident after you've been through the program of hot and cold thermal waters, stream treatment and finally—and not a moment too soon—the relaxation room. It's an experience not to be missed. The best part: A marvelous soap massage given

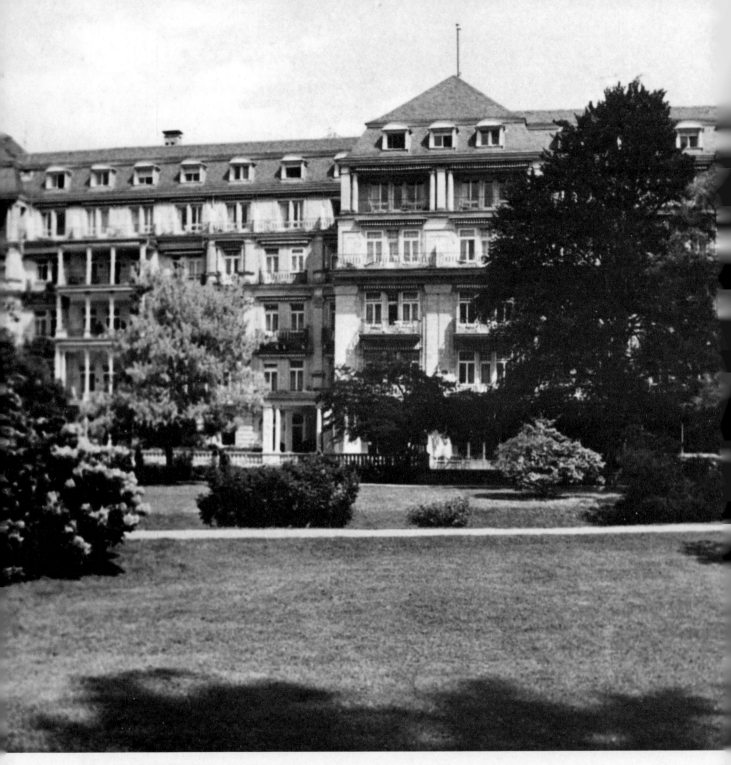

Brenner's Park Baden-Baden, Germany

by an attendant with muscles like Popeye who orchestrated with a bristle brush. The end result was the next best thing to growing new skin. I positively glowed—all over.

If your doctor's Rx is physical exercise therapy for heart and vascular disorders, head for the hills. Dr. Werner Hess has designed a network of Terrainkur trails in a beautiful mountainous area. There are different degrees of incline—from beginner's slope to what may seem to some, Mt. Everest heights. But what better way to build endurance than in the grand and glorious great German outdoors.

If revitalization is your quest, the Schwarzwald Clinic in the Villa Stephanie on the grounds at Brenner's Park under the excellent diagnosis and care of Dr. Claudia Melms offers many rejuvenating options with a program that seems to offer something for everyone. You can opt for the Neihans cell therapy, the Aslan Gerovital H3 injections, or the Kneipp water treatment to ease vein problems. Medical gymnastics and massage are available. Psychotherapy and mind control (the latter helps ease sleep problems) can also be on your agenda. The big plus: A variety of diet programs, including HCG injections and a 500-calorie-a-day regimen that promises to make weight on extra-heavy body areas do a Houdini disappearing act.

All of this at Brenner's Park and more—the marvelous Lancaster Beauty Farm Program for men as well as women. Since the farm was added to the hotel, there are some guests who start self-improvement programs even before they take the waters or leave Brenner's Park's portals.

Nina Walters, who directs the Lancaster program, is the best advertisement there is for the kind of beauty dividends a disciplined approach can pay. She's slim, trim, impeccably groomed, everything you'd like to be—and so you sign up for yoga, dip into the Roman pool for underwater gymnastics (don't miss the heated benches, a super touch of luxury!) enjoy the sauna, massages, the magic of facials, the relaxation of body packs. Then you indulge in glamorizing extras, such as manicures and pedicures. How else could you feel but fabulous? It is a great regimen. Best of all, you take away some of the how-tos, souvenirs of your stay that can serve you well.

Lancaster skin-care preparations and cosmetics are available for taking home, so you can keep the magic going with the techniques you learned during your stay.

The whole "Farm" atmosphere is pleasantly geared to self-improvement and new approaches to fitness, grooming, and diet. The healthful menu choices (available to all guests at Brenner's Park) are geared to making you think twice before you make an eating choice that isn't fresh, wholesome, good for your body, and great for your figure.

SUMMARY: Baden-Baden is irrefutable evidence that the Germans have a keen understanding of spaing. Everything here combines for a Super Spa stay. Schedules are as closely adhered to as a first baby's feeding schedule—and what baby ever got such pampering. The service is superb, the accommodations luxurious, the treatments, all that's promised, and more. And don't forget the extras: climate, culture, cuisine, casino-ing and the great fresh air, which you can enjoy, as the Germans do, by stepping out afoot. There are miles of scenic walks along the Lichtentaler Allee and the sparkling, Oos River plus the French architecture that lends a touch of Paris. Also there are other sightseeing attractions such as the villas that the Russian writer Turgenev and Prince Menshikov once called home. Such grandeur.

Brenner's Park prices start at $800 per week for room and three delectable meals a day on the Lancaster Beauty Farm Program. Book through Hotel Representatives, Inc., 770 Lexington Avenue, New York, N.Y. 10022.—E.W.

Kurhaus Vienna-Beauty Austria (formerly Dr. Lauda's Think-Beautiful Farm)

I took the crack Ljubljana Express train from Vienna to Linz and then a local train to Velden am Worther See where I was met by the new director, Mrs. Berty Buchacher, Dr. Lauda's long-time assistant, who took me to the beauty farm. It is from beauty farms such as this one that the American beauty spas could well derive additional inspiration.

"Farm" is the word. It was just that, rolling hills and pastures with tones of fresh air flowing in from the surrounding fir and pine forests.

Although the spa is open from the beginning of March through mid-November, the knowledgeable visitor usually elects a two- or three-week stay either in the spring or autumn or both. And although the currency situation is about as settled as a teen-aged girl in love, you can reasonably figure about $935 for a two-week visit (one week for half the price). That includes lodging, meals, and all beauty treatments except special correctives (such as capillary, vein, or brown spot removal).*

---

* Dr. Fillaferro, a medical doctor, removes brown spots and "spider" veins by injection. Facial veins are treated with an electric needle.

What I found so reassuring was Berty Buchacher's PERSONAL treatment. While I was there she had seventeen visitors, each of whom she gave a physical exam. The program and diet are geared to her diagnosis.

Patients reside in one of two guest houses on the farm. The main house is reserved for treatments only.

Dr. Lauda was an exponent of a mononutritional approach, sticking to just one or two things exclusively, such as a milk-and-day-old-rolls regimen, or a grapes-and-peaches regimen. One would not be given both milk-and-rolls and the fruit.

Dr. Lauda's notions of exercise have to do with ENTIRE BODY MOVEMENT, and her program usually results in an improved posture and carriage that often adds more than one inch to one's operating stature.

"Most people, in climbing stairs, move from the knee, but our exercise program involves swinging the entire body—arms, legs, the natural physiological movement."

There is also a serious attitude-improvement program, with its own instructor. The secret is a scheme whereby clients trade on each other's faults. (We're all experts in criticising others, but rarely perceive our own mistakes.)

The specialty is resurrecting lost or strayed personalities suffering from, say, the death of a spouse or a recent divorce.

"Such a woman is enclosed like an Eskimo in an igloo. Her eyes are small and narrow. Her face has fallen into a maze of lines. Her mouth is pinched. She is a tableau of withdrawal and anxiety. While we CAN'T enlarge her eyes, we CAN teach her to open up the muscles around the eyes to bear witness to the world's beauty. We CAN teach her to see beyond her personal problems to little things, like flowers."

After each patient's diagnosis, there's a special program, consisting of a daily body massage and facial. Every morning the treatments are given (using mostly German equipment), saving the afternoon for auto-suggestion training, makeup instruction, judo lessons, bridge lessons, and discussions on various beauty and health topics.

The farm hairdresser washes and sets clients' hair once a week. Comb-outs are given daily. There are also special hair-conditioning treatments employing electrical currents and vitamin packed oils. Vitamin E is used in almost all of the preparations. Manicures, pedicures, hair-bleaching and coloring are done for a small extra fee.

Berty Buchacher's secret lies in her insistence that every client leave the beauty farm with a fresh STYLE of comportment. Women usually sit so that their circulation is strangled—the abdomen protrudes, the breasts sag, the shoulders are rounded. They are taught (and reminded a hundred times a day if need be) to sit tall yet gracefully.

One of the most valuable gifts I received was instruction in instantaneously falling asleep. I refer to this in Dr. Lauda's auto-hypnosis method (see page 64).

Berty Buchacher endorses Dr. Lauda's approach to the old reliable positive thinking.

"We always say to our ladies, 'Look, you are our partners. You must be positive. You must learn not to think negative things.' That's the most important element in achieving the appearance of beauty."

Dr. Lauda herself was an example of her success. She was a most efficient-looking woman, with a fresh face and a firm body. One of her secrets, which she passed on to her clients, counteracts the pernicious effect of high heels on the legs and general posture. It's simplicity itself. (See page 58.)

Most of the Beauty Farm's clientele, ranging in age from eighteen to eighty, is Austrian. I found them most appreciative of the personal attention Berty Buchacher gave them, cherishing every nugget of advice and criticism they were getting from her.

Most of them were seeking smaller waistlines and relief from the cares that had been etched into their faces. The beauty farm was probably the one break in their routine, but one they strove to schedule at least twice a year, preferably during the high spring and autumnal seasons.

SUMMARY: Kurhaus Vienna-Beauty offers a cordial, sensible approach to better looks and sense of well-being. While the cosmetic improvement armamentarium (products and equipment) is quite up to date, clients also receive some old-fashioned instruction in basic relaxation and posture.—E.W.

Bad Gastein Austria

Snuggled in the bosom of the Austrian Alps, Bad Gastein is a picturebook village nourished by eighteen thermal springs that have been a favorite of visiting royalty since 1350. If you include the Salzburg festival on your next itinerary, you might set aside a few days for Bad Gastein. There's rarely a bother over accom-

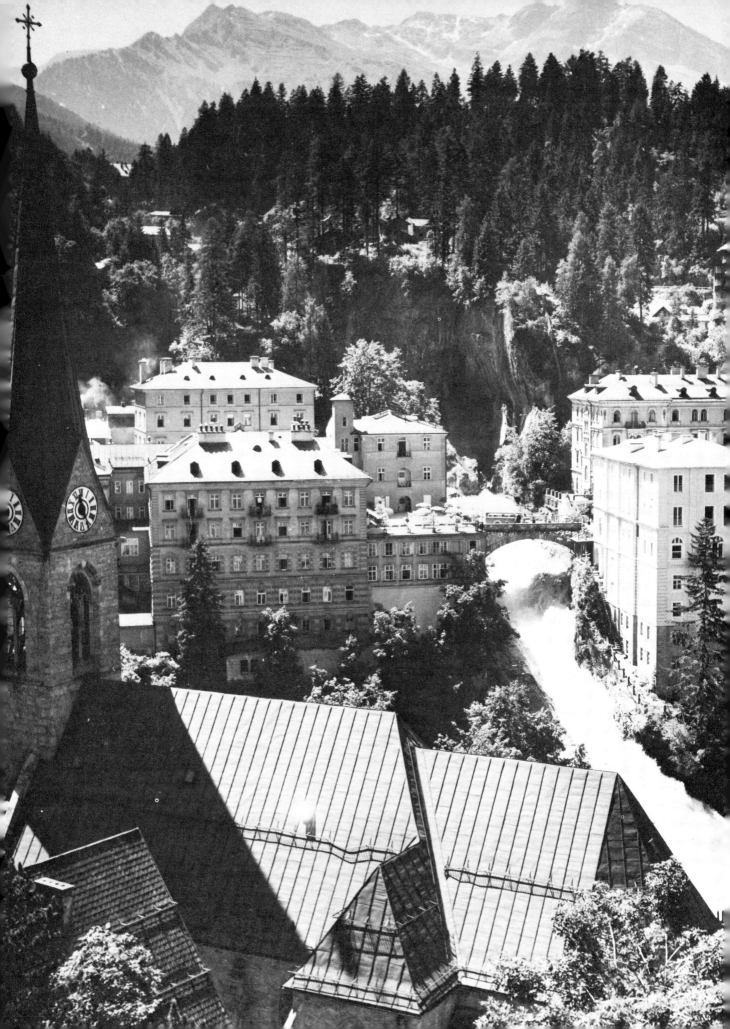

modations. The Kurhotels and other hotels (the KURHOTELS have thermal-water facilities) have a collective capacity of 7,000 visitors.

Bad Gastein is a little town with everything: casino, ski slopes, sleigh rides, iceskating, twenty-five miles of (dust free) promenades, every kind of swimming pool imaginable, tennis courts, miniature golf, a gondola-cable and railway, riding trails, fashion shows, theaters, cinemas, concert halls, and a plethora of beauty and health facilities. It is also fog-free.

The train ride from Vienna is like a trip through a child's Christmas mock-up railroad landscape of shepherd's chalets, unbelievably green grassy pastures, towering snow-capped mountains, sparkling little rivulets and cascades. And the olfactory experiences are heaven! That marvelous blend of pine resin, wildflowers, hearthfire smoke, leather, livestock, green grass, and melting snow! The air alone is an insomniac's cure.

I dropped off my luggage at the Salzburgerhof, a particularly inviting little chalet-style inn, and began to climb up a mini-mountain for my appointment with the renowned Marianne, whose beauty salon is at the top surrounded by pine trees.

Marianne is a cheery, rosy-cheeked woman whose intelligent face bespeaks tons of beauty and health lore. I couldn't wait to chat with her alone. She ushered me into a small, glass-enclosed room after handing me a crisp dressing gown and a cup of peppermint tea spiked with honey. I disrobed and lay down on the couch, while a contoured cushion cradled my lower torso. Then a fresh fluffy coverlet was placed over me.

I felt I wanted to fall asleep, but the sights outside kept me awake: guests bathing in a mountain pool, colorfully-garbed visitors climbing a mountain trail. After cleansing my face with a fragrant herbal milk, Marianne began to blend the special facial compound from oils, "earth" herbs, and plant and vegetable extracts. Hers is probably the world's finest five-dollar facial—and alone worth the trip to Austria!

Marianne gave me a wonderful take-home facial and some recipes for my readers. (To take advantage of her secret, see page 34.)

The bonus you get from a Marianne facial is that you can ask her anything at all about her diet and beauty secrets. Here is a really good-for-you luncheon soup recipe she gave me while toning my facial muscles:

Marianne's Good-For-You Soup
Simmer lean beef and bones in water, skimming off the

grease as it forms. Add any good soup herbs you have on hand. Fresh herbs give a more tingly taste, but dried will do. Then add onions, chives, parsley, and carrots.

This light, nourishing soup is Marianne's standard lunch. Sometimes, for variety, she strains it and has it as a consommé, followed by a meat dish (boiled or grilled) and a salad dressed with lemon juice and vitamin E oil.

Remember, Austrians consider their midday meal their main repast. In the evening, they have porridge or MÜSLI. There are 48,769 varieties of MÜSLI, by conservative estimate. Here's one of them.

Tyrolean Müsli
Soak oatmeal in hot water to cover for several hours, then mix in some honey and yogurt, fresh fruit, grated filberts or almonds.
      You'll love it—and it's filling.

Her favorite health dessert is a fresh fruit compote using a seasonal fruit, lightly steamed and sweetened with brown sugar. Here is one instance where she prefers brown sugar to honey because honey, when heated, may not agree with the tummy.

Marianne is an apostle of "seasonal dieting." She includes eggs in her diet for three months only, eliminating them altogether for the next nine months.

"When I'm eating eggs, I have three of them in the morning, and nothing else. These three eggs act like a chemical cleanser and purify my entire system."

When she's on her "egg quarter" (as she calls it) she occasionally eats them for lunch as an herb omelette. She suggests that omelettes are best when made with one tablespoon of water and nothing but fresh, sweet butter in the pan.

Marianne is my very favorite Bad Gastein phenomenon. As for the waters, I'm a bit diffident about them. I don't know if the claims are factual. I don't know if these radon-rich* thermal waters actually relieve gout, rheumatism, nervousness, stomach and intestinal, kidney and gallbladder disorders.

In 1940, when they tried to create a new mine at the site of the old Bad Gastein gold mine, they noticed very high temperatures in the recesses of the tunnel. It turned out that there were rich radon deposits—and workers suffering from rheumatism claimed to feel better as a result.

---

* Radon is a natural radioactive gas produced by the disintegration of radium. The story goes that radon's inertness and rapid departure from the body (four hours at the latest) make it quite safe to inhale.

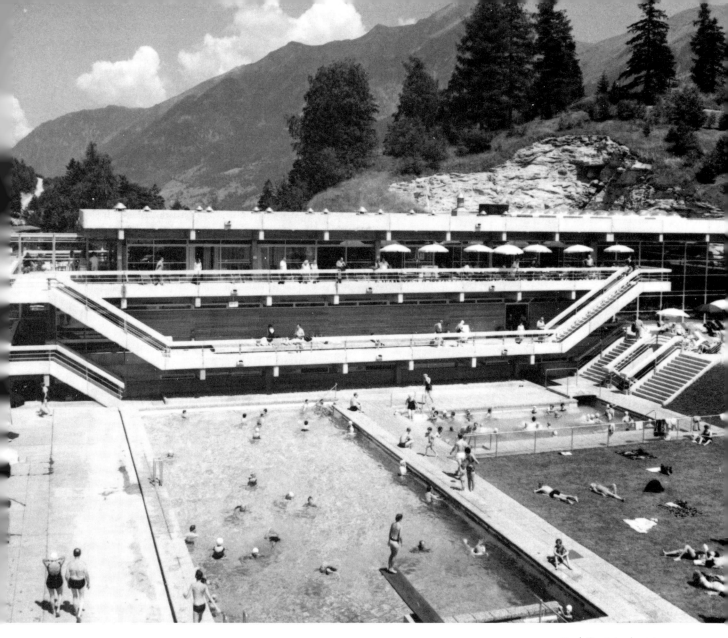

Bad Gastein Austria

Each of the STOLLEN (tunnels) is about a mile and a half long. The temperature inside is around 90 degrees Fahrenheit. The STOLLENKURHAUS—or Air Spa Building—is located just next to the thermal galleries. You are transported to your location via a small train in the company of special nurses.

None of the thermal baths may be taken without a medical prescription. Since these Heilstollen (healing galleries) were opened to the public in 1951, over sixty thousand patients have been treated in them.

The springs emerge from the ground at 110 degrees Fahrenheit and are directly available in 106 different Bad Gastein establishments, including the underwater therapy station, the thermal galleries mentioned before, natural vapor baths, and places where you can just rinse your mouth or drink the waters.

Cure lag hits you as soon as you leave your spa. It's a kind of lassitude and exhaustion that is very common with spa-niks, and the more sophisticated among them take ANOTHER week off for rest and relaxation from the treatments they've undergone.

Whether you're drinking or bathing in the waters, they have a way of draining you of energy. This puts you into another world. To return to the old pressures and stresses without a hiatus can be a mistake.

SUMMARY: If you are into radioactive waters as a way of fleeing radioactive hypercivilization, Bad Gastein can be the perfect place for you. Bed-and-board rates range from very stiff to ridiculously cheap. And there's the bonus of eye-boggling mountain- and valley-scapes that have to be among the Creator's most inspired layouts.—E.W.

Warmbad Villach Austria

Warmbad Villach's thermal springs are expressly intended for people whose resistance is low or who have simply "had it."

In Roman times, the springs were a sort of military spa. Soldiers found their wounds healing faster after washing them in waters from the three wells. While walking miles through clusters of chirping birds and leafy trees, I frequently noticed old chariot paths left by the Roman soldiers. Much later, Napoleon rehabilitated the spas for himself and his armies.

The town itself occupies a wide basin surrounded by regal mountains. It's easily reached, since it is located on the Munich–Trieste and Vienna–Venice–Rome rail- and roadways. Any time of year is fine, depending on your sports preferences. High summer season is from June 1 through the end of September.

I've been a spa lover long enough not to be too easily snowed by magical therapeutic claims. But I have to confess that I've never enjoyed a more refreshing and invigorating thermal water shower than the one I had in my hotel in Warmbad (the Warmbaderhof).

Warmbad Villach boasts the world's largest indoor thermal swimming pool: five feet deep, fifty feet wide, and eighty-two feet long.

The Warmbaderhof, the Karawankenhof and the Josefinenhof pay special attention to visitors with dietary restrictions, and the former invites guests to discuss their dietary problems with the assistant dietician. Generally, no animal fats are used. They favor olive, sunflower, and peanut oils.

Weight-loss luncheons at the Warmbaderhof exclude all fried dishes and carbohydrates and most fats. You might begin with orange juice, then go to plain veal (trimmed of all fat) with a side dish of green beans (from their garden) and asparagus salad with lemon juice. Dessert might be raspberries and yogurt.

The dinner menu I found more exciting. It began with a glass of fresh-squeezed carrot juice, poached flounder with vegetables, salad with lemon, and stewed peaches. A special fruit sugar is seved on weight-reduction diets.

Anyone who gets bored with the diet menu is always free to attack the buffet table, which has an interesting collection of salads and fruit.

One night I had a most sumptuous (non-diet) dinner. They served a very young chicken that had been breaded (à la Wiener Schnitzel), rolled in crumbs and eggs, and then popped into hot unsaturated oil. For dessert there were small pancakes, which looked exactly like French crepes, filled with white cheese, raisins, and cream.

The director of the Warmbad Villach showed me around. The thing I was most struck by was the mammoth indoor thermal pool that has so enthralled people they will neglect many nearby spas and travel hundreds of miles just to bathe here. After my first experience with the Warmbad thermal waters, I have to say that I appreciate their preference.

The Warmbad authorities are very specific about the contra-indications of their thermal and radioactive waters. If you have any of the following conditions, you will not be permitted to use the baths: acute rheumatism, heart and circulatory ailments where there is inadequate circulation, venereal or skin diseases, tuberculosis in an acute or sub-acute stage, or the flu.

SUMMARY: Warmbad Villach is a naturalist's delight. The spa's twelve acres of beautiful deciduous and spruce trees, natural meadows and flowerbeds and footpaths, make this an ideal place for contemplation and escape. It's a pleasant, five-o'clock-tea, concert-and-promenade gentility that's all too scarce in this busy world.—E.W.

While at Warmbad Villach, I took a side trip to visit the nearby Kneipp Institute, a mecca to worshippers of the famous naturalist and Bavarian priest, Sebastian Kneipp. Even the official American Medical Association debunkers have been relatively mild on Kneipp. Possibly because, as a priest, he did not himself gain financially from his water cure (although the parish church did rather handsomely). Kneipp espoused sparse diets, herbs and natural foods, and the use of water internally and externally to purify and strengthen the body.

Kneipp's system has outlasted hundreds of other hydrotherapy systems. It purports to stimulate the body's own defenses against disease and wear. The therapy includes (1) a water cure in which water of different temperatures is applied in various ways to stimulate the body; (2) phytotherapy, which employs plants or parts of plants to heal; (3) kinesotherapy (walking, sports, massage); (4) dietetics, which eliminates toxins (tea, coffee, tobacco) and high-caloric substances, and substitutes organic foods; and (5) a complicated "order-of-life" therapy to restore natural life rhythm and psychic harmony.

Monsignor Kneipp prescribed herbs such as chicory and thyme for his followers. Chicory, he suggested, "purified" the liver, kidneys, and spleen and was a particular balm for dyspeptics. Thyme in an infusion, he said, relieved stomach cramps and diarrhea.

At the Institute, I was shown a wonderful assortment of herbs used in the various baths—with eucalyptus predominating. The building was set way up in the hills. There is a dietary adjunct to this spa, which I shan't describe in any detail because it so closely resembles what I found at Bircher-Benner. I shall note only that the local Tyrolean wines are lovely, and I recommend in particular a Kalterer-Sec-Wein I enjoyed while I was there. You'll also find an abundance of herbal teas, and fresh fruit and vegetable juices.

The Bircher-Benner Clinic Switzerland

The mystique of the Bircher-Benner Clinic, near Zurich, does not come from radioactive douches, incredible cellular implants, puzzling herbal decoctions, or a magic shot where you sit down. It comes from a breakfast cereal.

With this cereal and a list of "do's and don'ts," this clinic has become one of the most prestigious of the Super Spas. Founded in 1897 by Dr. Max Bircher-Benner, its doctors and "sisters" treat victims of all kinds of systemic haywire: fat people, thin people, asthmatics, eczematics, allergics, hypertensives, cardiac types and headache types, arthritics and arteriosclerotics, the vitamin-deficient, as well as sick gallbladders, intestines, kidneys, and psyches.

Can a cereal REALLY be so all-fired terrific against all of these conditions? My opinion is that it possibly can be—when that magic bowl of cereal, called BIRCHER MÜSLI, becomes less a dietary supplement and more a substitute for your favorite booze, cigarettes, candy bars, coffee, and meat. What the old radio pitchmen might have called MÜSLI's "locked-in goodness" may be more what the Bircher-Benner regime eliminates rather than what it actually provides.

Whatever the goodness of Bircher-Benner is, this spa has never failed to please those hard-to-please friends of mine. Even the VERY hard-to-please Gaylord Hauser has gone back for seconds.

From either the 1,600-feet-above-sea-level treatment-and-research facility or the chalet-style residential villas, one can rejoice in the sight of glistening snow-clad Alpine peaks, the meadow-fringed Lake Zurich, and the city lights of Zurich piercing the brumal air. Surrounding the clinic are endless miles of woodlands, interrupted by tidy, weedless gardens. It is a walker's paradise.

A few go for the five-day physical checkup alone, while others settle in for a brief rest cure. The curists stay an average of three weeks.

If that MÜSLI is an essential part of the Bircher-Benner therapy, it is not the whole story. All treatments are carefully prescribed according to your individual physical and mental condition and personal proclivities.

The clinic is not cheap. (Reserve six months in advance, if you can.) Rooms with private bath run $135 per day; rooms without bath from $90 to $120. Deposits are required. The daily rate entitles you to full board, including any prescribed diet, service charges, and group gymnastics. Also included are baths, showers, ablutions, packs, compresses, and short-wave therapy.

NOT included are such items as underwater massage (ten dollars), massages (from six to eight dollars), carbonic acid baths (three-twenty-five), bath mixes such as fango (two dollars), aerosol inhalations (two dollars). (Only natural herbal extracts are used in the bath mixtures.) A psychotherapist's services run from thirty to fifty dollars per session. And if you want your medical report translated into English, that will cost an extra ten dollars.

The entire regimen is based on the postulate that diet (HEAVY on the raw fruit and vegetables which contain their own digestive enzymes) can help the body to heal itself of almost ANYTHING. And if you're overheard discussing your pills and injections, you'll win only scowls and frowns there. Their feeling is that the medical establishment's touting of injectable chemical treatments is shortsighted and destructive. Most of the seventy patients I saw were middle-aged, upper middle-class, and female. They appeared mainly to be seeking an escape from stress.

The dietetic dining room—the gravity center for the clinic—is not especially imposing. The service is traditional Swiss efficient, which is not bad at all: spotless linens, impeccable tableware, totally organized routine.

Now, as to the ECHT (the one, the true, the original) Bircher MÜSLI, I have the recipe for you! (See for yourself if there isn't a world of difference between it and the packaged stuff!)

The Original Bircher Müsli

For each serving, soak 3 tablespoons of oatmeal overnight in cold water and cover. In the morning, add a tablespoon of fresh lemon juice, a tablespoon of light cream, a grated (unpeeled) apple or two. Then sprinkle a tablespoon of grated nuts (almonds, hazelnuts, walnuts, or pecans are best, and fifteen seconds in a blender will fix the nuts as they should be). Add some honey, according to the sweetness of your tooth, and top with sliced seasonal fruits and berries. (And try using yogurt instead of milk or cream.)

This outrageously healthy looking and healthy tasting breakfast has become an addiction with health faddists around the world and is known in some parts as the "Swiss Breakfast."

In fact it is a centuries-old peasant meal that had almost become extinct with the Industrial Revolution and rustics' ill-advised mimicking of urban diets. The peasant's Müsli, however, demanded sharks' teeth to chew, since whole grains were used. Then the clinic's founder, Dr. Max Bircher-Benner, substituted oatmeal for the whole grains and proclaimed his version a total meal containing just the proper amounts of "all the nutrients."

Not everyone believed him. At the turn of the century, when he founded his clinic, most medical sophisticates believed that fruit knotted your alimentary canal in grannies and half-hitches. Bircher-Benner railed against this as nonsense, proclaiming fruit the absolutely INDISPENSABLE element in the Müsli. Today, still, Bircher-Benner doctors hold that Müsli as a weight-loss agent, is incomparably superior to any ephemeral "crash diet"—which they say is both ineffectual (in the long run) and destructive.

Max Bircher-Benner became fascinated with nutrition-qua-cure when a female patient with a gastric disorder lost her capacity to digest food. A colleague reminded him that Pythagoras healed digestive malfunction with a mixture of crushed raw fruit, mixed nuts, honey, and goat's milk. When he tried the recipe on his patient, she not only digested it but thrived on it—and became well again!

The answer, he decided, was RAW FOOD! It alone contained the maximum quality of "food energy" because it was so near the living state. In 1911, he inaugurated his "Life-Force Sanitarium."

The notion of paying a visit to Bircher-Benner had enthralled me for years. It seemed a good way of getting the best, freshest food, prepared with painstaking, scientific care. I confess being turned on by the fantasy of hobnobbing with such Bircher-Benner loyalists as Emilio Pucci, Gaylord Hauser, and Yehudi Menuhin.

When I arrived, I made straightaway for the kitchen. There I found a woman preparing the Müsli, tasting the preparation with a large wooden spoon at each stage. I was relieved that, after licking each spoon, she threw it into a nearby sink rather than back into the mixture.

Sinewy laborers were carting into the kitchen huge cartons of apples, which were squeezed for juice or grated for the Müsli. It struck me, as I watched this hive of activity, that Bircher-Benner was a perfect detoxification station. The ambiance seemed to generate the kind of cheery optimism that any good doctor knows can speed up the healing process.

In 1973, the Bircher-Benner Clinic went public, so to speak. Until then, it had been run by founder Max Bircher-Benner and, upon his demise, by his daughter Ruth Kunz-Bircher and her husband, Dr. Alfred Kunz-Bircher, who headed the chemical research and diagnostic department. Now the entire enterprise belongs to the canton of Zurich which administers it. Veteran visitors take comfort in the fact that the philosophy, treatments, and personnel remain unchanged under the medical director, Dr. Dagmar Liechti-Von Brasch, a niece of the late Dr. Bircher-Benner.

My typical day there began with an early morning stroll in the garden, followed by a Müsli breakfast.

Then I would take a sunbath, proceed to the gym for exercise, and take one of the many baths available (carbonic acid, aescusal, stanger, Scotch shower, fango, light, shuffle, thigh, knee, or a special one-hour shower). After the bath, a massage.

Lunch consists of three vegetables, a salad, and some fruit.

Bircher-Benner recommends a post-prandial rest, followed by free time, which you can spend swimming, skating, golfing, horseback riding, or playing tennis. Zurich, by the way, is one of the best places in Europe to shop; it is a fine cultural center and a university town.

Dinner is still more—but this time DIFFERENT—Müsli. They will use, for example, yogurt instead of cream, a different fruit, different nuts.

Bedtime comes faster at Bircher-Benner than at any other Super Spa. Chalk this up to Max Bircher-Benner's stiff-necked Calvinism. If you have a yen to paint the town and return after 8:30, you'll have

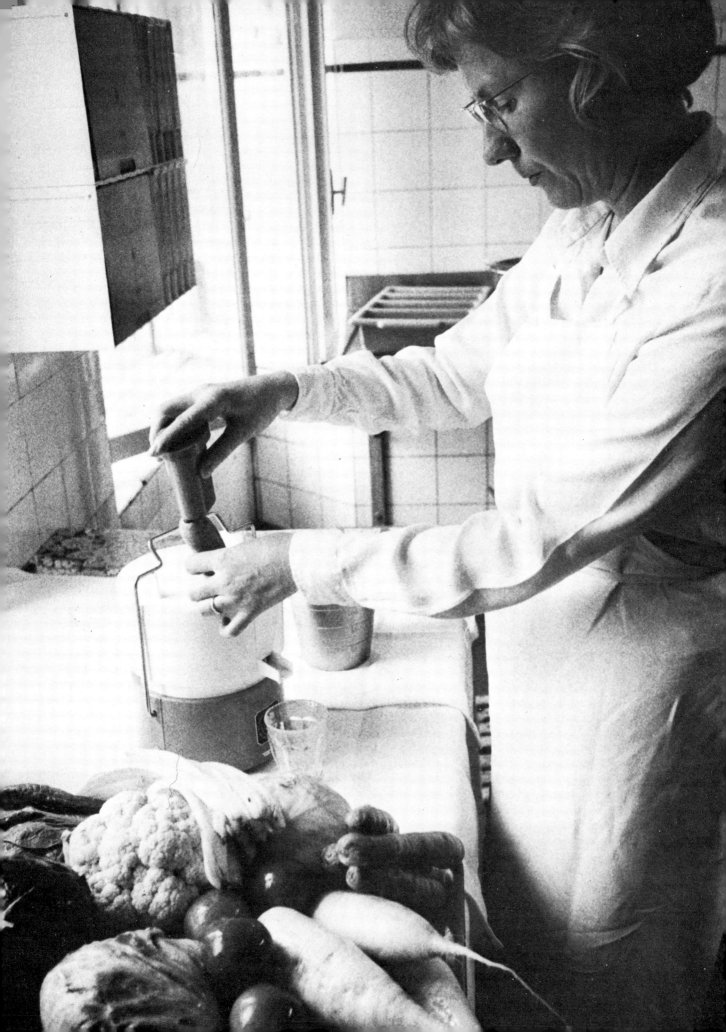

to get permission and a key to the front door. And you're allowed out evenings EXACTLY TWICE A WEEK. The entire program is a bit spartan—and don't go unless you're prepared to do without meat, fish, fowl, coffee, sweets, alcohol.

Let me just sum up the Bircher-Benner philosophy regarding slimming. While they tolerate the special situation of a fighter wanting to shave off twenty pounds for a championship encounter, or a panic-stricken actor trying to de-pouch himself for a younger role, they argue that repeated drastic weight-loss programs upset one's metabolic balance.

Here in a nutshell is their approach to weight reduction:

Bircher-Benner Hints on Weight Loss

Lower the amount of cooked food you consume and increase the amount of raw food (with which you should BEGIN your meal).

Be brutal in eliminating all fats, especially saturated fats, from your diet.

Natural fruit sugar should be your only source of carbohydrates, if possible.

Beware of high-protein diets, which can injure the liver, inflame the intestine, and provoke rheumatic disorders.

Restrict your intake of cooking salt, hot spices, stimulants such as coffee and nicotine.

No snacking.

Their slimming diet begins with one or two days in which you have nothing but juices*; two or three days of juice and protein (no fats); and two or three fat-free raw-food days. Then the patient goes on the classic slimming diet, which should be interrupted with one day of juices only or one day of juices-with-protein.

For Dr. Bircher-Benner's seven-day diet program, read his book, EATING YOUR WAY TO HEALTH (Penguin Books, 1972).

Medical director Dr. Dagmar Liechti-Von Brasch told me that her uncle, Dr. Bircher-Benner, discovered that a food's energy, or potentiality, was far more important than its calories, fat, protein, or carbohydrate considerations. This energy ferments enzymes and vitamins—and makes ALL the difference in its health-giving capacity.

Natural methods, she said, work better than

---

* STRICT JUICE DAYS, as they are called, are not to be performed at Bircher-Benner without bed rest and a weight check. The initial high weight loss is mostly dehydration. The later losses tend to be more regular and permanent.

medicines in most cases. For instance, in the winter, she has her patients run barefoot in the snow. (In the summer, they have to settle for a romp in the dew of the fields.) When they come back inside, they rub their feet until they're just as hot as they were cold. Their feet then feel prickly and comfortable. This technique brings blood down from the head, relaxes people, and allows a deep, peaceful sleep.

Dr. Liechti-Von Brasch went into the health spa business with more than genes inspiring her. At twenty-four the left side of her face became paralyzed following a bout with viral influenza. The paralysis destroyed her sense of taste entirely and the olfactory response in the left side of her nose.

She was a medical student, so she took her problem to her professor, an ear-nose-and-throat specialist. He told her that her chances of full recovery were nil, and that the best she could hope for was some minor improvement. His advice: "Don't catch cold again."

As a last resort, she consulted her uncle, who examined her thoroughly. His prognosis was more hopeful. She COULD recover, but ONLY if she followed his unorthodox prescription with an iron discipline.

She spent the next two weeks in bed, on a totally raw diet, perspiring for one hour daily, followed by a total body wrapping, having galvanic massage of the diseased nerves, and seeing no one.

By the fourth day, her numb facial muscles began to play again. The tongue began to perceive aromatic herbs. She could shut her left eye for the first time with ease. By the seventh day, she was totally cured!

She tells a story of another of her uncle's patients, a haggard, red-faced gourmand suffering from near total ptosis—a protruding abdomen with all the organs (stomach, liver, spleen, bowels) pouched low over his thighs. His muscles and tendons were dangerously stretched.

This patient not only went on the raw diet (which restored his digestive power), but heeded Bircher-Benner's advice to take long walks. In fact, he became a vagabond, tramping through Switzerland, Italy, Austria, Germany, and Sweden—working as a farmer's handyman for his meals and shelter, sleeping in haystacks, and eating the simplest foods. Two years later, he returned to Bircher-Benner, who did not recognize his former patient. His gait was erect, his body tanned and taut, his muscles lean and rippling; he was the picture of health.

The Bircher-Benner exercise director, Edith Risch, allowed me to work out in the gym with her. (She, incidentally, has a most youthful and relaxed-looking face for her age. For her technique for facial relaxation, see page 63.)

As a special treat, I'm going to give you a few of the best Bircher-Benner recipes.

Apple Müsli with Yogurt

Per person:

4 Tbs. yogurt	1 Tbs. honey or 1½ Tbs. brown sugar
1 tsp. lemon juice	
1 Tbs. rolled oats (or 1 Tbs. medium oatmeal) soaked for 12 hours in 3 Tbs. water	1 large apple (or 2–3 small ones)
	1 Tbs. grated filberts or almonds

Mix the yogurt to a smooth consistency with lemon juice. Add to the oats, stirring well, and mix in the honey or sugar.

    Grate and add unpeeled apple.

    Sprinkle nuts over the finished dish and serve immediately.

Vegetable Stock

1 Tbs. sunflower or soybean oil	Spinach or beet leaves
1 onion	4 or 5 qt. cold water
2 carrots or other roots	Lovage, basil or other fresh or dried herbs
1 cup shredded or diced celery or celeriac	½ bay leaf and salt (only for a normal diet)
Cabbage	

Vegetables according to season—for instance, celery, carrots, and other roots, some cabbage or kohlrabi, leeks, tomatoes, celeriac, and onions. The tougher but still sound parts may also be used, as well as scrubbed potato peel.

Heat oil. Halve onion, with skin, and brown cut surface in fat. Cut vegetables in small pieces. Add to the onion and stew gently for at least ¼ hour, covered with a lid.

    Add cold water, simmer for 2 hours. Season according to taste.

Clear Vegetable Broth

2½ qt. vegetable stock	1 level Tbs. butter
Marmite or other yeast extract to taste	Chives or parsley
	Salt

Pour hot vegetable stock over all other ingredients.

Orange Whip

3¾ cup milk	3 eggs
1–2 oranges	3½–5½ tsp. raw sugar
1 Tbs. cornstarch	½–1 cup cream
4½ Tbs. milk	

Peel oranges very thinly, and squeeze juice. Bring peel to the boil in the milk. Mix cornstarch with cold milk. Add to boiling peel and milk, and bring again to a boil.

    Whisk eggs and sugar, add a little of the boiling mixture, stir well. Pour back into the saucepan, stirring constantly, and bring again to near boiling point. Cool, then strain. Add a few spoonfuls orange juice and mix with whipped cream.

SUMMARY: A super experience for the Three R's—Rest, Relaxation, and Recuperation. If you've been yearning to try MÜSLI, the real thing, you'll find it here, plus unique helpful healthful therapies.—E.W.

Montecatini Terme Italy

If a consumers' group ever did a number on Montecatini, it would bulldoze this ninety-eight foot MONTE into a molehill. Its investigators would discover shocking instances of extortionate tipping and jubilant price-gouging and flimflams. Unless you'd actually BEEN to Montecatini or spent some time in Italy, you'd probably reckon it no more than just another tourist trap.

    But you'd be reckoning wrong. I mean, it IS a trap—Montecatini is Outstretched Palm country; all the goodies cost extra; and the posted rates are robust enough to make you think twice—and yet there's something so COMPELLING about Montecatini that people who know their spas go there year after year,

often several times a year. I'm talking about the names that have filled the golden guest books since 1905, such as the Princess Pahlevi, Rainier and Grace, the Queen of Morocco, Rose Kennedy, Anita Loos, Giorgio de Chirico, former Prime Minister Amintore Fanfani, and such past and present cinema greats as Katharine Hepburn and Spencer Tracy, Bill Holden, Vittorio Gassman, Vittorio De Sica, Rossano Brazzi, Walter Chiari, Marcello Mastroianni, Silvana Mangano, and Catherine Spaak.

    For me personally, Montecatini is truly the Queen of Spas. It is the one spa in the whole world I would take off for at the drop of a hat.

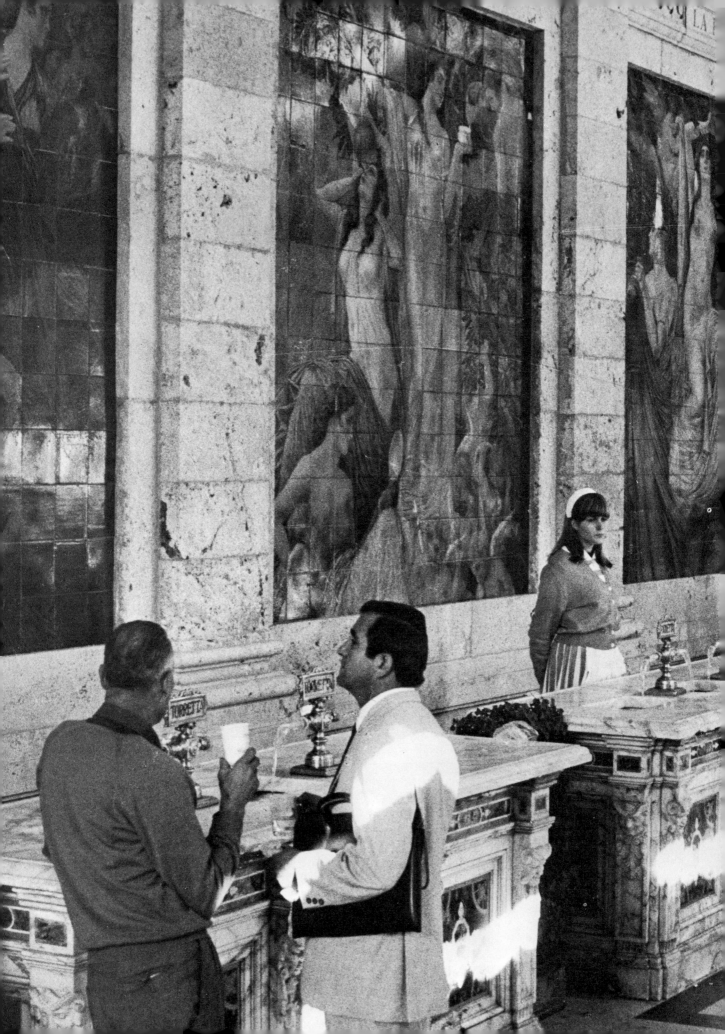

Hands down, Montecatini offers the easiest cure in the whole world—a 180-degree turnabout from the asceticism and masochism of the barbarian spas north of the Apennines. It has all the extras: racetrack, pigeon shoots, nightclubs, bars, tennis courts, pools galore, lean and dashing physicians—all in a frame of exquisite classical Roman architecture and three hundred square miles of intricately sculpted greenery and flowers.

Of the ten thousand people daily who take its waters, those who count may be classified either as BEAUTIFUL PEOPLE (Americans or Anglicized Europeans there for beauty treatments mainly) or LIVER PEOPLE (Continental cognoscenti who know to the fraction of a finger how far their self-indulgence has bulged IL FEGATO beyond their rib cages).

There are said to be some two hundred hostelries, ranging from palaces to modest PENSIONI. There is, however, only ONE place to stay—the Grand Hotel La Pace, known simply as "La Patch-eh." And while you can imbibe and bathe almost any old time, the people who KNOW save September for Montecatini. By then, ordinary tourists are back home hunched over their desks or selling their pots and pans or whatever.

The heart of the Montecatini cure is the hot natural springs, salty, sulfured, and immensely soothing. And you're not REALLY in business until you're found sipping them with a medicine glass calibrated in cubic centimeters.* But take them only as your DOTTORE tells you to. In all likelihood, he will prescribe a daily ritual for taking one or more or all of the purgative waters, ranging from the antitoxic, mild, tranquilizing TETTUCCIO, to the innards-stimulating TORRETTA, and the Roto-Rooteresque TAMERICI, which is principally for cast-iron colons toughened by at least several dozen cures. The REGINA waters are said to be great for animating your digestive enzymes.

My liver was just fine, but for research purposes I signed on for the full cure. It went like this:

My doctor, a gallant Florentine in his fifties named Pier Pieri took my medical history and blood pressure and palpated my abdomen. Without explanation, he compressed his brow into an authoritative frown and began to scribble into a notebook.

He prescribed a full course of three different waters and a program of mudbaths (with the stiff and aching areas to be massaged marked off on an anatomical diagram for the technicians).

My physician had ordained a severe regimen.

* If you're ever caught drinking the water with a porcelain mug inscribed RICORDO DI MONTECATINI you're liable to be whisked back to Grossinger's. In any event, that alone will quarantine you from anybody who IS anybody.

Boiled, non-oily fish, grilled meat—modest portions—with only the dull vegetables, boiled and mashed. No desserts, alcohol, or cold drinks. Nothing fried or cooked in butter. No eggs. None of those delicious Italian soft cheeses.

One of the "advices" inscribed by Dr. Pieri was "go to bed early." It was easy in that loveliest of bedrooms. The curiously large bed had a mattress of tufted cotton batting within silky linens and plump pillows. The pale green room was filled with Italian antiques and oriental carpeting. Bowls of fresh gardenias perfumed the air.

The bathrooms were lined with floor-to-ceiling, wall-to-wall Carrara marble and contained a matching, giant-sized tub. Unfortunately, a pedestrian plastic shower curtain detracted from the glamor.

Although rising time is 7:00 A.M., you can delay actually getting out of bed by having a waiter bring up your water in bottles to drink while walking about your room.

But the fun of the Cure is going to the springs. Even Princess Grace made the trek. Thermal establishments come first and second class, the difference being the trappings, not the water.

Each morning before breakfast, I attended one of the water stations, the most popular being the Tettuccio in a large neo-Greek temple adorned with piazzas, statuary, gardens, and fountains. The warm, mineral-heavy, sulfur-scented water reached my glass thanks to an elaborate pumping system culminating in a sort of sulfuric soda fountain.

I set out for Tettuccio. A season's ticket costs sixty-five dollars; a twelve-day "season" ticket, thirty-two dollars; the one-way ducat, two dollars. At any moment you may find yourself mingling with up to two thousand water-takers.

Women behind a mosaic marble counter drew my recommended dose into the glass. (The water can be sipped or gulped.) Then I strolled around the pavilion, waiting for signals that the water had begun to work.

My patience was never tried. Within minutes usually, nature urged me to run for one of the 1,600 gleaming-white GABBINETTI (cabinets) where I surrendered water and, presumably, soluble toxins accumulated during a previous spell of high-on-the-hog living.

It was cheering to think that somewhere down the line a princess or peer or playperson was squatting in a similar performance of this universal ritual which abolishes all rank and other distinctions.

Glancing at my notebook filled out by the doctor, I saw that my first prescription was for Torretta water at warm temperature. I put my glass up to the spigot, and—ECCO!—was into my cure. I carried the precious liquid to a little round table and drank it, as ordered, in exactly three minutes.

I refilled my glass and drank the second Torretta within the prescribed three minutes, and waited another ten minutes. The best way to wait is to walk. It seems to accelerate the water's activity.

Time flies as you stroll through the spectacular Tettuccio gardens filled with flowers, trees, hills, dales, steps, bushes. There are also open-air arcades filled with foreign newspaper kiosks, elegant shops, art galleries. Best of all is the music.

This pre-prandial purge leaves you very hungry. And nothing tastes as good as that strong, black, over-roasted Italian coffee with fresh-baked, flaky croissants served at a little table under those rich, blue Italian skies.

For many, that morning water is nothing more than a conscience-killer. They spend the rest of the day in gluttonous sampling and whatever other intemperance they can involve themselves with. I used to glance enviously over at them, breaking their fast with cappucino topped with billowing whipped cream and mountains of airy hot bread and slathers of mouth-watering CONFITURA.

My favorite blue denim pants suit, which I wore to the Tettuccio, was a mistake. It was so similar to the chic uniform worn by the girls dispensing water that I found myself hounded by men crying "SIGNORINA!" and snapping their fingers and waving empty glasses at me.

Occasionally, I wanted a REAL breakfast. And then I'd hasten back to La Pace where PICCOLE COLAZIONE would be served either in the garden or on my private terrace. I usually began with a delicious bouillon, which was the hotel's prized potassium broth made from an onion soup base.

The breakfast table is enticingly set with baskets of croissants, brioches, sweet rolls, lovely pots of strawberry and apricot jam, and preserved whole apricots from New Zealand, and the SPECIALITÉ DE LA MAISON: fresh ricotta cheese. Made from sheep's milk, this superb Italian cottage cheese is replenished twice daily at La Pace.

Breakfasting in the hotel garden gives you an opportunity to people-watch. La Pace, originally built in 1870, has had ten decades of celebrities mixing with the hoi polloi.

At 9:30 or 10:00, neck-craning comes to a halt. It's time to head for the Baths. The concierge at La Pace will make a reservation for you, because most of the bath attendants speak very little, if any, English. Just twenty words of Italian can be crucial. Practice saying: good morning (BUON GIORNO), please (PER PIACERE), thank you (GRAZIE), you're welcome (PREGO), too hot

(TROPPO CALDO), too cold (TROPPO FREDDO), stop (BASTA!!!), enough (BASTA COSÌ), too much (TROPPO), more (PIÙ), and, most important, how much (QUANTO?). If you can't master this little list, just remember lire talk! Frantically wave one of those super one-thousand-lire notes and the attendant will suddenly realize that the water's too hot, too cold, too much, or too too!

Continuing my recommended therapy, I was queued for a mudbath. Others were taking special treatments—thermal baths, hydro massages, skin treatments, inhalation therapy, mouth sprays, and electrotherapy.

Costs per session vary from two dollars for "humid inhalation" (on a hot day, simply stand in the street and breathe deeply instead) to seven dollars for an underwater manual massage. A mudpack comes in, during season, for roughly five-fifty (not counting tips).

At the baths, the sexes separate, and each guest enters a private room. Although the overall areas are spacious and luxurious, the treatment rooms themselves reminded me of prison cells with their spartan tub, sink, chair, and couch. I undressed and optimistically wrapped a muslin turban around my head to protect my hairdo. In vain! After my first mudpack session I learned that the only way to avoid a fright-wig appearance is to don a coverall hat with attached bandanna. This chapeau became my closest companion during the Cure. As I lay naked on the couch, modestly clutching an oversized towel, Julio, my "mud man," came in. He always looked so sad I used to tip him just to see him smile.

The custom was to take all your treatments and tip at the end of the series. But I found it friendlier and more rewarding to reverse the process. My bath attendant, Piera, not only slathered mud on the areas indicated in my guidebook, but literally covered me from neck to toe with mud. The amount of mud was directly related to the amount of tip: one thousand lire, I found, went much farther than the routine five hundred, and the more mud, the merrier the bath!

The stimulating mud stays on for ten or fifteen minutes, and then the attendant literally shoves the mud off. Next step was a bath in radioactive iridescent 88-degree water where I rested for five minutes.

Finally, I was hosed with a huge spray and daubed with a plump sponge to remove every last speck of mud. Piera quickly dried me with a gigantic towel, bundled me into a soft, unbleached muslin, one-size-fits-all pajama, and tucked me into bed. I dropped off quickly into a deep dream-filled erogenous sleep.

In these somnolent fantasies, one often sheds pajamas, sheets, and kerchief. It's very hot. The mud man often returns to reclaim his pail, shortly after you've kicked off your pajama bottom. (I found that Julio could smile even without a tip.)

I went to another floor for a facial mudpack. Here even less English is spoken, and I found myself in the hands of a capable, terse operator who gave a quick "tsk-tsk" look at my skin and promptly started treatment. Special creams were smoothed on first, then mud. After a brief rest, another dousing. Frankly I found this procedure excellent for oily skins, but a bit dessicating for dry skins.

And then, just before lunch, a massage in my room. For a few extra lire (the basic treatment costs eleven dollars), the masseuse used special camphorated cream. After a half-hour workout, my stomach was growling for food.

Whenever I left my room, the maids—directed by an efficient, Swedish housekeeper—came in to plump pillows, bring freshly picked gardenias, replenish towels, and mop the bathroom once more. The service is better than that of most other deluxe hotels, and the cost is only about fifty dollars per day per person, including meals.

The always-in-waiting waiter and the assorted RAGAZZI working as elevator boys and busboys are remarkably attentive. La Pace is such a marvelous training ground for service-with-a-smile, that Gene, of New York's gone-but-not forgotten Colony Restaurant, sent his two sons to apprentice in the kitchen there.

The luncheon meal is served by the pool and in the spacious dining rooms. The major activities are divided into resisting temptation and giving in to it. Although every busboy, waiter, captain, and certainly the maîtres d'hôtel are well aware of the Cure diet, they unremittingly suggest fantastic pasta and spiced sauces and hold devilishly attractive trays of pastries under your nose. If you really want the Cure to work, you should give total consideration to your liver. (See chart on page 135.)

My choice for lunch was usually a taste of boiled fish, followed by delicious bouillon. I skipped the pasta but enjoyed a roast chicken flavored with rosemary, or a special mixed dish of boiled meat and chicken—an Italian POT-AU-FEU. The fresh fruit and vegetables on the approved list are positively "alive" and delicious, all organically grown and newly gathered from the hills surrounding Montecatini.

The veal, chicken, and fish are prepared simply but stylishly. Sylvia Lyons, wife of columnist Leonard Lyons and a frequent visitor to Montecatini, really makes the Cure work for her by "turning off" all impulses for rich concoctions and turning her attention completely to the "right" food. For her, the no-no's

simply do not exist!

My suggestion for getting the CRAVING for sumptuous fare out of your system is to try it ALL the first day, THEN steel yourself for the Cure diet.

From July to September, particularly, an afterlunch nap is in order. Montecatini is hot then, and a siesta is a welcome refresher.

Incidentally, Montecatini thrives even when the tourists are gone. Upper-class Italians take the Cure when the seasons change—in April—May and September—October. Thoroughbred racehorses from all over Italy visit the spa in the winter to be dunked in gigantic tubs, swathed in mud, and given a cure much like the one I had. The Cure is considered a major element in some gamblers' handicapping.

On the late afternoon agenda of a typically busy Cure day is a visit to a hairdresser or barber. Tenderly manipulated blowers and brushes is a must after the mudbaths, massage, and other hairdo-wrecking activities. Happily, this luxury doesn't break the bank. If you're impatient, once again a generous tip will get you into the chair and past those who stand on a no-tip principle.

Newly coiffed, I used to get together with other guests for cocktails in the lower lounge and courtyard garden. Cool, informal dresses were the rule. Heavy drinking is NOT in at La Pace (or anywhere else in Montecatini). The most popular drinks were Vermouth Cassis and dry vermouth. Negrinos and Americanos are considered strong. Many sipped rosy orange juice and freshly squeezed carrot juice as APÉRITIFS. In fact, after dinner, some people sat around the hotel courtyard for hours sharing one large bottle of Pelligrino water with lemon wedges they squeezed into each new glass.

Dinner was served simultaneously in two dining rooms. Tables near the door were coveted since the rooms are not air-conditioned. The central show table was laden with outrageous pastries and desserts—twice as provocative and dangerous as the luncheon tempters.

I noticed that guests discussed their menus seriously. However, most of them ordered serving after serving since there was no limit on portions, and the chocolate mousse always seemed to find an inordinate number of samplers. Almost everyone began with the delicious, but forbidden prosciutto and melon or figs.

Montecatini is NOT a swingers' paradise. For the most part, night life consists of talk, shopping, walking, and café-sitting. Romances do blossom there, however.

Gambrino's is the favorite open-air nightclub of La Pace guests, since it's right across the street. Hun-

	Si!	Food	No!
Boiled fresh fish	**Appetizer**		Fat or salty foods
Vegetable or bouillon	**Soup**		Every other kind of soup
O.K. with butter and parsley	**Pasta**		Tomato, mushroom, cream sauces
White meat (veal or chicken)	**Meat**		All other, especially no fried meats or gravies
Fresh boiled trout	**Fish**		No shellfish, nothing fried
Tomatoes, lettuce with olive oil and lemon juice	**Salads**		Heavy dressings, mushrooms, spinach, cabbage, peppers
Ripe fresh or stewed fruit except for . . .	**Fruit**		. . . all melons, strawberries, figs, dried fruit
Fresh cheese only, such as ricotta, mozzarella, Bel Paese	**Cheese**		Nothing aged, dry, or salted
Biscuits or plain cake with milk and fruit	**Dessert**		No chocolate, spirits, cream, or ice cream
Slightly-charged mineral waters, light wine, light coffee, and tea	**Beverages**		No hard liquor of any kind, nothing ice cold

dreds of people cluster around little tables (and hundreds more stand on the sidewalks) to hear the small orchestra play pop tunes. The price of admission is puchase of a beverage—frozen coffee topped with whipped cream (GRANITA) being the favorite.

It's possible to find bargains among the overpriced items on Montecatini's so-called "Fifth Avenue." You might consider the linens, no-iron tablecloths, napkins, makeup capes, and monogrammed handkerchiefs. The perfumeries that sell cosmetics and toiletries charge mercilessly. A word to the wise: BRING YOUR OWN BEAUTY AIDS.

Men flock to tailors who turn out nifty-looking slacks at fantastically low prices. Some Beau Brummels wait all year to stock up on a dozen pair at a time. And knowledgeable Sylvia Lyons recommends the services of a talented dressmaker who will copy almost anything for about thirty dollars plus fabric. (Your hotel concierge can supply addresses.)

If troublesome feet are taking their toll on your beauty, you'll definitely find relief here. Italians specialize in foot care. Great pedicures are available at Tonfoni and they include a podiatric "clean-up" and a total leg waxing. They cost less than half what they do in the United States.

Beauty services can fill your time on your days off. Usually it's three days on the Cure and one day of rest for at least twelve days. It's tempting, however, to spend your free day driving the twenty-nine miles to Florence to splurge on shopping. Picturesque Pisa is thirty miles away and Livorno, Viareggio, and other spots on the Thyrrenian Sea are less than fifty miles from Montecatini.

The Cure at Montecatini is not the easiest to take. It can be tough going for some. I found my own pleasure and the sight of well-fed, well-rested, well-treated people strolling through the parks and gardens persuasive testimony of a most rewarding spa. As Anita Loos once wrote: "In Montecatini one finds everything which is most agreeable in life—health, beauty, hospitality, and charm."

Don't miss taking treatments at the spa in the Hotel La Pace. You will find spa treatments galore from head to toe—special health and beauty rituals not withstanding.

Daily rates at La Pace: single $68–$89; double $120–$147. All rates include continental breakfast.

SUMMARY: Montecatini is an appetizing broth and froth of an Italian-style water cure. But it tends toward a kind of vital intensity you may have trouble keeping up with. For sinfully opulent furnishings, food, and flunkies, Montecatini is unbeatable—a WHO'S WHO'S favorite for liver and lover resuscitation.—E.W.

Grayshott Hall England

To Grayshott Hall's forty-seven acres of Hampshire greenery, add the adjacent seven hundred acres of unspoiled countryside preserved by the National Trust. It is just forty-three miles from London and a favorite retreat for Ava Gardner, the Duke and Duchess of Bedford, and assorted Members of Parliament and diplomats.

It occupies a painstakingly reconstructed Victorian home, with some fifty new rooms added since Alfred Lord Tennyson lived there a century ago.

Although unmitigatedly "British," Grayshott is anything but stuffy. Visitors can be found strolling the gardens and halls, in their bathrobes, pink chenille nighties, and scuffy slippers.

Available treatments include high colonics, sauna, osteopathy, massages, electrotherapy, neuromuscular massages, and—above all—diet. They claim a visitor can drop a stone (fourteen pounds) in one week at Grayshott. Meat is served, but the weight-reduction regimen is fundamentally vegetarian.

The dining room table is loaded with goodies that include: a marvelous whole-milk yogurt; bowls and bowls of wheat germ; salad dressings; organically grown fruits and vegetables; honey pots; and Salads à Gogo, with nothing but the crispest, freshest fruits and vegetables. Vegetables are chopped or grated finely, as are the nuts. Fruit is sliced into small pieces. The cheeses are a mild white variety or cottage cheese. Ingredients are allowed to stand for thirty minutes together to permit blending of flavors. Salads are bound with a small amount of mayonnaise made from an egg yolk, an unsaturated oil, and fresh lemon juice.

Here is a list of the various Grayshott salad combinations:

cauliflower—cheese
celery—apple
carrot—coconut
apple—leek
pineapple—sultanas
tomato—pimiento
melon—red pepper—tomato
cottage cheese—prunes
millet (cooked or soaked overnight)—cabbage—carraway seeds—onion

aubergine (eggplant)—cucumber—onion—tomato
pineapple—watercress
egg—onion
cabbage—cheese—apples—nuts
sliced mushrooms (in lemon juice and oil)
chicory—sweet corn—apple
tomato—cucumber—cheese

Grayshott puts much stock in a detoxification program that appears quite effective for quick weight loss and general physiological rehabilitation. The program begins with a brief period of fasting and complete rest.

The diet starts with a few days of no more than grapefruit and hot lemon water, and graduates to a "light diet" of breakfast, a salad for lunch, and small pieces of fruit or cheeses for dinner.

There is a total and enforced taboo on excessive protein intake, all alcohol, caffeine, milk (except for the fermented variety, such as yogurt), white sugar, white flour, and salt. Four eggs per week are the maximum. The rationale here is to repose the body from its routine stresses so as to allow it to cleanse and medicate itself.

Grayshott has an enclosed swimming pool (with convertible top for sunny days), a golf course, tennis courts, a billiard room, a good health and general library, and lectures.

The staff-patient ratio is one-to-one, and their personnel and ambiance combine to assure you of a truly good rest cure.

Grayshott Hall England

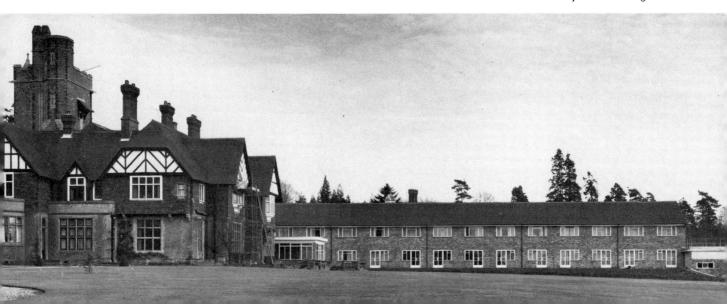

13
Middle
Eastern Spas

Hamei Zohar Israel

Hamei Zohar is one of the world's most fascinating spas—and the most cleverly concealed. Its therapeutic profile beggars most of the Continental spas, but you're one in a thousand if you even know where to find it.

If you look on a map of Israel, you'll find Hamei Zohar (pronounced ham-ay zo-are) located near the southern tip of the Dead Sea. It's a two-hour drive from Jerusalem—and what a drive! Until you get to the sea itself, you traverse the wild and mysterious Judean Desert.

As you follow the road along the Dead Sea, you can look over onto the beautiful snow-capped mountains of Moab on the Jordanian side. To your right, on the Israeli side, you'll find the Judean Mountains, with a sprinkling of kibbutzim on the hillsides, where farmers scratch out meager livings from small gardens.

Sunrises and sunsets in the Negev have an enthralling lunaresque beauty, as the sun and moon play light games with the crags, craters, and canyons that have been left unbothered since Biblical days.

For those of you who don't know, the Dead Sea is the lowest point on earth; near the Hamei Zohar resort area is the towering mountain of Masada, the site of the legendary stand of the Jews against the Romans in the year 73 A.D. At Hamei Zohar, there are five modern hotels, all catering to a spa clientele, but only the Moriah Dead Sea has its own built in spa.

Let me list the reasons why I believe Hamei Zohar deserves a superlative rating:

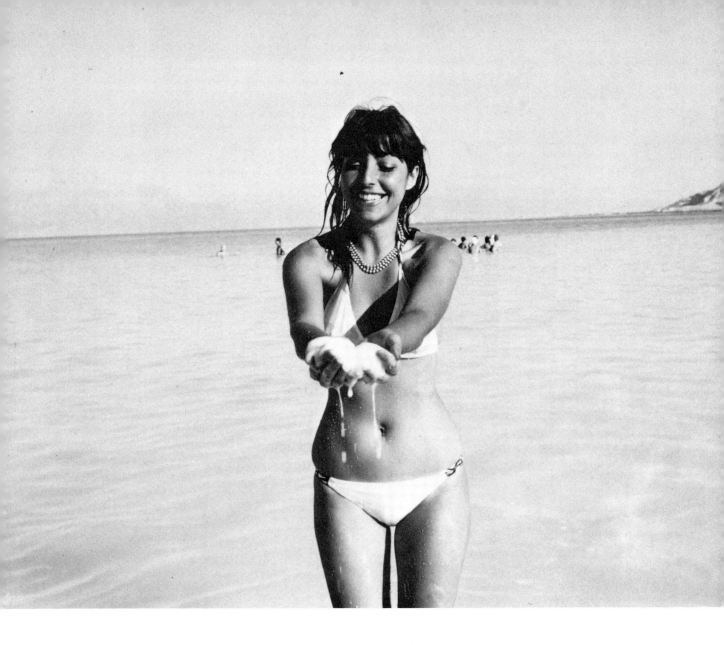

1. As the lowest spot on earth (some 1,300 feet below sea level), it has the highest atmospheric pressure (making breathing easy) and the greatest filtration of damaging sunrays (making sunburns hard to come by). This should be of special interest to those with super-sensitive skins and women who've undergone face-peelings or face-lifts.

2. Bathing in the Dead Sea, with its high magnesium content, gives your skin as good a beauty treatment as anything you've ever had in a salon. You emerge from the sea feeling not salty, but lubricated. And the softness of your skin, even after one dunk, stays with you for a couple of days afterward. (One is reminded that, however new the Moriah is, the Dead Sea area has been a resort for several millen-

nia and in pre-Biblical times had a thriving cosmetics industry owing to its mineral richness.)

3. The "dead" nomenclature refers to the fact that there is no life, fish or plant, in the Dead Sea. The same holds for the desert surrounding it. So, with no flowers, trees, smokestacks, or other pollutants, you've got a practically allergen-free atmosphere. It's a hayfever sufferer's paradise.

4. The combination of balnealogical treatments and filtered sun, the Dead Sea specialty, produce a tender, effective therapy for psoriasis patients. The extraordinary filtering of the sun's rays caused by the extra 1,200 feet or so of atmosphere through which they travel—takes almost all the burn out of the sun, leaving just its curative powers. Chronic

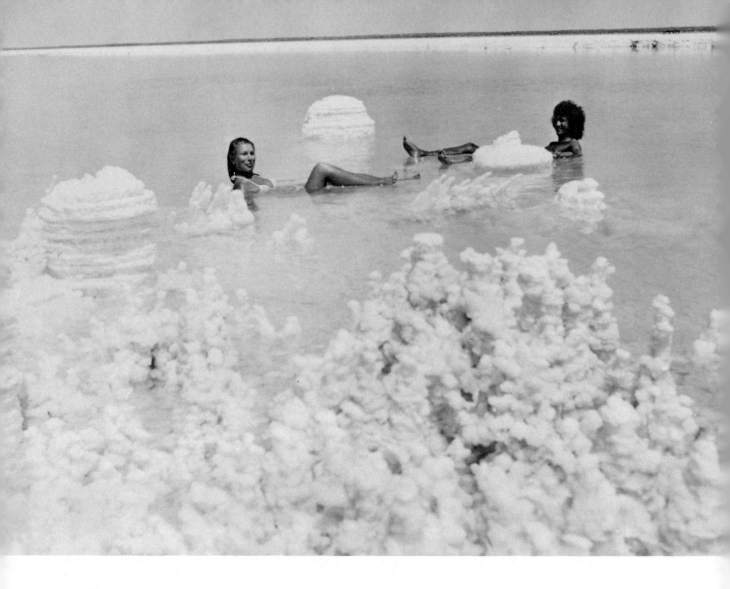

Dead Sea Israel

psoriasis patients spend four weeks a year at the Dead Sea, after which their skin is completely healed and the disease only returns in time for the next curative trip. The Danish national health system even covers the cost of the entire Dead Sea visit for their patients suffering from psoriasis.

The Moriah Dead Sea is rated 5-Stars by the Israeli Government, and while it does not always run with deluxe efficiency and charm, it has a bounty of amenities to please the spa-minded traveler. It is very reasonably priced, the service is good (if a little casual), and the 230 rooms are delightful, each featuring the sea and the "moonscape" beyond.

A large glass French door—window opens up onto a small terrace where you can sunbathe. The architecture assures privacy and freedom from daylong sunlight streaming into your room. And I recall the beatific exaltation felt in observing the sunrise explode over the Moab.

The room's lighting was modern and unobtrusive. The air conditioning (with mild, medium, and strong options) is sensibly located over the foyer entrance—and NOT targeted at your pillows as in so many resort hotels. The light ash furniture was just right, and I welcomed the floor-to-ceiling mirror near my bedside for both exercising and cosmetic enjoyment.

There is, however, a kind of busybodiness about the hotel. Within an hour of my arrival, two employees stopped by—separately—to ask me when I was leaving. They turned out to be the vanguard of a stream of unannounced hotel employees on various missions: replacing a piece of fallen plaster, doing head counts, making up the room (before either the sun or I had risen), and just having a peek.

On the other hand, the Moriah's desire to please cannot be gainsaid. A friend of mine who rang fruitlessly for room service called the desk clerk and was told: "Sir, give me your order and I'll have it sent up immediately."

"I'd like to have some breakfast," said my friend.

"Fine, sir. I'll send up our entire menu. You just select whatever you want from the table."

What breakfasts, by the way! I was forced to leave all sorts of mouth-watering morsels on my breakfast tray. I never got to the croissants, the porridge, or the rolls. I couldn't even BEGIN the grapefruit, since a basket of fruit had been left in the room the previous night. I did eat the limpid yogurt, and the cottage cheese and the sheep cheese. But I only dented the hillock of goat cheese they'd given me. I nibbled at the boiled egg and put away a dozen of the plump black and green olives. I sidestepped the herrings and tackled one of the tomatoes. The honeyed tea was excellent, as was the fruit juice. I shunned the marmalade in a feeble dietetic gesture. With breakfasts like these, and believe me, this one was TYPICAL, how does the average Israeli get STARTED in the day? How does he even manage to get UP from the table?

They tell you to bring a doctor's certificate before using any of the spa's facilities. Some asthmatics are said to thrive better in high elevations—such as nearby Arad, which is 2,034 feet above sea level, and which is dry and allergen-free as well. Accommodations at Arad, by the way, are plentiful and less than an hour's drive from the Dead Sea. Municipal authorities there have proscribed the planting of any tree or vegetation that produces allergenic pollen. Other asthmatics find the Dead Sea more congenial to their conditions. Find out from your doctor whether you'll be better off high or low BEFORE you go.

However, the "doctor's certificate" rule is not strictly enforced. One tourist, who dutifully went up to the Moriah's doctor's office before going into the baths, was startled to find loud moans and groans issuing from her room. When he opened the door, he found the German doctor lying in bed, a thermometer stuck in her mouth, shouting feverishly: "ICH BIN KRANK! ICH BIN KRANK! GEHEN SIE WEG!" ("I'm sick! I'm sick! Go away!")

When he then consulted the desk clerk as to how he should get his doctor's permission to visit the baths, the clerk told him not to bother about it.

When you bathe in the Dead Sea,* by the way, take a good shower first. I made the mistake of not washing off my makeup and perfume—and found myself attacked by flies who kept up a non-stop assault on

my lips and my eyes. If you go in clean, they leave you alone.

The balnealogical treatment building was built over the hot springs gushing from the underlying rocks. It has seven floors (including two cellars), with the upper four floors terraced and built right into the rock face.

The springs are radioactive thermal sulphur springs, with a natural heat of 91.4 degrees Fahrenheit. For special baths, they are further warmed to 100.4 degrees. The high magnesium content—so good for the skin—is a rare bonus, and that, plus the other minerals and radon and radium, seems to exert a pressure on the blood vessels and muscles, improving circulation and cleansing the body of wastes. Israeli doctors recommend these springs for rheumatism, joint diseases, allergies, and most especially psoriasis.

Probably the best time of the year to come to Hamei Zohar is the winter. Remember, 300 out of 365 days are utterly cloudless and fog has never been seen. And when it's snowing in Jerusalem (which it sometimes does), you can have 70-plus temperatures on the Dead Sea.

The hot springs center can provide up to six hundred treatments per day in its twelve bath cubicles, four massage rooms, two sulfur pools (with six seats attached to the side of the pool for special patients), two changing rooms, and two rest rooms with eleven beds each.

You can have any number of different private baths, including air bubble baths (in which air is added to the regular sulfur baths), carbon dioxide baths (in which CO_2 is added to a fresh-water or sulphur bath), mud (from the Dead Sea) baths containing organic and inorganic materials, electro-galvanic baths (in sulfur water), and vibration baths (fresh water with mechanical massage).

There are also facilities for short-wave, infra-red, ultra-violet, and ultrasonic treatments, and various massages and a manipulative experience called "spine and neck extension" that I, perhaps too timidly, passed up.

Despite the Muzak-style rhythms floating through the building (which I resent whenever and wherever I encounter them), I found the treatments excellent—most of them administered by recent emigrants from the Soviet Union, where physiotherapy is a fairly advanced science. The manager, Max Kleimatsky, is a fountain of lore about the Dead Sea, and he is most courteous. I should mention, too, the air conditioning throughout, the snack bars, and a clever alarm-bell system for patients in distress.

If you really want to be kosher about your visit to

---

*The Dead Sea's salt content is ten times that of any other body of water in the world; the bromine (which has a tranquilizing effect) is fifty times higher; the magnesium, fifteen; iodine, ten.

Hamei Zohar, you ought to stay the minimum two to three weeks they say are required for maximum therapeutic benefits. But I can tell you that only a few days there, which was all I could spend, leave you feeling just terrific!

My first dinner at the Moriah wouldn't win three stars from Michelin, but it was quite satisfactory.

The "Bat-Yam" bouchées, crisp MILLE-FEUILLES with creamed chicken, were an excellent appetizer. The St. Germain potage was made from freshly blended vegetables, which made me think that there HAD to be a good Jewish mother in the kitchen. Here was a soup to cure everything from warts to angina.

The curried chicken was unadventuresome but palatable, with peanuts, diced egg, and bits of otherwise unidentifiable flotsam. This was balanced with side dishes of rice, carrots, and eggplant, and a good green salad. The chilled melon was super. The Carmel Ardat wine was only fair.

The dining room is, as is the whole Dead Sea experience, very informal. The Moriah's guests are mostly Europeans and Israelis, with an evergrowing number of Americans. By the way, Israel is not, as often perceived, a country preoccupied either with its problems, or its religious heritage. The cities, ancient and modern, are vibrant and exciting; the scenery offers a spectrum from lush and tropical to arid and desolate. The country has miles of beaches along the four seas (the Dead, the Red, the Mediterranean and the Galilee)—with resorts by the dozen.

Israelis were not what I expected either. They come in all colors and shades, blond and blue-eyed, dark and black-eyed. They have a native charm and are very proud of their country and its not-unimpressive achievements. Yet they are interested in the visitor's views and reactions to them and their land.

SUMMARY: If you can dispense with draconian regimens, prissy diets, tank-suit exercise classes—and if the prospect of a slightly anarchic atmosphere doesn't turn you off—Hamei Zohar has much to give you. While research into the whys and wherefores is still rudimentary, it seems a good bet that the extraordinary mineral waters of the Dead Sea and the alluvial muds on its shore constitute a fabulous and inimitable therapy for tired skins, drooping faces, dermatological discombobulations, tired blood and the like.—E.W.

Tiberias Israel

Two hours north of Jerusalem lies the tranquil Sea of Galilee, a harp-shaped inland lake fed by the River Jordan. On the western shore lies the town of Tiberias, founded in the first century A.D. by King Herod, to honor Roman Emperor Tiberius Caesar. Tiberias has been a spa for more than 2,000 years, its hot springs pumping water from a depth of over 6,000 feet to the surface where it emerges at 144 degrees Fahrenheit. Tiberias' hot springs are surrounded by 15 acres of beautiful parkland, a haven for wild birds, fauna and flora, and 17 of the underground springs have been tapped for balneological use by the Tiberias Hot Springs Company.

Unlike Hamei Zohar, Tiberias is a lively town, one of Israel's true vacation-oriented cities. The city's spa is contained in a sprawling Las Vegas-style complex on the lake shore. The New Tiberias Hot Springs is a far cry from the old Turkish bath house described by the author of Cook's 1909 guide to the Holyland in the immortal words: "and, anyone who dares bathe in this filthy place, deserves to be cured." The new complex boasts indoor and outdoor mineral water pools, a massive hydrotherapy and physiotherapy wing, and a delightful fish restaurant overlooking the lake where the freshly caught local St. Peter's fish is delicious, plump and meaty—and very low in calories.

Tiberias bottles its own mineral water, which is all the rage in Israel—and available in health-food stores in certain U.S. cities. The water is barely effervescent and has a clean, fresh taste. The water is excellent for treating muscular and joint diseases (arthritis treatment is big here!); it is also wonderful for clearing the sinuses. A New York couple I know, who suffer dreadfully from sinus problems, spend three weeks every fall in Tiberias and return home breathing easily, their noses unstuffed!

I especially enjoy Tiberias' aerated mineral pools and baths, which soothingly massage aches and pains into oblivion. But the real joy at Tiberias is "Piloma", their own special mud treatment. A mixture of muds with a suspension of mineral particles is immersed in the hot spring waters to absorb their salt and warmth. Once it reaches 127 degrees Fahrenheit, it is cooled to the temperature specified by the physician in atten-

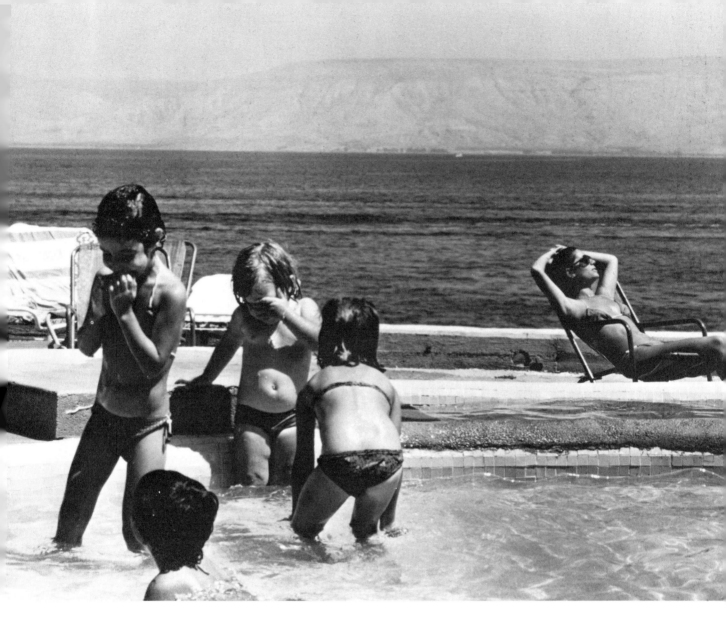

dance and then applied. It is so marvelous because the Piloma transmits its heat very slowly so there is no irritation to the skin and the heat, which would not normally be tolerable, penetrates comfortably and deeply into the body.

After the Piloma there is nothing to do but to whisk to the hotel and into bed. Tiberias is full of hotels, two of which are rated 5-Star. The Galeii Kinneret, built originally in the 1930's has all the atmosphere of a pre-war Swiss resort. While very pleasant, it is a little too staidly austere for my taste. I much prefer the adjacent Tiberias Plaza Hotel, a resort operated by the Canadian Pacific Hotel chain with international flair. It is a modern hotel, built in a pyramid of "steps", each step being the private terrace of a bedroom. The hotel has a delightful pool, a big airy restaurant, coffee shop, and a very pleasant lobby lounge. The rooms have every facility, and although somewhat garishly decorated, are very pleasant. The nicest touch is the bud vase with a fresh rose delivered to the room on Friday evening to usher in the Sabbath. The hotel's handsome general manager, Hungarian-born Bernard Cohn, runs the hotel like clockwork, from the glistening polished marble entrance hall to the starched linen napkins at the sumptuous Saturday buffet luncheon. After the treatments, the naps, the swims in the lake, Tiberias is a lovely town for touring. Its houses are built of the local black basalt stone (attesting to the valley's volcanic past) and the promenade along the shore is perfect for evening strolls. And Tiberias is just a short drive from biblical Nazareth, Capernaum, and the Mount of Beatitudes.

157

Cagaloglu Hamami Turkey

Turkey is a land of spas, with nearly three hundred, many of which have been in continuous use since ancient times. But no collection of the world's super spas can be considered complete without a visit to a Turkish institution that isn't exactly a spa at all—a real Turkish bath.

Right in the heart of old Istanbul, without so much as a sign, there is an ancient bath still in operation. A cherubic, smiling woman escorted me to a dressing room furnished with a towel-covered cot. There were additional towels and a pair of wooden clogs. I donned the towel and clogs, while a large, buxom, sweet-faced woman dressed only in black undies took me by the arm and led me over the slippery marble floor into a huge, domed room that resembled a mosque.

In the center of the room was an octagonal platform, from whose center rose a cloud of steam. The platform was rather broad, and several women—some accompanied by pre-school children—were washing themselves with water that was constantly poured into stone basins.

A woman doused me with water from a basin, asked me if I wanted a shampoo, and motioned for me to lie down on the steam platform. It was warm lying there, and she poured more water on me. Then she took a cake of soap and a small mop, draped herself over my body and began to soap me with the little mop. Then she massaged my entire body. Now and then she interrupted my reverie and asked me if I liked it. Yes, yes, yes. I felt like a tingling newborn baby. I'll never forget those blissful moments.

When I returned to my cubicle, a Turkish coffee and a sandwich were brought to me. After eating, I slumbered for a half-hour, dressed, and returned to my hotel. The next twelve hours I slept—probably the deepest, most refreshing sleep I've ever had!

Mediterranean and Middle Eastern women often have a problem of excess hair—just where they don't want it. An Istanbul beautician, Agda Kaptanoglu, keeps such customers looking feminine and beautiful with a centuries-old recipe for a natural depilatory. It's simple and easily prepared at home.

Secret of the Hairless Harem

In a frying pan, mix 12 level tablespoons of granulated sugar with 6 level tablespoons of water, and 3 level tablespoons of fresh (not reconstituted) lemon juice. Turn the flame medium and, stirring constantly, cook the sugar-water-lemon mixture, scraping it from the bottom and sides of the pan so it will cook evenly.

When the mixture becomes a light golden shade, turn it out onto a flat stainless steel surface or a kitchen counter. Be sure to wait for it to be cool enough to handle. Now comes the magic:

While it is still lukewarm—do not let it get cold or it will harden—knead with damp hands until the mixture forms a ball. Pull and stretch it, folding again and again, keeping your hands dampened so that the mixture won't stick to them. Continue until the mixture loses its transparency.

Divide the large ball into two smaller ones. Working with one at a time, press the ball against your leg, flattening it out, then yank out the hairs against the direction in which they grow. Reshape the mixture into a ball and apply to another area.

This lemon-sugar formula is extremely effective and can be used on underarms too. In between zip-offs, knead the ball constantly to keep the sugar-lemon mixture pliable.

The secret of this method is that it pulls the hair out by the roots, keeping legs fuzz-free for a month or more. Try this formula and enjoy the same results that harem beauties achieved in times past.

Here are two other Kaptanoglu recipes for skin correctives:

Dry Skin Enhancer

Mix 1 tablespoon of honey, a few drops of olive oil or almond oil, and an egg yolk until you have mask consistency. Apply to the face for 10 minutes. Then remove with a sponge soaked in rosewater. The Turks, by the way, use rosewater for practically EVERYTHING. Here it makes excellent sense.

Oily Skin Enhancer

Mix 1 tablespoon of honey, a raw egg white, 1 teaspoon of kaolin powder (your drugstore should have this), and 2 teaspoons of yogurt, until you've reached mask texture. Apply and leave on the face until you feel your skin tightening and "drawing." Rinse with lukewarm water; finish with a sponging of rosewater.

I can't resist passing on another hint to those of you who wish to do a little something for your black

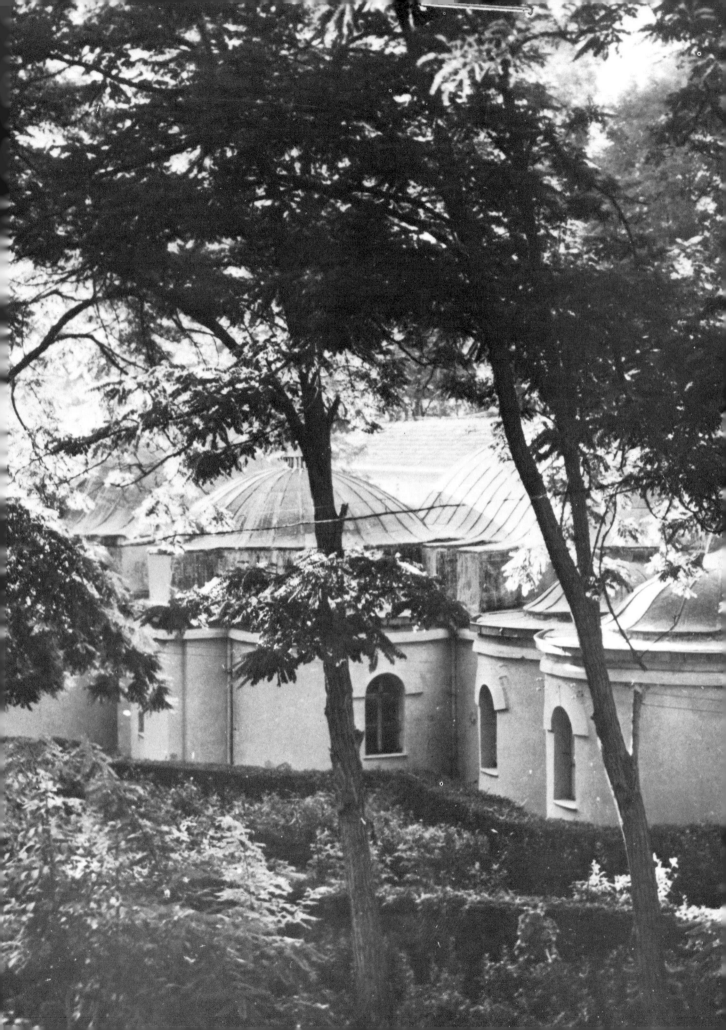

hair. It's just this: Take a small handful of bay leaves, pour boiling water over them, and let steep. If you use this as a setting lotion, you'll find it adds a delightful reddish tint to your hair.

SUMMARY: If you can't wait to have a super Turkish bath experience, don't miss the bath at Cagaloglu Hamami. Don't be surprised if you find me next to you enjoying the experience.—E.W.

14
The
Rejuvenation
Spas

La Prairie Switzerland

I decided to visit La Prairie, the clinic of the late Dr. Paul Niehans in Clarens-Montreaux outside of Lausanne.

You may recall reading, some years ago, about a trip Dr. Niehans made to Rome. He was called to the bedside of Pope Pius XII to administer sheep-cell injections to the ailing seventy-seven-year-old pontiff. The success of this treatment is attested to by an autographed picture of Dr. Niehans and the Pontiff together, displayed in the hall at the clinic.

In the 1920s, Dr. Niehans gave fresh animal-gland transplants to dwarfs. As a result, they grew as much as a foot taller. Later, a woman whose parathyroid was injured, was reported saved when Niehans prepared the parathyroid gland of an unborn lamb, added the gland extract to a saline solution and injected it into the patient. This treatment made news around the world. From that day on, celebrities have flocked to the clinic. Word spread that Dr. Niehans' experiments included injections that could turn back the clock and make patients look and feel younger.

La Prairie calls itself a clinic for internal medicine, specializing in cellular therapy with fresh cells. It is well known for treating sexual impotency. It also caters to overweight patients—but without using thyroid extracts or diuretics. Weight reduction is achieved with injections and diet. According to Dr. Eli Eddè the highest percentage of clinic patients are treated for stress, high blood pressure, circulatory disorders, arthritis, energy levels, and the side effects brought about by the aging process. The treatment is also beneficial as preventive medicine.

The youth treatment involves a nine-day stay at La Prairie. The cellular injections are given on Thursday of treatment week following extensive laboratory testing and consultation with doctors. The number of injections varies according to the patient's individual needs. Patients usually report feeling tired for several days after receiving the injections but, within a few months, some say they feel reborn.

There is more than cellular therapy involved in this treatment. Patients should observe these rules for

161

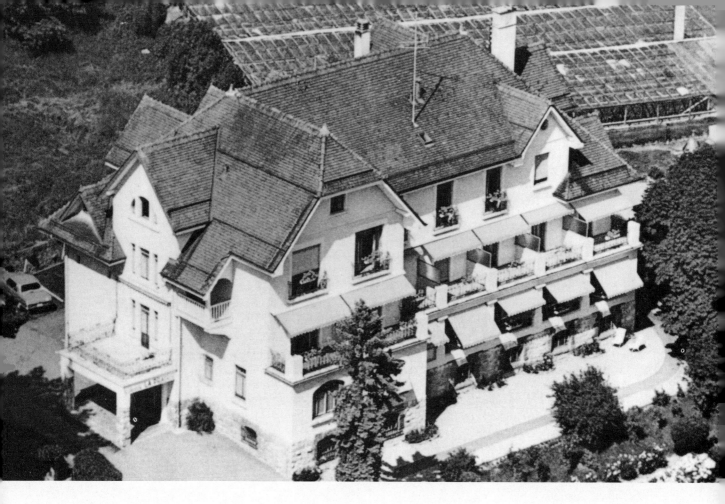

La Prairie Switzerland

three months following the injections.

No sunbaths, no Turkish baths, no saunas, no diathermy;
No X-rays without protecting the rest of the body;
No very hot hair dryers;
No short-wave treatment, no ultra-violet rays;
No drugs (if possible) and no hormones, no stimulants or sedatives;
No poisons, such as nicotine or strong alcohols.
No regular coffee (de-caf only)

A prescribed eating program should be followed strictly or the benefits of cellular therapy will not be attainable. Here are the rules of the diet:

STRICTLY FORBIDDEN: Everything fatty (butter, oil, lard) eggs, cheese, salt, boiled milk, fruit with pits, spinach, tomatoes, breads, patés, pastry, sugar, coffee, caffeine, strong alcohol.

TOLERATED: Milk that is warm but not cooked (boiled); lean grilled beef and veal; poached or grilled fish; a teaspoon of peanut oil on salad or on the grill.

One or two glasses of red wine daily. One glass of champagne on festive occasions.

RECOMMENDED: Raw or steamed vegetables and fruits, with the exception of peas, cabbage, spinach, tomatoes; rice, barley, enriched farina cooked with water; very weak tea (with a bit of uncooked milk and sugar if necessary). Regular intestinal evacuation.

NOTE: When boiling vegetables, you may add salt-free bouillon cubes to the water.

BREAKFAST: (a) A cup of tea (lightly brewed) with raw milk, biscuit; (b) Two tablespoons of crushed bran in water, cook for 30 minutes over a low flame, eventually filter). Bouillon cubes.

DINNER AND SUPPER: (a) Vegetable soup. Lean strips of beef or veal, grilled; (b) Broiled or steamed fish. (c) Boiled vegetables: artichokes, celery, turnips, carrots, red or green cabbage, endive, a few potatoes, white beets (recommended), chicory, lettuce. (d) Barley, millet, rice, semolina. (e) Fruit with pits, skinned apples.

These suggestions should be followed for three months after the treatment. A more moderate diet is allowed after this period.

Following the rules prescribed by La Prairie cannot always be easy, but this doesn't seem to deter those who want to recapture lost youth. The rich, the famous, and the beautiful flock to the clinic from all parts of the world. Hopeful, anxious, they want only one thing: to look young again. The late Duke of Windsor and the Duchess of Windsor, Marlene Dietrich, Charlie Chaplin, King Ibn Saud, Merle Oberon, and Greta Garbo have, like all of La Prairie's youth-seeking patients, waited derriere up, for cellular injections to be administered. Confidentiality is assured, however many famous personalities make known their satisfaction with Clinic La Prairie's treatment.

The trouble with cell therapy is that it has a way of falling into the hands of very suave, fast-talking doctors who have become rich from their rejuvenation injections—and who simply have not devoted any of their wealth to research that would explain how these injections work or IF they do.

Clinic La Prairie has a full scale research department and the cardiac surgeon, Dr. Christian Barnard, is now medical consultant. His team in South Africa performs cell culture studies and constant progress is made in diagnostics and results of the treatment. Dr. Barnard feels that La Prairie's Fresh Cell Therapy is one of the major breakthroughs in treatment of degenerative diseases, and this includes the aging process.

Dr. Walter Michel was a large, balding, Frenchified Swiss physician of the old school. He hewed faithfully to Niehans' techniques of injecting the clumps of embryonic cells shortly after (within one hour) the fetus was extracted. The so-called Sicacells, or lyophilized (preserved) cells, in their vacuum ampules, retain their potency indefinitely, but are far less potent. Dr. Claude Rossel, present Medical Director, and staff, have further developed the Niehans technique.

Thursday morning, I was to watch the operation. The fetus would be rushed from the abattoir to the Clinic La Prairie, where it would be dissected into its separate organs and tissues, and these, in turn, would be mashed and prepared so as to be able to pass through the syringe needles.

I was fascinated with the chalet-style clinic that greeted my eyes as the taxi drove up a long, winding path from the main road along Lake Geneva. That modest clinic is one of the last repositories of medical secrets in the whole world. The staff of six doctors and ten nurses go to exceptional lengths to conceal the identities of their celebrity patients, even from other patients.

A nurse led me upstairs to the laboratory. I slipped on a green gown and white face mask, such as those the technicians were wearing.

There on a table lay two black, woolly fetuses. Then, with knives, (now called "Niehans' knives"), technicians skillfully separated the organs and tissues and passed them on to others who diced and mashed them.

The placenta was also saved. For many, this tissue was the most important ingredient of a "cell therapy cocktail" that they believed would restore youthfulness and potency and good looks to their senescent bodies.

There was little waste. Only the male has testicular material for potency. Only the ewe has large enough ovaries. The advantage of the fetus (prenatal)—and this was a REAL Niehans discovery—is that its tissues cannot cause an anaphylactic (toxic protein) shock in the patient.

The entire dissection takes about fifteen minutes.

That lab scene was unforgettable. Somewhere between M.A.S.H. and Marcus Welby, M.D. I had a sneaking suspicion that this whole show was being put on for my benefit, it was so spectacular. The bloody tissues and trays of instruments and syringes were highlighted by mammoth surgical lamps. Each set of syringes was labeled by organ and tissue and stuffed accordingly.

As the doctors gazed at the list of patients waiting upstairs, they mixed clumps of cells with saline solutions and prepared injections, placing each filled syringe in the appropriate patient's tray. The assistants worked deftly and briskly, so that the least possible time would elapse.

I would not be permitted to watch the injections. The patients were paying for TOTAL privacy.

The clinic states that the sun is THE ENEMY. If you tan easily, you can take more than someone who does not. But, best of all, one should go for one's swim and then immediately seek shade.

Exercise is the best preventive measure against aging. To stay young, one should inhale a large quantity of oxygen each day. Otherwise, you are a pushover for disease.

Medication can be a curse. Instead, try fresh-air sports such as golf and hunting in the mountains and lake country.

For some, one cell therapy treatment is enough for a lifetime, if the accompanying diet is observed strictly, but many patients return in two to ten years, depending on their age.

I waited for a car to take me from the clinic to my hotel. Out of the clinic bounded a man who resembled Maurice Chevalier. As he strode jauntily down the walk, swinging his cane, tipping his bowler, radiating a JOIE DE VIVRE, and flashing a lascivious wink, I thought to myself that this amusing septuagenarian was the best ad Clinic La Prairie could ever ask for.

Incosol Spain

Where do you get cell therapy, outside of Vevey? Almost anywhere in Europe. Nowhere (legally, that is) in the United States, where the Food and Drug Administration has looked dimly at the research presented by the cell therapists. But thanks to the packaging of freeze-dried cells in vacuum ampules, many European pharmacies carry them.

One of the most pleasant spas for cell therapy is Incosol. Located near Marbella on the Costa del Sol, the gleaming new ten-million-dollar Incosol complex is the most up to date of the Spanish spas, offering all sorts of therapies, diet supervision (with optional human chorionic gonadotropin shots), and luxurious accommodations (most with terraces, all with air conditioning, TV, music). There are lounges, restaurants, bars, indoor and outdoor pools, waterskiing, golf, tennis, riding, a bowling alley, and a gym. And the price is not what you'd imagine—probably one-half what you'd pay for comparable facilities in the United States. Medical services include complete laboratory facilities, a coronary care unit (including monitoring system), radiology, physiotherapy (ozone baths, carbonic acid baths, Kneipp showers, mudpacks, etc.), dentistry, revitalization treatments (e.g., cell therapy and Gerovital). Swiss internist Dr. Augusto Gianoli has treated many heads of state with cell therapy. Gianoli charges (you and me) between $1200 and $1500 for his injections, and the room rates at Incosol are less than what an American hospital would charge. And American hospitals don't have a magnificent view of the Mediterranean and a chain of glorious, snow-capped Sierras. Dr. Gianoli is scientifically familiar with the sheep-cell therapy of the late Paul Niehans. At any rate, he boasts and caters to the same illustrious clientele.

The Wiedemann Kurhotels Germany

One of the most successful rejuvenation clinicians in the world—in terms of people treated—unquestionably is Fritz Wiedemann, M.D., of the Wiedemann Kurhotel in Ambach.

Wiedemann is to rejuvenation what Ford was to automobile production. He has standardized a gamut of therapies, brought the prices down several pegs from what some dazzling individual clinics charge, and regularly fills his two thousand-plus beds at the Ambach (Lake Starnberg) and Meersburg (Lake Constance) Kurhotels and affiliated institutions (operated by others but closely supervised by him).

Moreover, no other Kurhotel—to my knowledge—offers the range of rejuvenation therapies that Wiedemann does: organic diets, kinesotherapy, weight-loss programs, homeopathy, Bogomolets' sera, enzyme therapies, fresh and lyophilized cell injections, vitamin megadosages, Gerovital H3 injections, Cell KH3 pills, ozone therapy, neural therapy (which is a kind of acupuncture using slight amounts of procaine injections) and Ana Aslan's new H7 therapy.

He has also developed the organ-serum idea of Bogomolets into a regeneration serum of his own, to which he adds DNA from embryonic animal hearts.

Dr. Wiedemann sees six thousand patients per year for a range of ailments—everything from heart and circulation problems, arthritis, rheumatism, spinal troubles, and asthma to such relatively simple things as headaches, weight loss, insomnia, and fatigue.

Dr. Wiedemann believes a 'biological cure' is the answer to revitalization. His treatments aim to fortify the body's own defense system and power of recovery to cure or prevent, in a natural manner, the complaints and chronic diseases of aging. The normal "Regeneration Cure" takes three weeks, the fee ranging from $140 to $250 per week additional. Dr. Wiedemann believes, "more and more people who are not exactly

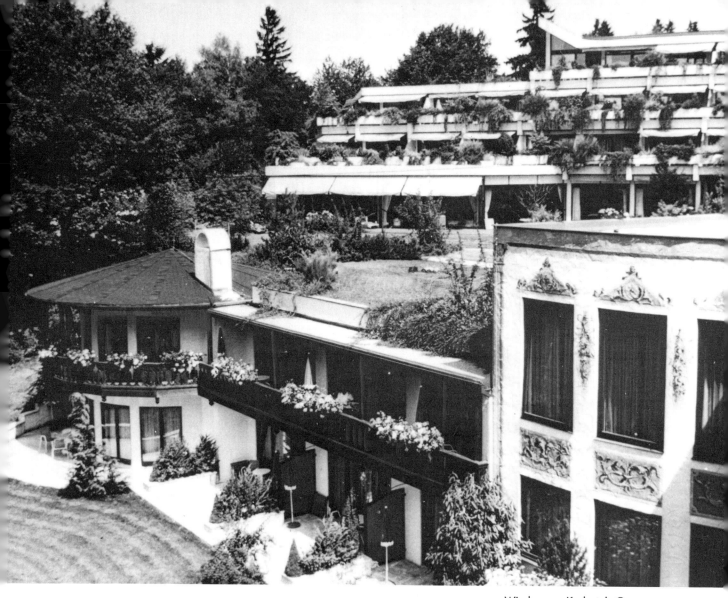

Wiedemann Kurhotels Germany

ill, but do not feel really healthy, or who feel exhausted, should make use of the facilities of an intensive health cure—in good time, before it is too late."

The Wiedemann Kurhotels are well equipped to provide all necessary services to achieve that end—sauna, heated swimming pool, health and cure facilities and dietetic cuisine. Prices are relatively reasonable. Room rates (with full board) range from about $30 to $70 per person per day; there are special accommodations for children and pets.

For information contact the German National Tourist Office, 747 Third Avenue, New York, NY 10016.

Dr. Wiedemann, in his 70's, is dynamic. He loves mountain climbing and thrives on vitamin-packed meals. He breakfasts on dark bread, sweet butter, natural honey and coffee, except when he personally takes the cure (twice a year). Then he abstains from coffee and alcohol and drinks the delicious rose hips tea and alcohol-free beer served in the sanatoriums' dining rooms.

The doctor is a firm believer in everything natural and thinks you should let well enough alone when it comes to face-lifts, bosom implants and such.

As to exercise, Wiedemann believes in walking and moving about generally to the best of one's ability—that is, a person with a heart attack history would not do a vigorous program.

From what I could observe, guests thrive on the Wiedemann diet—I know it made me feel vital and healthy. It differs according to "prescription" but there's no pepper, no coffee, no tea, and very little salt. Incidentally, dazzling white linen cloths give every meal the aura of a banquet.

The Wiedemann diet is worth trying. The menus have been a great success in the "old world" for many years.

165

A normal day's menu would include:

BREAKFAST

Cottage Cheese	Honey
Müsli	Soaked Prunes
Yogurt	Herb Tea
Rye Crisp (or other crisp bread)	Grain or Decaffinated Coffee
Butter	

	LUNCHEON	DINNER
MONDAY **(Dry Day)**	Chicken salad Veal knuckles (short pieces) in tomato sauce Whole veal knuckles (Italian style) Spaghetti (Milanese style) Mixed salad plate Cottage cheese with wild raspberries	Alsatian onion soufflé Veal meatballs with rice rings Cucumbers Chicory salad Sherbet

TUESDAY
 (Vitamin Day)
	Shredded red cabbage
	    with grated raw apples
	 Beef Tongue in Madeira wine
	 Green peppers
	 Mashed potatoes with chopped onions
	    and bacon
	 Creamy chocolate mousse
		Cauliflower
		 Fresh brook trout
		 Parsley potatoes
		 Salad of the season
		 Crepes (pancake) with nuts

WEDNESDAY **(Wet Day)**	Clear oxtail soup Veal steak in gravy and cream Mushrooms in cream Homemade noodles Tomatoes and watercress Peach melba	Hearts of palm Filet Mignon Broccoli Carrots Potatoes with tarragon and parsley Fresh fruit
THURSDAY **(Dry Day)**	Grapefruit Breast of veal with carrots Potatoes with leaf spinach Stewed apricots	Melon with ham Beef Stroganoff Tomatoes stuffed with rice Chicory salad with lettuce Raspberry pudding with vanilla sauce
FRIDAY **(Vitamin Day)**	Raw vegetable plate Pickled tongue Boiled potatoes with dill Lettuce with lemon juice Pineapple	Fresh blueberries Veal steak in wine Stuffed tomato Mashed potatoes Endive salad Cottage cheese pudding
SATURDAY **(Wet Day)**	Fresh mushroom soup Ribbed meat—French style Cabbage with boiled potatoes Lettuce Melon cocktail	Sour cherry juice Cheese platter with fruit Crepes with Brandy and orange juice
SUNDAY **(Normal Day)**	Stuffed avocado Leg of venison (deer) Potatoes (mashed with flowers —eggs cooked) Lettuce, braised Nut salad (Italian) Lemon mousse	Mixed vegetables with spicy sauce Veal sweetbread and vegetables Asparagus Buttered potatoes Endive salad Fresh fruit

The Fountain of Youth Romania

I am one of thousands of Americans who have discovered in the nicest way possible—while enjoying travel abroad—that Ponce de León was on the right track. There is something akin to the legendary Fountain of Youth. It is Gerovital H3, a once widely controversial drug (not yet on the FDA's approved list) that is gaining more supporters in medical circles every year. It was developed by Romania's remarkable Professor Dr. Ana Aslan to counteract many of the effects of aging.

GH3 has resulted in what must be the most unique tourist attraction in the world, the Romanian combination of treatment and travel. It is both beneficial and enjoyable. Once you have had your initial medical check in Bucharest and a custom-tailored course of treatments with GH3 has been prescribed, you are free to tour Romania while the treatments continue in doctor-staffed clinics along the way—at beautiful Black Sea beaches, in Carpathian Mountain ski resorts, near the curative mud baths—even in Dracula country which, judging from the standing-room-only crowds for the Broadway and off-Broadway versions of Dracula a few years ago, plus the sale of Dracula-printed sheets, towels and wall coverings, captured the imagination of Americans.

I have been to Romania three times. Each visit was fascinating. Changes and improvements are constantly being made in the tourist facilities. What's

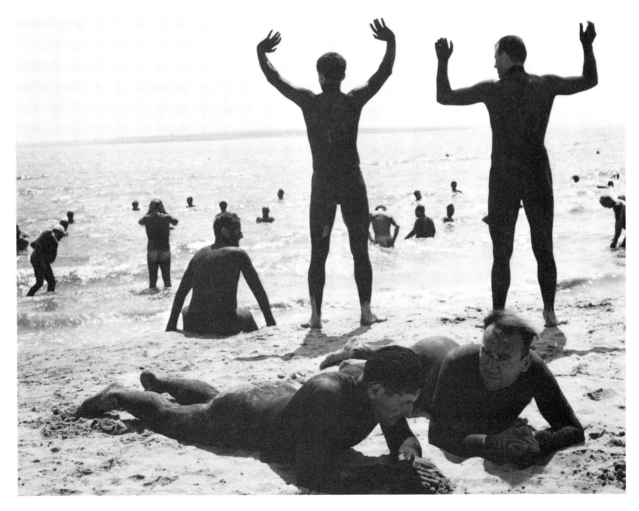

Lake Techirghiol Romania 167

more, any way you look at it, the Gerovital Tours are a travel and beauty bargain. A tour can cost as little as $1,434 (based on double occupancy) and including air fare, all meals, medical examination, lab tests, physiotherapy, and the GH3 injections for fourteen days. All this, plus a two-year supply of Gerovitol for $80.

With all the interest in rejuvenation—from spa visits to face-lift surgery—what does Romania have to offer that's different? Why do thousands of tourists from all over the world fly there each year specifically to follow the Aslan regimen?

The myths and myth-conceptions are many. In a way, to call GH3, hailed by many as a major medical breakthrough, a "youth drug", is to sensationalize it and perhaps suggest the ultimate in wrinkle removing and instant makeover. Yet what GH3 accomplishes is even more remarkable. Its effects, more internal than external, rejuvenate bodily functions, lift depression and anxiety, work to improve the memory. It also treats such old age ills as arthritis, neuritis, neuralgia, arteriosclerosis, and asthma.

Gerovital H3 not only is available in injection and tablet form (sometimes the prescribed course of treatment alternates the two) but in a hair lotion that has had marvelous effects in restoring hair or preventing its loss, and in a unique cream designed to ease wrinkles.

Another product formulated by Dr. Aslan is somewhat newer. Called Aslavital, it is being used in Romania to treat cases of cerebral and cardiovascular aging as well as problems related to intellectual over-exertion and loss of memory, concentration, and attention span.

One of the most spectacular results of GH3 treatments is the renewed interest in sex that many patients show. Dr. Aslan sees this as a fringe benefit. "When you don't feel well, sex is secondary," she remarked in a recent interview with me.

But sex is also youth, and when GH3 works its magic, that youthful urge returns, quickening the libido. The results aren't always exactly what patients or those who advise GH3 for them have in mind. For example, Dr. Aslan told me of a wife who sent her husband, an overworked man in his mid-50s, for the treatments. They were so effective that he divorced her and after a wild love affair, married a much younger woman.

"So I advise husbands and wives to take the treatments together," Dr. Aslan said, "that they can enjoy the benefits together."

GH3 does not bring on menstruation once a woman has gone through menopause, but Dr. Aslan does not feel this is significant. "A woman can be sexually active after menopause if she has the will for it," she pointed out. In some magic way, GH3 provides that will.

The energetic older people you meet in the Romanian clinics are remarkable. But they are no novelty to Dr. Aslan who has been witnessing "youth miracles" for the 30 years she has supervised the GH3 program in Romania.

I met an 86-year-old pianist who, since he has been on the program, feels vigorous enough to practice four hours a day. Another 93-year-old patient helps Dr. Aslan with her correspondence, translating in five languages. Such mental and physical feats are the norm. While she doesn't believe in eternal youth, Dr. Aslan does believe that aging can be retarded and that people can expect to have fifteen more years of "youth" on GH3 than they could normally anticipate without it.

What is interesting is that as word of the Romanian Fountain of Youth spreads more men are taking the treatment as well as more husbands and wives together. The clinics also are attracting a younger set, men and women in their 40s, who are anxious either to avoid normal or premature aging problems.

Dr. Aslan stressed that GH3 is not necessarily a crash course but should be taken for a period of time to energize oneself, and on a regular basis under medical supervision to allay aging symptoms. "No need to fear the ravages of time," she said.

In Dr. Aslan's words, "Aging is like a disease, sometimes you can heal it. Life can be prolonged—and more important—these years can be filled with vitality and the joy of life. We want to emphasize that geriatric clinics are not only for old people, but also for preventing diseases of old age and delaying the aging process, thereby prolonging biological youth. From age 45 on, most people need GH3, some even earlier."

When you arrive in Romania for treatment and travel, your first stop is Bucharest, nicknamed "a little Paris," an incredibly beautiful city of wide boulevards, trees, and flowers. I've been to the Romanian capital twice in the summer and, most recently, in late fall. In all seasons there is a special warmth and fragrance in the air.

On my other two trips, I stayed at the Athenée Palace, a lovely hotel. This time I registered at the Flora, a hotel-clinic combined. Everyone who checks into this modern facility isn't taking the treatments but most are.

Despite its magnificent red carpeting and oak paneling, the hotel has a casual air. Guest-patients on their way to the treatment rooms stroll through the halls in their robes, passing businessmen, attache cases

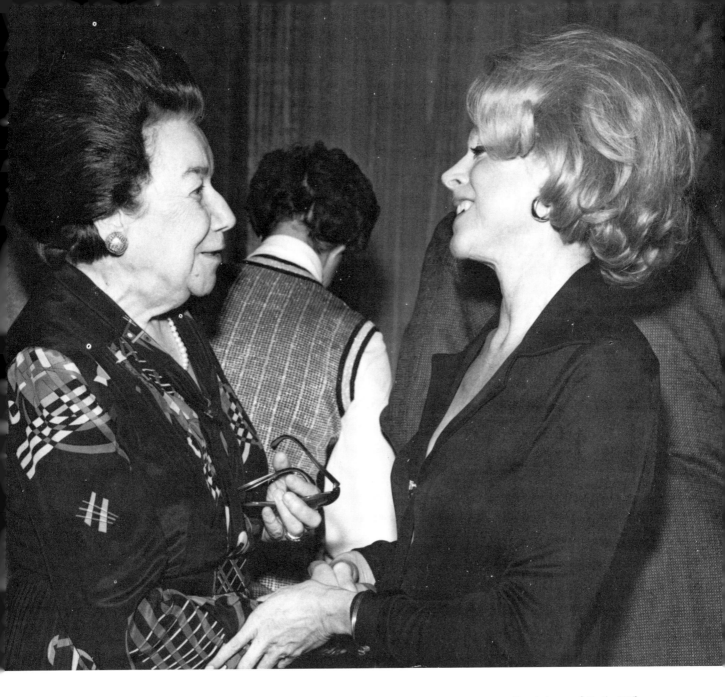

in hand, hurrying off to make import-export deals.

The clinic is a veritable Tower of Babel because interest in GH3 is worldwide. Yet, despite language barriers, there's great camaraderie. Smiles are exchanged and efforts are made at a phrase, a word or—all else failing—sign language. The mood is upbeat.

At the Flora, my room was clean and pleasant, with comfortable chairs for relaxing, a charming balcony so I could enjoy the view and the air. The towels were thick and plentiful. Best of all, I had my own small refrigerator to stock with fresh fruit of the season.

Dinner was served in the Red Salon. The bottle for every table turned out to be Borsec, a bubbly, reasonably priced Romanian mineral water that contains trace elements of potassium, calcium, magnesium and iron. Along with their superb wines, Borsec is the national drink because no one drinks tap water, not even the Romanians.

The Romanian wines can hold their own with the greats that France, California or New York State can produce. The Minion Restaurant in Bucharest, where I had a late lunch one day, had its own vineyard. The special wine was Dealvl-mare (The Daisy Mill), fresh

169

from the pressing. It was so good one was encouraged to drink more—but felt the effects less—except for pure enjoyment.

The other wines I sipped at the Flora were Muscade, a dry white, and Murfatlah 1971.

Menus at the Hotel Flora, and throughout Romania, offer interesting choices—fish from the Danube, including fresh sturgeon, and more chicken and pork dishes than beef. You can have boiled potatoes or thick french fries.

The Romanians use oil made from the seeds of the big and beautiful sunflowers that brighten the landscape in summer. This oil makes superb salad dressings and also is used for cooking. Sunflower oil not only lends great flavor but also vitamins. Combined with lemon, the oil dresses marvelously fresh lettuce, tomatoes, and cucumbers at every meal. Added attractions for this Romanian salad—black olives and dill.

At the Capsa Restaurant, one of the unusual features is a Surprise Salad. My companion and I were each served a different surprise in a large wine goblet. Mine was cabbage, lobster, carrot, and mayonnaise. My guess is that the "surprise" involves leftovers (a good idea for thrifty home cooks too because it was delicious).

Incidentally, you don't find fast food counters in Bucharest, but if you yearn for a snack while sightseeing, there are milk bars that serve delicious yogurt.

Musical entertainments are popular. Almost everywhere you go—at restaurants, theater performances, in parks and night clubs, you can expect to see folk dancers colorfully costumed like dancing dolls. If the program features "The Wedding," each guest can be sure to receive a flower on the way in. One of the most popular numbers that invariably is performed is "The Little Horsemen." The male dancers gallop and prance in a production that aptly and colorfully lives up to its name.

"The Skylark," played on a Romanian reed instrument, is No. 1 on the local hit parade. It is a tradition to hear it at least once an evening.

Most often the peasant dancing is professionally done. Sometimes, however, you're invited to join in as you are in Greece and Israel. If you really want to dance, there are charming restaurants, including the one on Lake Tescarus Herestrau, where you can dine and dance outdoors. Don't expect too many foxtrots. The beat may very well be rock. Disco is catching on in Romania as are single spots such as the elegant dining room at the Athenée Palace.

If you like the romantic sound of violins, you'll find violin music featured in many restaurants. It does give dinner an extra dimension. Call it romantic.

You can swim, ski, sightsee, take the mineral waters, enjoy the night life replete with belly dancers in all parts of Romania. For shoppers, there are colorful arts and crafts. Wonderful hand-woven rugs and wood carvings are designed to give your decorating scheme at home a touch that's peasantly appealing. Embroidered blouses and boleros make great gifts.

There is lots to see in beautiful Bucharest but, once the course of treatments has been prescribed, which takes a few days, many visitors choose to see more of Romania or to take a weekend side trip out of the country to Odessa, Athens, Istanbul, or Kiev.

One of the trips I enjoyed in Romania was to the famous mud lake at Lake Techirgiol where men and women, separated by a seethrough fence, strip and bathe in the mud lake that is believed to have great curative powers. They look as if they are engaging in some strange tribal rite but everyone is too intensely involved with mud-packing that no one gives a thought to appearances.

On my next trip, and I'm looking forward to enjoying yet another sip from the original Romanian Fountain of Youth, I plan to head for Felix, a Romanian Super Spa. It's definitely on my agenda.

For information contact the Romanian National Tourist Office, 573 Third Avenue, New York, N.Y. 10016.

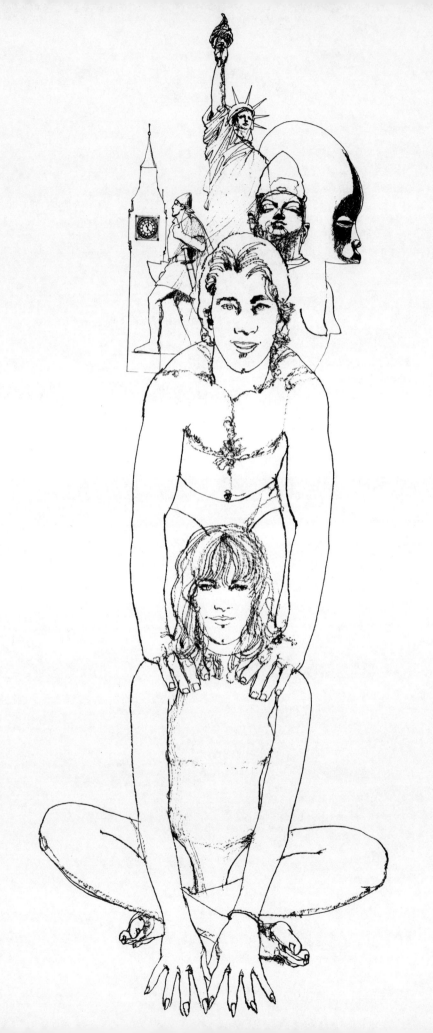

Part Three:
Spavelogue

United States

There are 2,000 spas in the United States, and several times that number worldwide. I have already discussed the major spas that combine beauty and health programs, with which I'm personally familiar.

The following is a list of prominent spas that have either health or beauty facilities or both.

The list does not include every spa, but it does give you a hefty grab-bag of opportunities at a wide price range.

Alabama

FOR INFORMATION: Ms. Caroline Cavanaugh, Director, Bureau of Publicity and Information, 532 S. Perry St., Montgomery, AL 36130, (205) 832–5510

Olympic Spa (Dothan)

With honey-sweet Southern hospitality, the Olympic Spa offers forty-eight luxury rooms, golf, entertainment, fishing, surf bathing, and boating, along with its spa. The latter is manned by physicians and a physical therapist who supervise a hot mineral-water pool with twelve whirlpool jets, well-equipped exercise rooms, steam rooms, saunas, massages, and paraffin baths.

Alaska

FOR INFORMATION: Mr. Don Dickey, Director of Tourism, Alaska Travel Division, Department of Commerce & Economic Development, Pouch E. Juneau, AK 99811, (907) 465-2010, FTS: 8–0–206–442–0150

American Samoa

FOR INFORMATION: Mr. Moaka Mua, Director, Office of Development & Planning, Government of American Samoa, Pago Pago, American Samoa 96799

Arizona

FOR INFORMATION: Mr. John A. Marks, Director, Arizona Office of Tourism, 3507 N. Central Ave., Phoenix, AZ 85012, (602) 255-3618

Canyon Ranch (Tucson)

If fitness is your game, the name may very well be Canyon Ranch—five miles out of Tucson, spread over 28 acres in the foothills of the Santa Catalina Mountains. An inspiration of Mel Zuckerman, a businessman, Canyon Ranch boasts of twenty-one individual casitas, tennis and racquet-ball courts, swimming pools, hiking, jogging, bicycle and horseback riding trails.

The fitness and diet programs are keyed to the guests and supervised carefully. The 28,000 square foot fitness center offers every type of exercise plus herbal wraps. All types of massages, Swedish, Shiatsu, reflexology, to name but a few, are offered.

Men as well as women can enjoy plant extract facials or mineral packs from the "Dead Sea" area as well as lubricating and toning treatments.

Nutritional offerings appear on all menus. Canyon Ranch believes in nourishment for the body as well as the mind. Consultations and lectures by experts in a variety of fields are available. Here, the "whole person" is taken into consideration!

The "Intensive," a one-week program, is limited to 10–16 guests. One must be willing to engage in eight hours of structured programming, which includes a detoxification diet plus raw natural food, fruit, vegetables, and grains. The intent is to improve one's physical, mental and spiritual well-being from head to toe.

Arkansas

FOR INFORMATION: Mr. Terry Smith, Director, Arkansas Department of Tourism, 1 Capitol Mall, Little Rock, AR 72201, (501) 371–1087

The Arlington (Hot Springs)

The name "My Health and Beauty Spa" truly describes the program. Enhanced by its superb location in the elegant Arlington Hotel—the surrounding Hot Springs National Park with the Quachita Mountains in the background offers invigorating walks and hikes—this spa is a unique weekend experience. Many guests lose pounds and inches while being pampered.

I recall enjoying the world-famous hot thermal baths—they made me feel revitalized from head to toe. A fabulously relaxing and stress-dispelling massage helped release all my tensions.

At the spa you will feel like a "Queen for a Weekend" rather than "Queen for a Day." Under the supervision of Dr. Rick Guyton, co-author of BREAKING THE HABIT, your nutritional needs are seriously studied. Along with the elegant meals, you are encouraged to establish sensible and nutritious eating habits that you can rely on when you return home.

The fitness program features aerobic dancing, stretching and toning exercises, and water exercising—all aimed at helping you lose inches as well as pounds.

"My Health and Beauty Spa" weekends are available by advance reservation only.

Hot Springs National Park (Hot Springs)

Dixie's answer to all those highly touted radioactive, mineralized watering places in Europe, Hot Springs has attracted some seventy physicians to prescribe thermal treatments at fourteen hydrotherapy institutions. Standards are high owing to federal regulation of the forty-seven springs, whether they're operated by hotels or on the public Bath House Row.

Just write to the local chamber of commerce describing your needs, and they'll tell you which hostelry best meets them. Definitely in the spa tradition, complete with loofahs, cabinet vapor baths, reclining thermal baths, hot packs, whirlpools, underwater massages.

The Quapaw Bath House offers "after-hours" bathing on Saturday afternoons and Sunday mornings, and the bath-massage combinations are geared to the specific effect you seek: regular, sedative, or stimulating.

Hot Springs also offers good restaurants, golf, nightclubs, excellent supper clubs, fishing, camping, carriage rides, a wax museum, Animal Wonderland with dolphin acts, and a petting zoo. Be sure to sample the Mountain Valley water, a true native treat.

California

For Information: Ms. Barbara Klein, Director, California Office of Tourism, 1030 13th St., Suite 200, Sacramento, CA 95814, (916) 322–1396

The Ashram (Calabasas)

The Ashram, more a retreat than a spa, is situated slightly west of Los Angeles, close to the Pacific Ocean and surrounded by mountains. It is an oasis of peace and solitude far from the problems and stresses of modern life. While most other spas attempt to offer their guests every comfort and luxury, The Ashram goes to the other extreme. There are no private rooms, no beauty treatments, and the diet is mainly raw fruit and vegetables washed down with juices and herbal teas. The Ashram day is long—beginning at 6:00 A.M. with meditation, followed by long, arduous hikes through the mountains, intensive exercise programs and finally ending with yoga at 7:00 P.M. The Ashram accepts only 6 to 8 guests—men and women—for one-week sessions. If you have the stamina for a rigorous, unpampered routine, you should find The Ashram a unique and revitalizing experience.

Hidden Valley Health Ranch (Escondido)

Hidden Valley, operated by its owner and founder, Dr. Bernard Jensen, is self-styled as "designed with your mental, physical, and spiritual health in mind." Diet principles are stressed, but there is no trace of fanaticism.

The Ranch boasts its own organically grown fruit and vegetables, butter, milk, eggs, and grains—all served in copious portions. Meat is not served every day.

Outdoor activities include hiking, sunbathing, swimming, exercises, miniature golf, and shuffleboard. Evenings bring nutrition lectures, television, movies, guest presentations, bingo. Bedtime at the cottages is 9:30 P.M.

For an inexpensive look-see, you may drive to Hidden Valley for Sunday dinner. The meal is served at 12:30 P.M., and several activities are available afterwards. Be sure to phone ahead for a reservation.

Esalen Institute (Big Sur)

Interested in rejuvenating your psyche? Then Esalen may be your cup of tea.

(Warning: Esalen is not for sissies, weaklings, or squares. It is a heady experience and unforgettable if you've never "encountered" before.)

The glorious Big Sur landscape and seascape, rugged and primeval, is only a backdrop for the psyching that goes on during the various programs. Esalen will send you its catalogue of prices and programs, for which you'll do well to book as far in advance as possible.

A lot of informal rapping goes on at the two sulphur baths (one for women, the other for anybody of either sex, both nude) looking out over the cavorting seals on the rocky Pacific Coast. The Esalen massage is by now world-famous; it is basically Chinese in origin and can be exceedingly erotic. Exercises are highly eclectic, and run the gamut from Jack LaLanne to Hatha Yoga, and include "sensitivity" and "T-group" classics.

Dress is strictly what you care to make it, highly informal. The food is generally simple, but delicious. Although young people predominate, older guests are not made to feel uncomfortable in any way.

The Oaks (Ojai)

Located in the secluded artist's colony at Ojai, 80 minutes from Los Angeles, The Oaks is a small world unto itself.

It includes a swimming pool and spa on the terrace; gymnasium, indoor saunas, and steaming whirlpool; a smart galleria with beauty salon, cosmetics and gift shops; a mini art gallery and relaxing garden room.

It presents a healthful variety of gourmet low-calorie menus featuring natural food, fresh fruit and vegetables, homemade salad dressings and soups—all without a touch of additional salt, white sugar, or white flour in preparation.

And it presents a world of rejuvenation activities that gives you a choice of up to 12 optional fitness classes per day, ranging from light exercise to vigorous workouts, including water exercises, body dynamics, body contouring, yoga, and dance; plus evenings of entertainment, games, arts and crafts, and lectures.

Rates range from $89 per person per day single; $72 per person per day double; $64 per person per day triple. The Oaks offers massages, facials, hair and nail care, but at an additional cost.

The Palms (Palm Springs)

At Palm Springs, the internationally known resort, The Palms is a health spa in residence. You can tone up, wind down, lose weight, rest and relax—all in a sunny, fun vacation atmosphere. You'll enjoy The Palms' tasty diet cuisine, along with your choice of 12 fitness programs each day—all designed to tone up your muscles, raise your spirits, and help you lose as much as a pound a day safely.

The Palms offers escape from stress, poor eating habits, and lethargy. You can loosen up, lose weight, and lose yourself in a sun-soaked atmosphere that can be invigorating or tranquilizing, depending on your mood.

The Palms offers three-mile morning walks, 12 different exercise and dance classes a day, aqua-calisthenics, cellulite wraps, massages, facials, and 750-calorie gourmet meals.

The Palms is located in a setting of incomparable beauty and climate less than a two hour drive from Los Angeles.

Special weekend and mid-week packages are available. Shiela Cluff is owner as well as director of The Palms as well as The Oaks at Ojai. She is above all a true fitness expert in every way.

The Spa (Sonoma Mission Inn)

Located in the heart of the California wine country 40 miles from San Francisco, The Spa, attempts to provide a very personalized program.

Recently, all new spa facilities were installed just a few steps away from the main building complex.

The chef's spa menu is tempting, balanced, and healthful. Whether you are on the 850-calories-a-day reducing plan, or the 1,200-calories-a-day maintenance diet, you will never feel deprived. There is also a once-a-week Cleansing Day liquid diet.

The spa accommodates 30 women at a time on a six-day, three-day, or weekend program. Men's weekends are scheduled throughout the year. Couples weeks are in the planning stages.

At the Sonoma Spa each guest is given personal attention and an individual program to follow. These programs are devised by fitness director Gary Chlad and supervised by staff members.

The Spa offers the most up-to-date gym equipment, including pneumatic resistance machines similar to Nautilus equipment, except that they use compressed air rather than weights and pulleys to create the resistance factor. A spinal-alignment gravity device gives you a sense of weightlessness, sends blood rushing to your brain and gently moves your vertebrae into natural alignment. A Dynavit electronic bicycle measures your cardiovascular abilities by monitoring your pulse rate as you pedal.

The Spa programs also include warm-up exercises, morning hikes, spot-reducing exercise, indoor running, trampolines, rowing machines, stretch and water-exercise classes and stress-management sessions. They also offer hydrotherapy and herbal-wrap therapy.

Hospitality and comfort have always been the by-words of the Sonoma Mission Inn. From the moment a guest enters the exquisite, marble-fountained spa atrium until the time she walks out, she realizes an exceptional experience.

Colorado

FOR INFORMATION: Mr. Harold L. Haney, Program Director, Office of Tourism Information & Services,

Division of Commerce and Development, 1313 Sherman St., Denver, CO 80203, (303) 892–3045

El Dorado Springs
Just over a mile high, El Dorado Springs has a radium pool, rental cottages, and is open from May 30 through Labor Day. Just twenty-five miles from Denver.

Glenwood Springs
Famous Western Slope resort, seventy miles west of Denver on U.S. 6. Claims world's largest outdoor hot mineral-water pool; open year-round; baths, pool, massage, lodge.

Radium Hot Springs Spa (Idaho Springs)
These radium hot springs have been used ever since Chief Idaho brought his wounded and sick braves here for recuperation. At the Blue Ribbon Tunnel, one can drink refreshing mineral waters. Reasonable rates for sauna, massage, radium baths.

Manitou Springs (Manitou)
At the Gateway to the Pikes Peak region, Manitou Springs has seventy-five motels, thirty-five restaurants, ten campgrounds, a heated municipal pool, riding stables, historic castles and Victorian homes, and some pretty fair entertainment. There is radioactive soda water, various baths, physiotherapy treatments, massages.

Ouray Swimming Pool (Ouray)
Ouray has more than the name would imply—radium hot springs baths, vapor caves, massages—all just 305 miles southwest of Denver. Lodging for five hundred. Old Indian baths.

Connecticut

FOR INFORMATION: Mr. Barnett Laschever, Director, Tourism Division, Connecticut Department of Economic Development, 210 Washington St., Hartford, CT 06106, (203) 566–3385

Delaware

FOR INFORMATION: Ms. Jan Geddes, Acting Manager, Delaware State Travel Service, 630 State College Rd., P.O. Box 1401, Dover DE 19901, (302) 736–4254

District of Columbia

FOR INFORMATION: Ms. Mary Walker. Director of Visitor Marketing, Washington Convention and Visitors Assn., 1575 Eye St., NW, Washington, DC 20005, (202) 789–7000

Florida

FOR INFORMATION: Mr. Edward Gilbert, Director, Division of Tourism, 107 West Gaines St., Tallahassee, FL 32302 (904) 488–5606

The Palm Beach Spa (Palm Beach)
The philosophy here is that attaining health is tantamount to achieving beauty, so the accent is on the former: dietetic counseling, exercise in a mirrored gym, whirlpool, steam, sauna, indoor or solarium massage, two pools, nearby beach, tennis, golf. Check the chef for recipes of delicious, low-calorie, salt-free, low-fat menus, including paella, veal marsala, Chinese pepper steak, shrimp creole, and rack of lamb. Two-week cures, among other plans.

Warm Mineral Springs (Venice)
Located twelve miles south of Venice on U.S. 41, Warm Mineral Springs has fango baths as well as its natural warm waters with eighteen parts of minerals per thousand of water. Its ten-million-daily gallon flow is more than four times that of Vichy, Baden-Baden, Hot Springs, or Aix-les-Bains. Treatments for arthritis, rheumatism, muscular ailments, and skin disorders. Bed down at Warm Mineral Springs Apartments or Warm Mineral Springs Motel and you get a 50 percent reduction on the normal admission charge to the baths.

Georgia

FOR INFORMATION: Mr. Doug Weaver, Director, Tourism Division, Georgia Department of Industry & Trade, P.O. Box 1776, Atlanta, GA 30301, (404) 656–3550

Warm Springs Foundation (Warm Springs)
For better or worse, these lovely thermal baths have been pre-empted by the state for its special patients. One of them was the late Franklin D. Roosevelt, who found relaxation and relief in those mineral waters over the years. Generally not open to the public.

177

Guam

FOR INFORMATION: Mr. Joseph Cepeda, Acting General Manager, Guam Visitors Bureau, P.O. Box 3520, Agana, Guam 96910

Hawaii

FOR INFORMATION: Mr. Kennett Char, President Hawaii Visitors Bureau, P.O. Box 8527, Honolulu, HA 96815 (808) 923–1811, FTS: 8–0–415–556–0220.

The Royal Door Health and Beauty Spa (Honolulu)

For a real ring-a-ding vacation, you'll have to look far and wide to beat Hawaii's Royal Door Spa in Honolulu—and the likes of Canadian Prime Minister Pierre Trudeau, film director John Schlesinger, and American Bar Association head, Chesterfield Smith have looked no further.

Here you'll find a congenial mix of residents and tourists using the spa facilities of the Royal Hawaiian Hotel—or the Pink Palace.

Where else does the exercise list include belly dancing, hula lessons, and scientific stretches? And where else can you get cellulite massage, thalassotherapy, acupressure massage, water exercises, facials, pedicures, manicures, saunas, and whirlpools—all together in one place?

You're pretty much on your own, free to split for the beach when you wish, or have a seaside sand sauna. But you'll get as much pampering as you can stand for your money.

The Door diet is heavy on such goodies as papayas, pineapples, guava juice, bamboo-shoot salads, MAHIMAHI, and the like.

Idaho

FOR INFORMATION: Mr. Stephen Wilson, Manager, Visitor Services Section, Division of Economic & Community Affairs, State Capitol Building, Room 108, Boise, ID 83720, (208) 334–2470

Lava Hot Springs

One of some fifty mineral and hot springs in the state, Lava Hot Springs has the warmth but none of the bad smells of many mineral-water springs. In fact, as you stand on the pool's soft sand, the hot water bubbles up at a comfortably hot 110 degrees.

It's a swimmer's paradise, with nearly a million gallons of 86-degree water filling Olympic- and AAU-sized pools, with fifty-meter racing lanes and a ten-meter diving platform. Also shallow depths for small-fry. Has hosted as many as 3,500 guests in a day.

Illinois

FOR INFORMATION: Ms. Marjorie Beenders, Acting Managing Director, Illinois Office of Tourism, Dept. of Commerce & Community Affairs, 222 South College Street, Springfield, IL 62706, (217) 782–7139

St. Joseph's Health Resort (Wedron)

If the idea of a modestly priced religious retreat-cum-sulfur-springs appeals to you, visit the lovely, tranquil spa operated by the Missionary Sisters of the Most Sacred Heart of Jesus. (No religious restriction for guests.)

Medical care is handled by the Sulphur Lick Springs Clinic Medical Director, T. G. Hiebert, and Donald Fruendt, R.P.T. The staff is affiliated with the Chicago Medical School and Schwab Rehabilitation Hospital, so you're in excellent hands.

Some one thousand gallons of pure sulfur water per minute rise up from great depths through 175 feet of sandstone at a temperature of 52 degrees.

With special diets to rejuvenate the body, and the message of the sisters to rejuvenate the spirit, you can't go far wrong on an authentic get-away-from-it-all retreat.

Original Mineral Springs Hotel and Bath House (Oakville)

Called the Little Hot Springs of Illinois, this spa gives you mineral springs and skilled hands for its famous Swedish massage. Its cozy size and homey atmosphere have made it a marvelous hideaway for rat-race-fleeing exeuctives. Rates reasonable, food aplenty.

Indiana

FOR INFORMATION: Ms. Jan Louise Diggins, Director, Tourism Development Division, Indiana Dept. of Commerce, 440 North Meridian Street, Indianapolis, IN 46204, (317) 232–8860

French Lick—Sheraton Hotel and Country Club (French Lick)

This is a stately turn-of-the-century hotel that once boasted of Whitneys, Morgans, Vanderbilts, and the like, before a long decline set in. At its nadir a couple of decades ago, Sheraton bought it, expanded the plant, and revamped and refurbished the hotel.

The French Lick occupies 1,600 valley acres flanking Hoosier National Forest and offers sauna, whirlpool, massage, steam, exercise equipment, a beauty salon, and their famous Pluto spring-mineral waterbaths. (Remember when they used to drink that stuff?)

The hotel now has a three-days-and-two-nights "New Leaf" reshaping program with a beauty retreat for women. If you detest the forcible chumminess of some spas, this one might be for you. You can enjoy your dietary "gourmet" menu in a special private dining room.

Programs begin on Monday and Wednesday—some women electing to do two or more programs consecutively. Don't forget swimsuit, slippers, sportswear, and dressy dinner apparel. The hotel provides leotards, but recommends toting your own for maximum comfort.

Extras: tennis, golf, biking, surrey rides, skeet and trap shooting, and bowling.

Iowa

For Information: Mr. Harold Morgan, Director, Tourism and Travel Division, Iowa Development Commission, 250 Jewett Building, Des Moines, IA 50309, (515) 281–3401

Kansas

For Information: Ms. Cathy Kruzic, Director, Travel Marketing Division, Kansas Department of Economic Development, 503 Kansas Ave., Sixth Floor, Topeka, KS 66603, (913) 296–3481

Kentucky

For Information: Ms. Lois Mateus, Commissioner, Kentucky Department of Tourism, Capitol Plaza Tower, Frankfort, KY 40601, (502) 564–4930

Louisiana

For Information: Ms. Cornelia Carrier, Asst. Secretary, Louisiana Office of Tourism, P.O. Box 44291, Capitol Station, Baton Rouge, LA 70804, (504) 389–5981

Hot Wells Resort Center (Boyce)

Interested in legends of healing miracles? Here's one for you:

Back in 1913, an oil-drilling crew found a well they weren't looking for. Instead of oil, up gushed hot mineral waters from deep within the earth. A crewman washed his hands in the water and the very next day a skin rash that had plagued him for years began to clear up.

Soon others began using the waters as a balm for their skin ailments, and some of them were cured.

The state of Louisiana operates these mineral bath treatments, which are said to heal not only skin disorders, but also circulatory malfunctions, fatigue, tension, and other conditions. The water is supposed to be a terrific complexion perker-upper.

If you plan to stay overnight or for a few days, there are reasonably priced motels in the vicinity.

Maine

For Information: Mr. George Stobie, Director, Maine Publicity Bureau, 97 Winthrop St., Hollowell, ME 04347, (207) 289–2423

Maryland

For Information: Mr. Kurt Alverson, Director, Maryland Office of Tourist Development, 1748 Forest Dr., Annapolis, MD 21401, (301) 269–2686

Massachusetts

For Information: Mr. Francis J. Shaw, Director, Division of Tourism, Massachusetts Department of Commerce and Development, 100 Cambridge Street, Boston, MA 02202, (617) 727–3205

The New England Conservatory of Health at Magnolia Manor (Magnolia)

Although I've never been there, I'm inclined by hearsay to credit the conservatory's boast of being "the largest institution in America dedicated to improving health by natural nutrition and naturopathic procedures."

Just forty-five minutes from Boston on the North Shore and overlooking the ocean, it gives you a variety of weight-reduction and dietary programs: fasting, juices and herbal teas, vegetarian, high protein, et al.

Cynics take note: the Conservatory GUARANTEES

you a minimum one-pound-per-day weight loss. (My advice, though, is to take it easy and settle for less.)

It features exercise, massage (including facial massages and zone therapy), sauna and steam, nutrition and health lectures, nature walks, ocean-water pools out of doors, yoga, sleep therapy, music/color therapy, and physiotherapy.

You'll also find what the more orthodox might consider a gamut of fringe practitioners. There's a regular physician on hand, as well as a naturopath, a reflexologist, a hypnotist, and a yogi.

Michigan

FOR INFORMATION: Mr. Jack S. Wilson, Director, Michigan Tourist Council, 300 S. Capitol Avenue, Suite 102, Lansing, MI 48909, (517) 373–0670

The Kon Tiki Spa (Riverside)

If you've tried all the fad diets, see if the Kon Tiki's latest appeals to you: totally liquid meals.

The Kon Tiki is a small spa close to Lake Michigan that profits from this proximity and uses the beach for swimming and walking exercises. Also a good gym, sauna, whirlpool, and the usual facilities.

Minnesota

FOR INFORMATION: Mr. Henry Todd, Jr., Director, Minnesota Tourism Bureau, 419 N. Robert St., St. Paul, MN 55101, (612) 296–5027

Mississippi

FOR INFORMATION: Mr. George Williams, Director, Mississippi Division of Tourism, Box 849, 1504 Walter Sillers Bldg., Jackson, MS 39205, (601) 354–6715

Missouri

FOR INFORMATION: Mr. Charles L. Boyd, Director, Missouri Division of Tourism, P.O. Box 1055, Jefferson City, MO 65102, (314) 751–4133

Montana

FOR INFORMATION: Mr. John Wilson, Director, Travel Promotion Bureau, Montana Department of Highways, Helena, MT 59601, (406) 449–2654

Fairmont Hot Springs Resort (Anaconda)

Not exactly a SPA spa, but Montana's entry for a change-of-pace vacation. Located at Discovery Basin Ski Resort, its muscle-soothing après-ski activity includes swimming in outdoor and indoor (odorless) hot mineral-water pools and soaking in "swirlpools." A "cure"? Well, with clean, fresh mountain air, vigorous exercise, hot mineral-spring bathing waters, you're almost sure to feel better afterwards.

Nebraska

FOR INFORMATION: Ms. Diane Johnston, Director, Nebraska Division of Travel and Tourism, P.O. Box 94666, State Capitol, Lincoln, NB 68509, (402) 471–3111

Nevada

FOR INFORMATION: Ms. Leslie Sluman, Director of Tourism, Capitol Complex, Carson City, NV 89710, (702) 885–4322

New Hampshire

FOR INFORMATION: Norman Vandernoot, Director, New Hampshire Office of Vacation Travel, P.O. Box 856, Concord, NH 03301, (603) 271–2666

New Jersey

FOR INFORMATION: Mr. Stephen B. Richer, Director, N.J. Division of Travel & Tourism, P.O. Box 400, Trenton, NJ 08625, (609) 292–2470

Harbor Island Spa (WestEnd)

Harbor Island Spa gives ocean lovers an opportunity to breathe fresh air filled with negative ions.

As sea air stimulates your appetite, Harbor Isle provides non-fattening meals that taste delicious. The green-and-white dining room is very attractive. Candles and crisp linen make the dining table look festive. Portions are moderate, salads are fresh and crisp, the diet dressing good. Harbor Isle is famous for its exceptional mousses with calorie counts only 40 per serving—your choice of chocolate, mocha, butterscotch, lemon, even pineapple-coconut, to name a few.

Stuart Paskow has whipped up a colorful jello cake for guests' birthdays or other festive occasions. High-protein main courses include fresh fish, chicken, veal, egg dishes—all satisfying (salt and fat-free) accompanied by a small salad with a tasty dressing. The popular De Bole sesame bread sticks are made from artichoke flour (one per meal suggested). De Bole also makes a rusk that has a licorice-like flavor to go with your beverage instead of a high-calorie cookie.

Fresh vegetables are steamed—and herb-seasoned soups skimmed. Red meat thinly sliced, is served twice weekly.

There are separate exercise rooms for men and women where one can work out plus steam, sauna, and whirlpool facilities. Harbor Island Spa is especially convenient and healthful for people in the New York Metropolitan Area.

The Original Englewood Cliffs Milk Farm (Englewood Cliffs)

Just a brief distance from the Jersey side of the George Washington Bridge, the Milk Farm helps its small clientele fleeing the city for weight reduction or just plain relaxation. The reducing program, under supervision, includes a range of diets, from liquid to high protein. The salads, which I haven't tried yet, sound and look particularly scrumptious.

While the Milk Farm is earthy, it does offer daily massages, steam treatments, facials, pedicures, and hair styling. There are also exercise machines, a solarium, and an outdoor swimming pool for the warm months. Informality is the keynote.

A bus from New York City's Port Authority Terminal stops only a block away.

New Mexico

For Information: Mr. Fabian Chavez, Jr., Director, Tourist Division, New Mexico Department of Development, 113 Washington Avenue, Santa Fe, NM 87501, (505) 827–3101

In New Mexico, there are three hot-bath health resorts: Ojo Caliente Mineral Springs in the Jemez Mountains, fifty miles north of Santa Fe; Radium Hot Springs in south-central New Mexico, near Las Cruces; and the Truth and Consequences area in the southeast of the state boasts numerous springs, bathhouses, motels, restaurants.

If these don't strike you as worth a special trip, you might wish to pause at one or all of them for a therapeutic—or at least relaxing—dip on any trip to Far West. At any rate, this state is a splendid land of mountains, deserts, purple sunsets, Indian crafts, and abandoned cliff dwellings.

New York

For Information: Mr. Joseph J. Horan, Director, Travel Bureau, New York State Department of Commerce, 99 Washington Avenue, Albany, NY 12210, (518) 474–4116

Saratoga Spa (Saratoga Springs)

Basking in the glory of its Gay Nineties heyday when it had guests like Diamond Jim Brady and Lillian Russell, the Saratoga Spa is still—believe it or not—in business.

The once glittering casino is now a museum, the grand hotels are no longer so grand, but the mineral waters still flow, and the Saratoga Performing Arts Center offers ballet, concerts, and popular entertainers.

The racetrack is open July and August.

It's sort of sad to see my parents' favorite spa decline to an out-patient resort. But I recommend highly the waters for bathing and drinking. Massage and other treatments available.

Pawling Health Manor (Hyde Park)

Natural hygienists and fasters seem to cherish Pawling Health Manor as a "retreat devoted to the living of natural health principles." Sunbathing, exercise, fasting, controlled diets. No smoking. One-week minimum.

North Carolina

For Information: Mr. Charles Heatherly, Director, Travel and Tourism Division, North Carolina Department of Commerce, P.O. Box 25249, Raleigh, NC 27611, (919) 733–4171

North Dakota

For Information: Mr. Michael Foster, Director of Tourism, North Dakota Tourism Promotion, Economic Development Commission, Bismarck, ND 58501, (701) 224–2525

Ohio

For Information: Mrs. Pat Brown, Manager, Ohio Office of Travel and Tourism, P.O. Box 1001, Columbus, OH 43216, (614) 466–8844

Kerr House (Grand Rapids)

The Kerr House, just 30 miles south of Toledo, is quaintly picturesque—situated along the wooded tow path of the historic Erie Canal with a fine view of the scenic Maumee River. The ambiance there is conducive to a new peace you can sense that refreshes and revitalizes both body and spirit.

Your week at the Kerr House, a beautifully restored Victorian mansion, offers luxurious guest accommodations. Only eight guests are accepted (the week runs from Sunday to Friday). They receive full individual attention starting with breakfast in bed, stretching, breathing and yoga exercises, and aerobic dancing. Throughout the week you'll enjoy whirlpool, saunas, facials, beauty treatments, herbal wraps, massages, foot reflexology, as well as delicious meals of natural food nutritionally balanced and calorie controlled. An excellent chef prepares the gourmet food served at the Kerr House.

Explaining why the Kerr House is devoted to women only, Laurie Hostelter, the Director, says, "Women give so much to their families, their husbands and their careers, they need an opportunity to give something back to themselves."

Oklahoma

FOR INFORMATION: Mr. Eugene Dilbeck, Director, Division of Marketing Services, Oklahoma Department of Tourism and Recreation, 504 Will Rogers Memorial Bldg., Oklahoma City, OK 73105, (405) 521-2406

Shangri-La (Afton)

A sort of spa-i-fied resort, Shangri-La has a marina, golf course, tennis, indoor and outdoor pools, whirlpool, boating, and fishing. Park your private plane on their private airstrip. A few condominium homes, regular guest accommodations, and three restaurants (one with orchestra and dancing). Men and women have massage, sauna, steam, gym, yoga, and diet services—at extra charges. Limousine service and babysitting.

Will Rogers Hotel (Claremore)

This quaint old hostelry brags that it is the place "where the world bathes itself to health . . . with an Eastern Atmosphere, Western Welcome, and Southern Hospitality." Radioactive mineral baths stake claims for improvement of rheumatism, alcoholism, dandruff, athelete's foot, poison ivy, and poison oak.

Oregon

FOR INFORMATION: Ms. Shirley Eads, Manager Director, Travel Information Section, 101 Transportation Building, Salem, OR 97310, (503) 378-6546

Kah/Nee/Ta Vacation Resort (Warm Springs)

Most luxurious of the Oregon thermal resorts is the Kah/Nee/Ta Vacation Resort, north of Warm Springs, with a modest spread of 564,000 acres! It is owned and operated by the Confederated Tribes of the Warm Springs Reservation of Oregon.

Campers can haul in their trailers, bed down at the ultra-modern lodge, or settle into a teepee.

Swimming pools are heated to 95 degrees by the natural mineralized spring waters—while the Roman-style bath springs come up at 145 degrees. Follow your bath with a stimulating massage. Also available: golf and miniature golf, babysitters, Indian Crafts Shop and boutiques, a riding stable, three cocktail lounges, three restaurants, Indian festivals and ceremonies, rodeos, and movies.

Breitenbush Hot Springs Resort (Detroit)

For someone seeking a modest-budget spring-and-summer resort, Breitenbush might be the ticket. Cabins, camping facilities, bathhouse with mineral baths (up to 178 degrees), and massage. Treatments for arthritis, gout, goiter, and "nicotine habit."

Pennsylvania

FOR INFORMATION: Mr. Skip Becker, Director, Bureau of Travel Development, Pennsylvania Department of Commerce, 416 Forum Bldg., Harrisburg, PA 17120, (717) 787-5453

Puerto Rico

FOR INFORMATION: Frances Rios de Moran, Executive Director, Puerto Rico Tourism Company (PRTC), GPO Box 3072, San Juan, PR 00903, (809) 754-9292

El Conquistador

El Conquistador, the Caribbean prototype of the complete-facilities luxury resort, was built on the cliff-top northeast point of the island (three-quarters of an hour from San Juan), overlooking the Caribbean on one side and the Atlantic Ocean on the other.

Accommodations are built on three different sections of the hill (rooms on the MIDDLE level are straight out of a decorator's snazziest portfolio). Transportation for the three levels is by cable car and funicular railway. There are three swimming pools (one saltwater), a well-kept golf course, tennis courts, scuba diving, good food, entertainment, gambling casino, marina, and an entire spa building for health-conscious vacationers.

The spa offers daily check-ups, special diets, saunas, steam rooms, whirlpools, gym, solarium, massages, "Turkish" wraps, and exercises. There are special Spa package rates.

Rhode Island

FOR INFORMATION: Mr. Leonard J. Panaggio, Asst. Director, Rhode Island Tourist Promotion Division, 7 Jackson Walk Way, Providence, RI 02903, (401) 277–2614

South Carolina

FOR INFORMATION: Mr. Robert G. Liming, Director, Division of Tourism, South Carolina Dept. of Parks, Recreation and Tourism, 1205 Pendleton St., Suite 113, Columbia, SC 29201, (803) 758–2536

Sea Pines Behavioral Institute (Hilton Head)

Dr. Peter Miller, director of Sea Pines contends that dieting has become a national obsession. Being overweight is simply the result of overeating and inactivity. You need to alter your habits for permanent weight control.

Dr. Miller does this by taking limited groups through a 26-day in-residence program consisting of behavior modification training, dieting, nutritional education, and controlled physical activity to unlearn poor behavioral patterns.

The Institute conducts 12 sessions a year. Guests are exposed to a serious course of daily exercise, a 700-calorie-a-day food plan, and a routine of daily behavioral seminars.

An added bonus is the Institute's location at the Wakeley House in the heart of Sea Pines Plantation, one of the country's leading resorts. Guests are encouraged to utilize the resort's 4,500 acres of wooded recreation area, nature preserves, bicycle trails, golf courses, tennis centers, and Atlantic beachfront.

Institute participants live in spacious, condo-style villas located within walking distance of the center. All meals are eaten together as each group takes part in the daily, personalized, planned regimen, to meet the specific weight-loss needs of the individual.

Each month's session is limited to 20 participants exclusively. Fees for the 26-day session include private room and bath, all meals, complete hospital medical examinations, daily workshops, supervised exercise programs, and consultations. Enrollment is based on a first-come, first-served basis.

Further information may be obtained by writing Dept. P-1, Sea Pines Behavioral Institute, Sea Pines Plantation, Hilton Head Island, SC 29928

South Dakota

FOR INFORMATION: Ms. Susan Edwards, Director, Division of Tourism, 221 South Central Avenue, Pierre, SD 57501, (605) 773–3301

Evan's Plunge (Pierre)

Strictly speaking, Evan's Plunge doesn't qualify as either spa or resort, but I couldn't omit mentioning "the world's largest natural warm-water indoor swimming pool" (fifty by two hundred feet) where the 87-degree water is changed sixteen times daily and has calcium, sodium, and potassium mineralizing the H_2O. The Sioux and the Cheyenne tribes used to bicker over ownership of the springs, which they used for both drinking and bathing.

If you're ever touring the Badlands, you'll find Evan's Plunge and ideal place to slake thirst and soak your weary bones. Open summers from 8:00 A.M. to 11:00 P.M.

Tennessee

FOR INFORMATION: Mr. Mark Onan, Commissioner, Tennessee Department of Tourist Development, P.O. Box 23170, Nashville, TN 37202, (615) 741–7994

Texas

FOR INFORMATION: Mr. Frank Hildebrand, Executive Director, Texas Tourist Development Agency, Box 12008, Capitol Station, Austin, TX 87811, (512) 475–4326

Falls Motor Hotel and Health Spa (Marlin)

The Falls Health Spa is the hub of a wheel whose spokes are roads from Dallas to Austin, Houston to

Fort Worth, and Galveston to Abilene—ergo convenient to any Texas traveler. Simple accommodations, heated pool, beauty parlor, mineral-water tub-bath, vapor bath, steam, sauna, salt rub, hot room with hot packs, exercise equipment, cooling room, and massage.

Utah

FOR INFORMATION: Phillip Keene, III, Director, Utah Travel Council, Council Hall, Capitol Hill, Salt Lake City, UT 84114, (801) 328–5681

Vermont

FOR INFORMATION: Mr. Donald A. Lyons, Director Vermont Travel Division, 61 Elm Street, Montpelier, VT 05602, (802) 828–3236

Green Mountain at Fox Run (Ludlow)

America is very involved with physical fitness, but diet and nutritional concerns lag well behind. Most who act to improve eating habits wander blindly through a maze of fad diets in search of miracle benefits.

This is not the case at Green Mountain at Fox Run, an Educational Community for Weight and Health Management. Since 1973, 2,000 women from 49 states and 22 countries have found something unique. There are no set diets and no guilt feelings allowed on the premises.

The Green Mountain philosophy, lifestyle repatterning, is a three-part program of nutrition education, exercise physiology, and behavior and attitude awareness. Designed for the long term, it emphasizes building self-esteem by promoting conscious choice.

It includes all the facilities and activities of a mountain resort—a swimming pool, sauna, golf course, and the Okemo Mountain ski area—but women do not go there for a pampered vacation. They go for lifestyle repatterning.

Lots of physical activity—for strength, flexibility, and aerobic fitness—lets you shed inhibitions along with pounds. Individualized attention and the rationale for specific exercises used are key features of the program along with group participation. Lecture and discussion groups provide further support. There are three meals a day with an optional snack.

Thelma Wayler, director of Green Mountain says, "We want our women to leave here with the ability to make choices and the confidence to continue the Green Mountain experience at home. Most of all, we want them to leave here feeling good about themselves."

Virgin Islands

FOR INFORMATION: Ms. Leona Bryant, Director, Virgin Islands Division of Tourism, P.O. Box 6400, Charlotte Amalie, St. Thomas, Virgin Islands 00801, (809) 774–8784

Virginia

FOR INFORMATION: Mr. Marshall E. Murdaugh, Commissioner, Virginia State Travel Service, 6 North Sixth Street, Richmond, VA 23219, (804) 786–2051

The Homestead (Hot Springs)

Presidents from Thomas Jefferson to Dwight Eisenhower have picked the Homestead for unbuttoned relaxation and repose.

The seventeen thousand acres have three eighteen-hole golf courses, seven tennis courts, a stocked trout stream, indoor and outdoor pools, skeet and trap shoots, miles of horseback-riding trails.

Open year-round, the Homestead features skiing and sleighing in the winter, surrey or buckboard riding during the summer.

The health spa portion of the Homestead offers mineral baths, ultra-violet and ultra-sonic treatments, saunas, steambaths, whirlpools, massage, and special exercises.

A special two-week spa package is available, otherwise it's entirely American plan—and not cheap.

Warm Springs Inn (Warm Springs)

One of the rare sulphur springs where the water emerges from underground at almost exactly body temperature, Warm Springs has a long and good reputation for energizing and revitalizing you. The 98-degree water has a way of creating a special euphoria and spiritual catharsis in the most pressure-dogged executive or housewife. The Inn's rooms and meals are reasonably priced. Its facilities include golf, fishing, horses, trap shooting. Informal and down-home atmosphere.

Washington

FOR INFORMATION: Mr. William Taylor, Assistant Director, Travel Development Division, Department of Commerce and Economic Development, General

Administration Building, Olympia, WA 98504, (206) 753–5630

Soap Lake (Soap Lake)

Located near the geographic center of the state, Soap Lake is so-called because of the suds that form along the shores on windy days. The Indians called it SMOKIAM (meaning "healing waters")—a label stemming from its content of sixteen minerals and its traditional use as drinking and bathing water. Bath salts are also extracted from the water and sold commercially.

The thirst of the Soap Lakers for their lake water is so strong that many have conduits pumping it into their homes, motels, and bathhouses to supplement the local well system.

Many resorts abound in the area, and the McKay Memorial Hospital has not only regular, qualified physicians, but also osteopaths, chiropractors, licensed masseurs, and hydrotherapy facilities.

This is a casual, settle-and-board-where-you-please resort that's awfully kind to ANYBODY's pocketbook.

West Virginia

FOR INFORMATION: Mr. Joseph Fowler, Manager, Travel Development Division, West Virginia Department of Commerce, 1900 Washington Street, East, Charleston, WV 25305, (304) 348–2286

The Greenbriar (White Sulphur Springs)

This mountain resort's variegated 6,500 acres (gardens, woodlands, lawns) have attracted princes, presidents, and prime ministers, as well as people like you and me who wish to combine a sporting vacation in a rugged setting with good professional spa therapies.

The Greenbriar Clinic offers an out-patient three-day check-up, using blood tests, cardiograms, X-rays, blood pressure and metabolism tests, consultations, and other modern diagnostic tools.

The sports available include golf, tennis, riding, shooting, bowling, swimming, and carriage rides.

The spa itself offers Swedish massage and, of course, sulphur springs (yes, it does smell like rotten eggs, but feels so good).

Berkeley Springs (Berkeley Springs)

This delightful valley thermal station's first public relations man was George Washington, who not only slept here, but lolled about in the Roman baths, surveyed, and summered here. The waters are fresh, sweet and hot (74.3 degrees), and are taken for gout, diabetes, arthritis, and rheumatism.

Take your pick of an ordinary bathtub or one of fourteen Roman sunken pools lined with tile or marble, which hold up to four hundred gallons of water. You can adjust the temperature of the water and afterwards try out infra-red, ultra-violet treatments or massages. Hotel rates are quite reasonable.

Wisconsin

FOR INFORMATION: Mr. Donald A. Woodruff, Executive Director, Wisconsin Division of Tourism, 123 West Washington Avenue, Room, 650, Madison, WI 53702, (608) 266–2147

Wyoming

FOR INFORMATION: Mr. Randall H. Wagner, Director, Wyoming Travel Commission, 2320 Capitol Avenue, Cheyenne, WY 82002, (307) 777–7777

Thermopolis (Thermopolis)

Did you know that the world's largest mineral hot springs is located in Wyoming? Yup. Every twenty-four hours, some 18,600,000 gallons of 135-degree water flow from this source in Hot Springs State Park. It offers year-round swimming, a public bathhouse, several small spas with special bath and massage services, as well as all the outdoor and water sports. Thermopolis houses the Gottsche Rehabilitation Center with its fifty-bed hospital that has bonuses of mineral-water hydrotherapy, electrotherapy, exercises, and so on.

Saratoga Hot Springs (Saratoga)

You've got your choice of hot (115 degrees) and cold running mineral springs and baths, with private or public bathing facilities. The Saratoga Inn pumps hot mineral water directly into several of its bedrooms. Great vacation spot.

Canada

FOR INFORMATION: Canadian Government Office of Tourism, 1251 Avenue of the Americas, New York, N.Y. 10019

Canada's famous spas are all located in and around the Rocky Mountain national parks. Any itinerary of this majestic part of our continent should include a stopover at one of them.

Banff Hot Springs

In Alberta's Banff National Park, there are three sulphur springs that empty into a large pool, which is open from May to September. Further up Sulphur Mountain, there is another large sulphur pool with 100-plus-degree water temperatures.

There's something for almost everyone here: camp sites, motels, mountaintop chalets, and ski villages. The sprawling old Banff Springs Hotel gives its guests a panoramic picture-postcard view of the mountains that leaves them breathless. The hotel is set in a ravine, framed by mountains and lush greenery.

The springs themselves are especially glorious on a fall night when steam rises from them as from a witch's cauldron.

Banff Springs offers all the services of a lavish resort: nightclub, discotheque, beauty salon, indoor pool, summer and winter sports, and a host of entertainments. Your free time can be spent visiting the Banff National Park, nearby Lake Louise, trading posts, art exhibits, and skiing.

Miette Hot Springs

These springs, at 129 degrees, are the hottest in Canada. Located in Jasper National Park, the area couldn't be better suited for hiking, horseback riding, mountain climbing. You also have steam rooms and a pool lit for nighttime dips. Miette Hot Springs Bungalows offers hotel rooms and suites—as well as classic bungalows complete with living rooms and delightful kitchens.

South America and The Caribbean

Argentina

FOR INFORMATION: Argentine Consulate General, 12 West 56th Street, New York, N.Y. 10019

Rio Hondo

A mammoth vacation resort and spa located in the north of Argentina, Rio Hondo's hot springs are piped to all of its hotels, and even many private residences in the area. The busy season is from May through October. Remember that their seasons are the opposite from ours.

In season, there are added attractions for tourists, with festive carnivals and the casinos luring huge crowds, many of them Argentinians, as this is a favorite vacation spot for THEM, too. You have a wide variety of accommodations to choose from, including some extremely lush and fashionable hotels.

Cormillot Clinic

The Cormillot Clinic is just a few minutes from downtown Buenos Aires. Housed in several staid old brownstones, it is one of the most sophisticated diet clinics in the world.

Read "starvation" for diet. But never fear: Dr. Alberto Cormillot, an internist, heads a qualified staff of doctors, psychotherapists, and nutritionists who will monitor your every waking and sleeping moment as the pounds slice from your torso.

One 417-pound patient lost 136 pounds in 120 days during her first stay, and 101 pounds in 180 days during her second. On her third visit of fifty-five days, she lost another 50 pounds.

Not surprisingly, I'm told that nine of every ten patients are women. The twenty-five patients accepted by the clinic are given regular blood-pressure checks, urine analyses, EKGs, blood tests, and basal metabolism tests. Cormillot believes that the head is mainly to blame for body weight, and if you detect a strong psychotherapeutic atmosphere there, it's quite intentional.

Under this severe fasting regimen, as you peruse your book or crochet or watch television, you will lose .7 calories for every pound you're carrying. If you dance, you'll lose 2.2 calories. Ping-Pong will remove 2.5 calories.

If you insist on this type of reducing, figure an average loss of 10 percent of your weight each month you spend at Cormillot's Clinic.

———

Brazil

FOR INFORMATION: Brazilian Tourism Authority, 230 Park Avenue, New York, N.Y. 10169

Encouraged by the great variety of their natural mineral springs, the Brazilians have recently redeveloped older spas, and large, modern, new ones are under construction. Tennis, rowing, riding, swimming, and hiking are generally available at Brazilian spas. Some offer skiing and skating as well.

Araxa

Araxa is an elegant, older spa that has been renovated to accommodate over one thousand guests, all cared for superbly. Araxa could be a convenient antidote to over-indulgence at the Rio Carnival, since it's only a two-hour flight away. The area is beautifully scenic, with magnificent floral beds and wooded grounds, and a picturesque lake. The climate is perpetually sunny and warm; the waters, good for diabetics; the mud-packs, given by the beauty salon and used by South American ladies for centuries, beautifying.

There are sulphur-mudbaths, a hot, slightly radioactive pool, other swimming pools, a gymnasium, a nightclub, movies, boating, and fishing facilities.

Pocos De Caldas

Another top Brazilian spa is Pocos De Caldas, said to be the biggest watering place in Brazil, with spring water piped directly to your room in the deluxe Palace Hotel, 160 miles from São Paulo. You can explore the countryside in pony carts.

———

Chile

FOR INFORMATION: Chilean Consulate General, 666 Second Avenue, New York, N.Y. 10017

If you are a pathological ski enthusiast, you winter in Switzerland or Austria, then "summer" in Portillo in Chile. If your batteries need recharging after all this strenuous exercise, you may welcome the idea of checking into one of Chile's health resorts located in the Andean foothills.

Panimavida

Panimavida, located 170 miles south of Santiago, may be just the spot. The climate is warm and sunny all year, with very little rain. The hotel offers different thermal baths, mud treatments, riding, fishing, hunting, and tennis. As in most spas in Chile, the rates are extremely modest.

———

Bermuda

FOR INFORMATION: Bermuda Government Official Travel Information Office, 630 Fifth Avenue, New York, N.Y. 10020

Deepdene

A New Zealand physiotherapist and Olympics team trainer named Stanley Paris has transformed a rather standard Bermuda resort hotel into a recreational and health resort—and the closest thing Bermuda offers to a spa. It boasts a freshwater full-fledged pool, a bit of a beach (bigger ones nearby), sailing, fishing, tennis, golf, cocktail lounge, afternoon tea (Bermuda is very British).

There is an emphasis on shaping up via physical activity and sensible eating. Guests can choose a Continental menu, a low-calorie diet, or health food. All fruit and vegetables are grown organically on the premises; meat is not chemically tenderized. A spa complex includes a saltwater whirlpool, sauna, thalassotherapy, massage, and what's billed as "Bermuda's most complete beauty salon." Exercise and yoga classes are offered, too. A physiotherapist and physician are available. A "Day of Beauty" plan lets you sample all these sybaritic goodies. Deepdene is geared to family vacations: Dad relaxes and tones up; Mother emerges slimmer and prettier; and the kids just have a ball. Rates vary with the season and the accommodations, and there are several interesting "Health Weekend" specials.

———

Jamaica

FOR INFORMATION: Jamaica Tourist Board, 2 Dag Hammarskjold Plaza, New York, N.Y. 10017

Although the beautiful beaches and wonderful climate of this island have long lured vacationers, Jamaica has only recently offered spa facilities and exploited its natural springs.

The Fairfield Golf and Tennis Club

Opened by a team of five doctors from Montego Bay, this resort offers so-called revitalization therapies. In the midst of lush vegetation, there is an excellent clinic with lab and X-ray facilities. Your check-in includes a physical, and the daily regimen comprises vitamins, enzymes, and/or cellular therapy. Golf, tennis, horseback riding, pool swimming, billiards, and Ping-Pong are available. Take time to stroll through the citrus orchard and the gardens, which boast 150 varieties of wild orchids, hibiscus, and other tropical blossoms.

Mexico

838-2947

For Information: Mexican National Tourist Council, 405 Park Avenue, New York, N.Y. 10022

Mexico has countless hot springs that, for centuries, have been deemed highly therapeutic. The quality range is vast—some for intrepid backpackers only, others no more ornate than a Tom Sawyerish "ol' swimming hole," and still others with extremely plush, well-developed bathing resorts.

Ixtapan

Ixtapan is far and away the most popular with North American tourists. It is a gleaming white resort-hotel in a breathtaking mountain landscape ninety miles from Mexico City. It is also close enough for excursions to cobblestoned Taxco.

Here you have swimming in fresh or thermal pools, golf, tennis, badminton, concerts, Mexican folk ballets, movies—even charming horse-drawn carriages.

And all that is a mere backdrop for a really good health and beauty program that promises to revitalize tired, tense, out-of-shape women.

A typical day begins with 6:15 A.M. breakfast in bed, followed by exercises, massage, spot-reducing, a fresh-fruit facial, a mineral bath, a nail treatment (feet, too), and a scalp treatment. Meals may be taken in a dietetic dining room—so as to avoid the pitfalls of rampant gourmandise that prevails in the main dining room. On your last day, you go home with a fresh manicure, pedicure, and hairdo.

If you're at all inclined to male company, bring your own along. There's a special health club for him, too, and most evenings are spent dancing and nightclubbing.

Puerto Salud

Puerto Salud (Port of Health) is located in the El Dorado Hotel in San Patricio (a thirty-minute drive from Manzanillo, five hours from Guadalajara) on the shores of a secluded bay on the Pacific coast. Greatest emphasis is on diet here (mostly fresh tropical fruit and vegetables and some fresh-caught ocean fish). "Cleansing" fasts and special juice diets are used for revitalization and for weight reduction.

Puerto Salud also offers deep-nerve massage, colonics, electrotherapy, Indian herbs, and other "natural" therapies. Some of the treatments are unavailable (i.e. unapproved) in the United States.

Rio Caliente

The Rio Caliente Spa, just twelve miles north of Guadalajara on the Nogales Highway, offers a natural volcanic sauna, large outdoor swimming pool, yoga classes, a beauty salon (facials, scalp treatments, etc.), and the "absence of telephone, television, radio, traffic, plastic food, social competition, neon signs, clocks, pollution."

The hot mineral waters of the Rio Caliente (Hot River) springs, used both for drinking and for thermal baths, come from an underground depth of one mile and are pumped into each guest's bathroom.

The diet is vegetarian, largely tropical produce. Activities include exercises, hikes, yoga, massage, health lectures, musical entertainment, and dancing.

The spa has no medical staff and does not undertake to perform medical services.

Europe

Austria

FOR INFORMATION: Austrian National Tourist Office, 545 Fifth Avenue, New York, N.Y. 10017

Considering the size of this country, there is an overwhelming number of spas and health resorts (more than fifty), so that if you're visiting any part of Austria and require "rest and rehabilitation," it won't be far away. Moreover, you can be sure of top quality since there are stringent government regulations regarding all spas and health resorts in Austria. Only approved remedies are offered to patients of these spas, and spa treatment may only be given on a doctor's prescription written not more than three days before your stay. All spas have resident medical staffs, and cures are under their strict supervision.

Baden bei Wien

Situated in the midst of the magnificent Vienna Woods, sixteen miles south of Vienna, this spa has long been a meeting place for Europe's "finest." Beethoven finished his Ninth Symphony here. Established as a watering place by the Romans some two thousand years ago, it is both opulent and homey. The splendor and charm of the Austrian past is evident everywhere. Baden bei Wien has been redeveloped into an up-to-date medical diagnostic center, with laboratories and modern therapy techniques. The fifteen sulphur springs are recommended, especially for rheumatic complaints. Treatments consist of underwater therapy for paralysis rehabilitation, sulphur mudpacks, massage, electrotherapy, saunas, and medically supervised diets. The recently rebuilt Congress Hall offers convention facilities for get-togethers of high-pressured American executives.

The wide variety of sports available includes skiing, cycling, golf, riding, tennis, iceskating, and swimming in thermal water beside a beautiful beach or in the indoor pools. For those less sports-oriented, there are scenic walks, concerts, operettas, a casino, an open-air theater, museums, crafts courses, nearby vineyards to visit, and the art treasures of Vienna only a half-hour away.

Bad Hofgastein

Actually part of the Bad Gastein complex, Hofgastein is nevertheless worth separate mention because of its Gastein Research Center clinic. Its mild but bracing climate is beneficial year-round, with sun in winter, and moderate temperatures at all times.

Traffic and noise restrictions in the area assure a peaceful stay. Skiing is considered therapeutic here, and the ski school is carefully supervised to prevent over-exertion. The water with its radon content and the climate combine for therapeutic results, and modern physiotherapy techniques are employed. There are doctors, dentists, a dental surgeon, and chemists in residence.

Belgium

FOR INFORMATION: Belgian National Tourist Office, 745 Fifth Avenue, New York, N.Y. 10151

The three watering places of Belgium are among the best-known spas in Europe, but the town of Spa, one of the most fashionable resorts in the world for centuries, has overshadowed the others.

Spa

Spa's history dates back to the sixteenth century; it is the original one after which all others get their names. Its tiara-studded list of regal patrons includes Peter the Great, Austrian Emperor Joseph II, German Emperor William II, and many more. Spa has been called the "Café of Europe," and really WAS the place where the elite DID meet.

The thermal establishments give the impression of a holiday center. Extensive facilities include X-rays, diathermy, and hydrotherapy. They claim the mineral waters and mudbaths are especially beneficial for heart and vein ailments, rheumatism, gout, and anemia. Patients are only accepted on a doctor's recommendation, and the cost of the cure can be covered by medical insurance.

Non-medical diversions include golf, tennis, bowling, riding, boating, and fishing. Spa's night-life is still considered fashionable, with a casino, theater, concerts, song and dance festivals.

Ostend

Ostend is proud of its famous baths—and properly so. The medical center is one of the best equipped anywhere, with an examination center, a bathing area, a sunbathing section, an electric-therapy division, a gymnastic-massage center, and respiration terrace.

Many people enjoy Ostend winters that can be enhanced by gastronomic weekends at the Kursaal-Casino, fresh sea air, the Folklore Museum, the Marine Museum, and the lovely and picturesque dock area.

Chaudfontaine

This seven-hundred-year-old spa town is five miles from Liège in the romantic Vesdre Valley on the fringe of the Ardennes. Here you find the only natural mineral hot spring in the country, which bubbles up from volcanic depths at 98 degrees Fahrenheit. Its slight mineralization makes it eminently drinkable and it seems to be good for unresponsive bowels. Rheumatics and people suffering from accidents use the waters in thermal baths, needle showers, reeducation pools, and whatnot.

Bulgaria

FOR INFORMATION: Bulgarian Tourist Office, 161 East 86th St., New York, N.Y. 10028

This East European country is spa heaven. For years it was the watering spot almost exclusively for the Communist Bloc. Then, about ten years ago, some bright apparatchik decided that an invitation to Western tourists might bring in some much-needed hard currency. It did. Today the Bulgarian resorts are highly touted by travel agencies all over Western Europe—and don't miss the yogurt.

Hisarya

This ancient Roman town offers bath and mineral waters, plus exercise programs and physiotherapy. The Balkan tourist hotel is recommended. And from there you can enjoy this enchanting town with its multitudes of gardens, restaurants, cafés, Roman amphitheater, beaches, and archeological museum.

Bankya

A year-round mild climate, just eleven miles from Sofia, and general-purpose mineral water (including inhalation systems) make the Bankya baths a local and foreign tourist attraction. Its balneolhospital with indoor and outdoor mineral-water pools offers foreign tourists the same medical examinations and physical therapy programs that the natives enjoy—i.e., excellent. Stay at the Lyulin Hotel.

Velingrad

There are thirty mineral springs in the Rhodope Mountains' Chepino Valley. They feed four balneolhospitals' bathing facilities, which include baths, pools, paraffin treatments, gymnastics, and general medical check-ups. Stay at the Zdravets Hotel.

Czechoslovakia

FOR INFORMATION: CEDOK, 10 East 40th Street, New York, N.Y. 10016

The opulent spa towns of Marienbad and Carlsbad have retained their palatial aura—despite the Czech socialist system.

Marienbad

So you saw the enigmatic LAST YEAR AT MARIENBAD, and now you want to see the dazzling settings here in person—well, forget it. The filmmakers, unable to get their stars and equipment into the real Marienbad, actually photographed the stunning splendor of the summer palace of the former Electors of Bavaria in Nymphenberg, Germany (on the outskirts of Munich).

However, the real Marienbad has much to recommend it, and it is considered one of the most impressive spas in the world. My friends who know it say that Marienbad is overwhelming, positively majestic, with ornate white buildings set along wide boulevards, esplanades, and the majestic architecture of a far grander period. There are wonderful arched pavilions—promenades where you can bump into famous personalities from all over the world. A century or so ago you might have rubbed elbows in any Marienbad café with Beethoven, Chopin, Johann Strauss, and Henrik Ibsen. Goethe is reported to have had his final romantic encounter in Marienbad, at age seventy-two, with a nineteen-year-old girl.

A minimum therapeutic visit is twelve days, all presided over by a resident medical staff. Marienbad is in the vicinity of forty curative mineral springs, a sulphurous spring, and healing mud. It's 2,044 feet above sea level, which is regarded by many as therapeutic.

Carlsbad (Karlovy Vary)

Founded in the fourteenth century by Emperor Charles IV, this fashionable resort has been attracting world visitors ever since. At the foot of a mountain range in a charming wooded valley seventy-eight miles from Prague, Carlsbad is a dream spa. Its twelve saline thermal springs have been visited by, among others, Bach, Wagner, Goether, and Karl Marx.

The main hot spring at Carlsbad yields over two thousand quarts of water (at 158 degrees Fahrenheit) and gas every MINUTE. Here, too, the treatments are medically supervised. Therapy also comprises fun and games. At Carlsbad you'll find golf, tennis, water sports, fishing, hunting, horseback riding, and excursions to nearby historic towns and castles. Evenings are lively and social. The cuisine has an excellent reputation.

Piestany

This is the best known of the Slovak spas, some 231 miles from Prague. It offers warm mineral springs that have existed for four centuries, plus "miracle" healing muds from a dead branch of the Vah River.

Piestany takes its therapies very seriously and maintains treatments for nervous-system malfunctions and motor-system disorders such as polyarthritis.

Frantiskovy Lazne

Frantiskovy Lazne's twenty-four mineral springs are located on a small flat park-studded plain surrounded by mountains. The muds are shipped to all of the West Bohemian spas for treatment of cardiovascular diseases, traumatology, disorders of the digestive tract, obesity, gynecological diseases such as sterility, and several types of arthritis.

Denmark

FOR INFORMATION: Danish National Tourist Office, 75 Rockefeller Plaza, New York, N.Y. 10019

Although springless, Denmark does have a few peaceful retreats offering general health resort facilities for rest and rehabilitation.

Silkeborg Bad

A large resort complex nestled in scenic parkland and wooded areas, Silkeborg Bad is designed for convalescents. It has some thermotherapy, indoor swimming, electrical baths, massage, and gymnastics.

Sködsborg Sanatorium

Not really what the name suggests, Sködsborg is really the largest vegetarian health resort on the Danish Riviera. Its medical clinic has facilities for EKGs, X-rays, electrical and medicinal baths, and massage. Sports include rowing, gymnastics, tennis, badminton, golf, riding, and walks in the beech woods.

Finland

FOR INFORMATION: Scandinavian National Tourist Offices, 505 Fifth Avenue, New York, N.Y. 10017

The land of the sauna is, predictably, very big on physical fitness—with one sauna for every six people in the country! Before you go, check on whether there'll be English-speaking guests and personnel. It could get lonely.

Savonlinna

An enormous tourist area with accommodations ranging from first-class hotels to cottages and bungalows. A popular spa since the turn of the century, Savonlinna has baths, clay treatments, rehabilitation, massage, paraffin treatments, ultra-sound treatments, heat treatments, and, naturally, saunas. There are sports activities ad infinitum, nightclubs, restaurants, a national park, theaters, cinema, and, in midsummer, an opera festival. And if you find its modest rates leaving you a mite flush, there is a gambling casino to help you part with any excess.

Haikko Health Spa (Porvoo)

Near Haikko Manor, dating back to the fourteenth century, is a completely modern Finnish health spa that offers a full program of health and beauty treatments.

The spa features a heated sea-water swimming pool in the sauna bath area and a Solarium that allows for a safe tan. Here is the list of additional therapies: log sauna; regular and underwater massage; herbaceous, medicinal, and effervescent baths; deep heat treatments; and rigorous, supervised exercise programs. Face, hand, feet, and hair treatments make every woman feel like a beauty queen.

There's plenty going on at the spa all year round. Organized activities are available throughout the year, both outdoors and indoors. In summer there are cruises, exhibitions, swimming, volleyball, and tennis; in winter, ice-fishing, sleighing, and skating.

France

FOR INFORMATION: French Government Tourist Office, 610 Fifth Avenue, New York, N.Y. 10020 or Syndicat National des Établissements Thermaux, 24 rue du 4 September, 75009 Paris, France

An American physician named Martin H. Fischer once said that hospital management could only be reformed by doing away with all dietitians and resurrecting a French chef. And yet, with all that good food, every Frenchman worth his or her salt finds it necessary to spend a few weeks annually recurperating from super viands and wines.

The assumption is that really good food devastates the liver. And this devastation can be reversed only by a water (i.e. drinking) "cure." Last year nearly a half-million people did their "cures" at one of hundreds of springs and spas.

Vichy

This is probably the best known of the water-cure spas in France—its reputation soiled by its selection by the Nazis as the capital of the puppet French state during the occupation from 1940 through 1945.

Three establishments offer every variety of internal and external hydrotherapy, from waters that flow cold, warm, and steaming hot. All of the waters emerge GAZEUSES (effervescent) and they are all allegedly marvelous for digestive problems, including gastric ulcers. Its famous casino, however, probably undoes a lot of the benefits the water imparts to ulcer patients.

Thousands annually drink the water, repose in the revolving solarium, enjoy the therapies, and socialize in the animated resort ambiance. There is also a first-class medical laboratory which many of the local physicians seem to put to serious employment.

Vichy's "in season" runs from May to October, and the municipality thoughtfully schedules festivals, tournaments, galas, horse races, water sports on the lake, and cultural events.

Eugenie Les Bains

Eugenie Les Bains derives its name from the Empress Eugenie who is said to have preferred its waters to any other. The spa is unusual in that it combines all the usual European treatments and therapies with a marvelous low-calorie French cuisine. Michel Guérard who created the "cuisine minceur" runs the spa. It offers every luxury, but manages to retain the charm of a French country home. The beautiful people come from all over the world to relax, revitalize, and diet on such delicacies as crayfish soup, canard au poivre frais, and fruit souffles. The thermal baths and the cuisine minceur are designed to bring about a weight loss of from 8 to 12 pounds during a half-cure of 11 days; and from 12 to more than 20 pounds during a full-cure of 21 days. The waters are said to be a curative for everything including cellulite, excessive weight, urinary and digestive disorders, rheumatism, and arthritis. While there may be some skepticism about these claims,

there is none about the fact that Eugenie Les Bains provides an excellent fitness program in the most luxurious surroundings possible.

Évian-les-Bains

Évian, like Vichy, is mainly known for the bottles of water bearing its name that have made their way into American supermarkets recently. Although I have trouble telling Évian water from any reasonably fresh water, the French swear that it has special healing properties—expressly beneficial for gout and diabetic patients. And now they've even put it in an aerosol can for spraying your face.

The spa itself offers dry massage, mudbaths, sauna, gymnastics, and a delightful beauty salon. You'll find the lake a lot of fun, particularly if you're a devotee of sailing or water sports. Land sports include tennis, golf, roulette, and baccarat—chemin de fer.

Vittel

Practically hugging the Vosges Mountains, Vittel's thermal establishment offers excellent drinking water, an Old World pace and ambiance, various massages, a host of sports, and superb (or dietetic) eating.

Quiberon

In a lovely little corner of the rugged, rocky Brittany Coast stands the Hotel Dietetique—a three-star hotel for prospective weight-losers and unwinders.

Starvation diets are "out" here, and you can work out your menus with the help of local physicians.

The Hotel Dietetique discourages alcoholic beverage consumption and nightclubbing is non-existent. But many notables have found the diet-seawater-massage-bath-and-relaxation routine much to their liking.

Germany

FOR INFORMATION: German National Tourist Office, 747 Third Avenue, New York, N.Y. 10017

Germany has over 250 spas, or KURORTS. The German people take their spa-ing seriously and offer modern diagnostic centers, treatments, and "the waters." You'll find that most spas are also super-fashionable resorts, with casinos, theater, opera, and sports activities.

Wiesbaden

Wiesbaden is a town near Frankfurt, principally devoted to spa activity: gymnastics, mudpacks, and thermal waters to drink and bathe in. Renowned for its twenty-six brine springs, these sophisticated German cure-folk should certainly work you into shape if anyone can. Take time to enjoy the town, with its outdoor cafés, shops, ballrooms, theaters, concerts, and beautiful hotels. The most marvelous way to arrive here is by Rhine steamer cruise.

Gertraud Gruber Kosmetik

For women only, this is a true beauty farm. It is presided over by Germany's first lady of cosmetics and is forty miles south of Munich. A perfect segue from the Oktober Fest. Frau Gruber offers a one- or two-week beauty program including treatments, rest cures, twice-daily water-gym sessions, cellulite massages, and general make-over regimens.

Sylt

A North Sea island linked to Germany by a causeway, this is one of the Germans' favorite vacation spots. Perhaps you've heard of its nudist colonies. But Sylt is much more. Here, thalassotherapy (seawater therapy) is the mainstay. Patients with high blood pressure and respiratory ailments often appear to benefit from the pleasant inhalations and showers of fresh seawater. Breathing that invigorating air, bathing hot and cold, having mudpacks applied to your taut body, and soaking up the sun on the beaches can calm anyone's jangled nerves. Sylt also offers pleasant boardwalk promenades, concerts, dancing, a cordial ambiance, excellent food—and even casinos for those whose blood-pressure levels can take the strain. Special rates are available for "anti-stress" package vacations.

Great Britain

FOR INFORMATION: British Tourist Authority, 680 Fifth Avenue, New York, N.Y. 10019

British spas tend to be terribly British. If you tend to be a "carry on" type, skeptical of bloated Continental spa cure claims, and yearn for less harried times or for boarding-school life, then take a look at the United Kingdom's "hydros."

The accent falls on RELAXATION AND REHABILITATION, rather than on TREATMENT. Weight-loss programs—in some—are excellent. But prepare yourself for puritanical early-to-bed, toxin-free, no-finery observances almost everywhere.

Advantages of the English spas:

They're easily reached from London, public transportation being rapid, clean, and ubiquitous.

Most of the spas are happily located in sightseeing havens (except for Bath, which is too near London), featuring stately homes, crumbling castles, beautiful parks, and charming landscapes that make you wish you'd been born there.

The fare, generally, is simple and palatable—despite a tendency to what one observer has branded as a suspicious plethora of "cruets and sauce bottles."

An abhorrence of "cures." Blue, nitrogenous thermal baths, for example, haven't been advertised as therapeutic for over a decade. Today they're for swimming. Period.

A sweet residue of the old days when spas were laid out for courting and spooning, for good talk and garden walks, and ritual tea-taking.

Forest Mere

Liphook, Hampshire, is a lovely scenic region in south England and the setting for Forest Mere, which, as the name suggests, is a country estate embedded in beautifully landscaped forests, grounds, a lake, and ponds.

Regarded as a "health hydro," it boasts reducing and nutritional diets geared to reconstructing victims of big-city blahs. Among its esteemed guests are actors Sean Connery, Maggie Smith, Stephen Boyd, and Alan Bates.

A variety of treatments is prescribed by medical consultants and administered by registered nurses. There are facilities for "colonic lavage" (an English hydro specialty), osteopathy, electrotherapy, massage, exercise machines, hydrotherapy, steambaths, saunas, and physiotherapy—all with up-to-date equipment and techniques.

Forest Mere's ambiance is relaxed, low-key. Its nutritional regimens are quite similar to Grayshott Hall's—and departing patients are given follow-up diets with recipes, as well as exercise remedies. Sports include golf, boating, sailing, riding, tennis, swimming, and billiards.

A mite bolder in some of its aspects, Forest Mere has a resident hypnotist and yogi, a visiting chiropodist, and several beauticians and hair stylists.

Bath

Somerset's Bath (seat of the Royal National Hospital for Rheumatic Diseases) is the oldest, most famous spa in Britain. Built by the Romans two thousand years ago, chunks of the original Roman fixtures and rooms can still be seen around the hot springs.

Rediscovered and rebuilt in the eighteenth century, the old baths became a mecca for the Royal Court and high society. The city has kept much of its antique charm with its quaint parks, terraces, riverside gardens, floral beds, Regency architecture, and a conscientiously preserved period ambiance.

The Bath water is used for both drinking and bathing. Today Bath is more of a pleasure resort than spa, with bustling shops, restaurants, cinemas, theaters, concerts, and the celebrated June festival.

Droitwich
From rock salt beds two hundred feet below the earth in Worcestershire rise the briniest of brines. Droitwich's water, used mainly for rheumatic ailments, has been channeled into immersion baths and pools. The spa itself is small and peaceful, and close enough to Shakespeare country to serve as a base of touring operations. The staff purportedly addresses itself to what is known as "general debility"—and if you've got that, their salt water might just help.

Greece

FOR INFORMATION: Greek National Tourist Organization, 645 Fifth Avenue, New York, N.Y. 10022

A Greek spa almost always gives you a special sightseeing bonus, since most are located near historic or archeological sites.

Loutraki
Fifty miles from Athens on the Gulf of Corinth, this may be the perfect side-trip if you've become a ruin climbing up the Acropolis. Loutraki has a cooler, drier, and more moderate climate than Athens; it has beautiful beaches and good swimming, and "the waters" for internal aid and comfort. It is the largest of the Greek spas, and the resort life also offers a casino, theater, golf, and evening entertainment. Temple ruins invite your exploration.

Kammena Vourla
On the shores of the Gulf of Euboea on a mountain foothill, this spa features warm radioactive brine springs, especially recommended for arthritic ailments. It has a beach, one hundred private marble baths, and twelve pools. More a spa than a pleasure spot, its ambiance is peaceful and serene, perfect for serious spa-goers.

Hungary

FOR INFORMATION: Consulate General to the Hungarian Peoples Republic, 8 East 75th Street, New York, N.Y. 10021

Budapest is virtually a spa city and has proclaimed itself "the richest capital in medicinal baths on the continent."

Budapest
Budapest spas dot the banks of the Danube, and the visitor has a large selection of luxurious hotels with excellent cuisine and night life. There are 170 thermal springs supplying medicinal waters, most of them recommended for arthritis, "female ailments," and general rejuvenation. The waters contain calcium, magnesium, and other valuable minerals. Among the therapies, you'll find baths, massage, mudpacks, hydrotherapy, and diets. Most treatments must be medically prescribed by resident physicians.

The major bathhouses-cum-spa facilities here are the Gellert, Kiraly, Imre, and the Rudas.

Heviz Spa
Located on the largest hot-water lake in central Europe, Heviz Spa is awash in radioactive sulphide water and mineral deposits. Bathing, mudbaths, diagnosis by the attendant physician, and up-to-date therapeutic methods are available. Recommended especially for bone and joint diseases, the nervous system, and back ailments, the spa also has traction baths.

Hajduszoboszlo Spa
This spa too has Hungary's typical saltwater-iodine baths, but with "hyper-thermal" water (ranging from 154 degrees up to 167 degrees Fahrenheit). Baths, mudpacks, massage, and inhalation therapy are available. Contra-indicated for persons with hypertension or heart conditions, but probably beneficial for joint diseases.

Iceland

FOR INFORMATION: Iceland Tourist Board, 75 Rockefeller Plaza, New York, N.Y. 10019

Hveragerdi
Here's a little secret spot known only by the locals and just a few tourists—nearly always full and hard to

crack. About thirty miles from Reykjavik, Hveragerdi is termed a "nature health association." It is a complete health resort: diet (organic foods), exercise, hot mineral baths (natural springs), steambaths, and mudbaths. Since there's rarely a room available, they don't bother with brochures or other advertising. For information, you have to speak to a representative at their mission to the United States in New York.

Hotel Loftleider

The Hotel Loftleider is located outside the capital, and is en route from Reykjavik to the airport. The hotel offers spa facilities: saunas, sun rooms, massage, hot-springs pool, and beauty salon (facials as well as the usual manicure-pedicure-hairdo routine).

Ireland

FOR INFORMATION: Irish Tourist Board, 590 Fifth Avenue, New York, N.Y. 10036

Ireland's mineral springs in Burren, a vast, rocky region in County Clare, are certainly worth a visit. Amateur geologists love to probe its petrified limestone formations on its moon-like landscape. If botany interests you, go in the spring and summer when the desert blooms riotously with rare and beautiful flowers. You'll enjoy exploring the megalithic tombs and hundreds of pre-historic stone forts. Motorists will enjoy the area's spectacular mountain passes and ocean coast excursions.

Lisdoonvarna

The small spa town of Lisdoonvarna is worth a visit, since its recent modernization. Waters from two sulphur springs, containing iron and iodine, are taken internally, heated or cold, and in baths. There are also saunas, massage, beauty therapy, and physiotherapy. Lisdoonvarna has facilities for bathing and boating, fishing in the rivers or the sea, and golf. Book well ahead for the summer months.

Italy

FOR INFORMATION: Italian Government Travel Office, 630 Fifth Avenue, New York, N.Y. 10111

Italy, the cradle of the spa, has inherited awesome bathhouses and pump rooms established by the Romans two thousand years ago. In fact, the Roman bathing fetish that eventually fascinated about half the world has never diminished. The country is literally sprinkled with spas and thermal resorts, with accommodations as varied as your desires—from spacious, elegant hotels in the classical tradition to cozy and modest villas and pensions. Many of the Italian spas offer gardens for strolling, spouting fountains, and huge baroque thermal establishments—altogether an Old World grandeur.

Ischia

Twenty-five miles from Capri, in the Bay of Naples, is a spa playground of jet setters, with gorgeous foliage; groves of orange, chestnut, and palm trees; smooth volcanic-sand beaches; pleasantly warm surf; and mild climate. Along the cliffs, hot springs gush from the rocks.

You'll find super-luxury (and comparable prices) at Lacco Ameno, a little town with charming, service-oriented hotels, including Regina Isabella—Italian-elegant, boasting a modern saltwater pool built right into the ocean. Here the hydrotherapy treatments are self-contained in the hotel.

Ischia (which you can reach by hydrofoil) offers everything, including thalassotherapy, inhalations, thermal-mineral baths, massage, and mudbaths. There are abundant hot springs and vapor grottos, and of course, traditional Roman baths. The warm sand on the beaches inspires some health-seekers to bury themselves up to the neck for its supposed therapeutic value. There is a very active and very social night life, if that is what you want.

A permanent colony of the wealthy is springing up around the coast. Among the famous visitors have been Sophia Loren, Gina Lollobrigida, and Sir Laurence Olivier.

Merano

Merano is a lively spa center at the foot of the Alps, with aesthetically conceived buildings and bathhouses and a perfect climate that allows it to remain open year-round (unlike most Italian spas, which close from late fall to early spring). The town holds frequent wine and agricultural festivals, making for non-stop conviviality. Skiing is always good. Hotels range from lavish to modest—and many have spa facilities. You can count on good mineral-mud treatments, inhalation therapy, and radioactive baths.

Fiuggi

Between Rome and Naples, 2,500 feet above sea level, lies Fiuggi with robust fresh air and an ideal climate. Michelangelo recommended it to his friends, and that's good enough for me. The waters are said to be beneficial for kidney and bladder conditions, and it's a vacationer's paradise with almost every imaginable recreational facility: swimming, tennis, golf, mountain hiking, fishing, and evening enjoyments that include movies, theater, dances, and fabulous Italian cuisine. It's also the source of a famous bottled water.

Bagni de Bormio
Located in the Lombardy region not far from Milan, this resort area is very proud of its vapor grotto, a cave fed by hot springs that resembles a natural steambath.

Luxembourg

FOR INFORMATION: Luxembourg National Tourist Department, 801 Second Avenue, New York, N.Y. 10017

Mondorf-les-Bains
At Mondorf-les-Bains, Luxembourg's lone spa, you have the Marie Adelaide and the Kind hot springs. The latter has had a new pavilion built over it recently. In conjunction with the springs, there are all manner of hydro-electro-physio-therapeutic treatments, gardens for strolling, and a complete rehabilitation institute for the seriously ill. The State Medical Institute has a well-equipped laboratory and X-ray facilities. Water (drinking) cures are available only under medical supervision.

Norway

FOR INFORMATION: Norwegian National Tourist Office, 75 Rockefeller Plaza, New York, N.Y. 10019

The health resorts in Norway are really convalescent hotels. Perhaps not for a jolly vacation, but if your needs are medical, the Norwegian government has approved health facilities that may be worth looking into.

Sandefjord
Here is a quaint old whaling town, on the Oslo fiord, seventy-six miles southwest of Oslo. Facing the fountain stands the new Park Hotel, with mineral baths, indoor swimming pool with heated seawater, medicinal baths, an elaborate gym, saunas, and a staff to show you how to use it all. There's a wonderful Whaling Museum, and a Whaling Fountain that revolves every hour.

Poland

FOR INFORMATION: ORBIS, Polish Travel Office, 500 Fifth Avenue, New York, N.Y. 10036

Here spa-going is a venerable tradition, and the country offers a hearty brew of inexpensive cures, fun, and beautiful scenery. Over one thousand doctors are in the employ of the thirty-six Polish health resorts.

Krynica
Located in a valley in the Carpathian Mountains, this is one of the largest and most modern Polish health resorts. It has fourteen sanatoria and three clinical centers, treating urological, gastric, and gynecological ailments. The sanatorium routine is rather strict. For greater freedom, stay at a local hotel.

Six mineral springs provide waters for bathing and drinking. The Krynica Therapeutical Establishment offers "dry gaseous bathing" in carbon dioxide from one of the springs and mudbaths.

Many budget-minded Americans have discovered the joys of carriage rides and boating on the Poprad River. Winter sports include ice hockey, skiing, and toboggan runs. Your aches and pains can be eased away afterwards by a skilled Polish physiotherapist and hot mineral baths.

Ciechocinek
The nearest spa to Warsaw, Ciechocinek is famous for its mudbaths and briny water. Here you can blend a cure with night life. There are movies, a theater, a library, beautiful gardens, a huge pool, and beaches. Parrafin therapy, medical gymnastics, and occupational therapy are also offered.

Portugal

FOR INFORMATION: Portuguese National Tourist Office, 548 Fifth Avenue, New York, N.Y. 10036

The Portuguese are making the most of their 114 mineral springs. There are twenty major thermal establishments. Some are for simple peace and quiet, others for bolder pleasuring. The phrase "everything under the sun" is particularly applicable, since the climate is cheery and sunny year-round, the temperatures are ideal, the scenery is breathtakingly beautiful, and the sea and sand and thermal waters are always nearby. Portugal's abundant mineral springs contain deposits of radium, fluoride, sulphur, sodium, and chloride.

Moncao and Melgaco

Just fifteen miles apart, these two thermal resorts are rather like "twin spas," located on the northern border with Spain. Aside from its spring water (taken internally and externally), Moncao offers great opportunities for sports afficionados, including an excellent golf course and fishing in the Minho River. Melgaco, with good tennis courts, seems the perfect vacation spot for those who wish to take their relaxation energetically in a scenic spot.

Monforthino

The lovely fashionable resort town of Monforthino is known for its curative facilities (specializing in dermatological treatments), tennis, hunting, fishing, boating, and animated social life. All categories of hotel are available, the largest being a thermal establishment with resident capacity for six hundred.

Romania

For Information: The Romanian Tourist Office, 573 Third Avenue, New York, N.Y. 10016

Situated on the coast of the Black Sea, Romania enjoys a wide variation in climate. Resorts and thermal treatments have a long history, dating back to the discovery of sulphur springs at Herculane. Today, the country boasts more than 160 health resorts and spas offering treatment of digestive ailments, respiratory complaints, cardiovascular and metabolic diseases, dermatological problems, and allergies.

The Ministry of Tourism recommends that, whenever possible, patients come with a letter of medical recommendation. Diets and treatment are prescribed by the spas for the respective diseases, and there are attendant physicians.

The Romanian spas do not purport to treat any kind of cancer, infectious diseases, tuberculosis, epilepsy, or serious heart diseases.

Most Romanian spas offer the now famous Gerovital developed by Dr. Ana Aslan and licensed in 1957 after a long period of research.

Eforie Nord

Emphasizing the therapeutic mud from Lake Techirghiol, Eforie Nord is in a region of relatively dry climate, thermal stability, salt air, and scorching sun. There is a constant breeze, which mitigates what might otherwise be excessive heat.

Eforie Nord also offers sand baths, sea baths, and heliotherapy. A special concentrated mud extract has been developed here for treatment of rheumatism, psoriasis, and varicose ulcers.

Felix

A balneoclimatic resort recommended for locomotory afflictions and for problems involving the peripheric nervous system, the Felix spa is situated in northwestern Romania, surrounded by wooded hills. The spa is accessible by plane to Oradea, then by train or bus to Felix. The climate is hot in summer and mild in winter.

Otopeni

Next time I try Dr. Ana Aslan's Gerovital H3 treatments, I will take them here. Her place in Bucharest is a mite too geriatric, if you know what I mean. Otopeni is ten busable miles from beautiful downtown Bucharest. It absolutely bowls you over, coming across like Versailles East in its spaciousness, sumptuous wines, delicious Romanian cuisines, and thirty acres of flowering trees, fountains, and promenades.

Spain

For Information: Spanish National Tourist Office, 665 Fifth Avenue, New York, N.Y. 10022

Spain has over two hundred spas, most of them near rich mineral springs. The sheer natural beauty of the land and the seascapes is worth the round-trip ticket.

La Toja

Lying adjacent to the northwestern point of the Iberian peninsula, La Toja is an idyllic garden-littered island set in the Bay of Arosa. A bridge connects it to the mainland. Here you'll find a wonderful selection of accommodations, from fashionable hotels to quaint chalets and villas. Some oceanfront hotels offer a dizzying schedule of recreational facilities and water sports for you to enjoy while taking the spa's warm waters.

Sweden

For Information: Swedish National Tourist Office, 75 Rockefeller Plaza, New York, N.Y. 10019

The main Swedish spas are retooling themselves to handle convention business, figuring perhaps that businessmen will want to tumble out of their smoke-filled rooms into mineral baths. Not a bad idea.

Ramlosa Brunn

Here is one spa that is ready for your convention and your tired, gaunt, neurasthenic, tic-ridden bodies. Ramlosa Brunn has shed its early eighteenth-century trappings for total modernity and now has meeting rooms, projectors, audio systems, visual aids, and other convention paraphernalia.

Remeber that old Philosphen Weg in Heidelberg, where the great thinkers used to hike in quest of fresh air and the muses? Well, Ramlosa Brunn has a similar footpath. Also medicinal baths, concerts, tennis, dancing and parks à GOGO.

Mossebergs Sanatorium

Mossebergs is a pretty well kept secret beyond the North Sea and the Baltic. But high and mighty Swedes dig its combined hospital/general-resort facilities. Its climate is recommended for patients with respiratory conditions, allergies, rheumatic ailments. It offers short-wave treatments, radar treatments, baths, massages, and the like. Near rubbernecking pre-historic and medieval sites.

Saltsjobadens Badhotell

Stockholmites have this gem conveniently located just twenty minutes from their city by car. It is open all year for medical treatment, convalescence, and recreation. You'll find the usual prime-quality Swedish diagnostic facilities, X-ray treatments, massage, medical baths, and dietary supervision. Perfect for summertime boating enthusiasts, and anytime for golf and tennis mavens.

Switzerland

FOR INFORMATION: Swiss National Tourist Office, 608 Fifth Avenue, New York, N.Y. 10020

Each of Switzerland's 250-odd mineral springs must undergo rigid government tests before making it a spa—and fewer than one in ten does. If you write, the Swiss National Tourist Office will send you a free POCKET GUIDE.

"Climatic health resorts" is the preferred terminology. This is based on the premise that air cures. But Swiss mountain air is different, and with that land's serenity, outdoor activities, and water, you may consider the whole country a health haven.

Baden

Baden, after centuries of enjoying high esteem for its thermal and sulphur- and gypsum-laden briny waters,

remains a perennial favorite. Near Zurich, its spa facilities are open year-round. Pick a spell from May through October if you like company.

Bex-les-Bains

Bex-les-Bains was blessed with salt mines that, with a little rain, a little well-digging, and a little piping, suddenly became a saline spa. Fold in Bex's dry (for Switzerland) sunny climate, lush scenery, and wooded promenades, and you have an unbeatable recipe.

St. Moritz

Although you may think of St. Moritz as a sky-high ski resort with sky-high prices for briefly grounded jet setters, it once was JUST a famous spa town. The thermal springs have been gushing ironized soda water (the most fortified carbonic iron water in Europe) since a thousand years before Christ. And none less than the old rebel alchemist Paracelsus in the sixteenth century described the waters most favorably.

Bad Ragaz

This delightful garden town is heavily into the health aspects of spa-ing, and the Quellenhof offers a good SWISS KUR: diet, thermal pools and baths, numerous therapies, golfing, tennis, riding, and fishing.

U.S.S.R.

FOR INFORMATION: Intourist, 630 Fifth Avenue, New York, N.Y. 10020

In the tradition begun by Peter the Great, spas in Russia are some of the grandest anywhere. Many are former palaces on the Russian Riviera (i.e., the Black Sea Coast).

Sochi-Matsesta

The largest health resort in the Soviet Union is actually a series of resorts along a ninety-mile stretch of Caucasian shore, of which Sochi is the most luxurious. Truly an international pleasure spot, with palaces, lush vegetation, wonderful parks, and pebbly beaches. Here you'll have seven hotels to choose from. Mineral mud, mineral springs, sun, and an energetic—if unsexy— night life.

Yugoslavia

FOR INFORMATION: Yugoslav State Tourist Office, 630 Fifth Avenue, New York, N.Y. 10020 or Generalturist, Medical Tourism Department, Zagreb, Praska 5/111, Yugoslavia

Most of Yugoslavia's eighty spas are geared to cope with specific physical ailments, although some of them offer cosmetic and slimming cures. There are even special spas for insomniacs.

Yugoslav health resorts are generally equipped with the newest facilities and medical supervision. Thanks to a moderate seaside climate, many are open all year. The rates are suprisingly low. Proof that they regard spas very seriously is their unique Medical Tourism Department.

Opatija

A lovely resort town on the Adriatic, Opatija offers both deluxe and modest hotels. Whether you select an elegant, older establishment or an ultra-modern spa depends purely on personal preference. All of them seem to be of a high quality, thanks to the long Balkan tradition.

Thalassotherapy is prescribed for heart and lung diseases and for rheumatism. The resident staff includes experienced diagnosticians and medical consultants. There is a clinical and biochemical lab with X-ray, EKGs, physiotherapy, and gymnastic facilities. Sounds somewhat pathologic, but in fact is not. You have beautiful bathing beaches, elegant dining, and an active and stimulating night life.

Rogaska Slatina

An older health resort—almost decadent in its splendor—Rogaska Slatina lies on the Alpine slopes just north of Zagreb, in the lovely, wooded Boc area. Its three-hundred-year-old pump room and bathhouse are still breathtaking. The grounds encompass rolling countryside, the woods, a park, and swimming pool. The climate is ever mild, its three major mineral-water springs provide saline and alkaline water, with carbonic acid and other beneficial mineral deposits. For WHAT, you ask? Well, ulcers, hepatitis, and diabetes for starters. Good music, good sports, and very good hunting.

Niska Banja

This eastern Serbian spa, once exclusively devoted to treatment of heart and rheumatic disorders, recently constructed new beauty parlors featuring cosmetic treatments employing radioactive mud and vapors.

Asia

India

FOR INFORMATION: India Government Tourist Office, 30 Rockefeller Plaza, New York, N.Y. 10020

Indian health resorts are truly tranquil retreats where many people from all over the world have gone for total escape, peace of mind, and a culture 180 degrees different from their own. They're called ASHRAMS.

If you want to more than dabble with yoga, you might consider an Indian resort—which you can do on an out-patient basis, operating from a nearby residential hotel in Delhi, Bombay, or Calcutta.

By the time you arrive, the Indian government may have revived some of the old JALACHIKITSA (hydrotherapy) establishments, which had been allowed to fall into ruin. Try the carbonated waters of Bakreswar Spring, an hour's drive from Visva Bharati University, near Calcutta. Or Manikaran in the Kulu Valley on the lower slopes of the Himalayas. Also in the Himalayan foothills, you can try Ranikhet, Almora, and Naini Ral—easy to reach from Delhi.

Yoga is a centuries-old Indian philosophy whereby an individual learns to control his mind and body, thus inuring him to life's ups and downs. Hatha Yoga is the most popular form in the West, consisting of thousands of exercises—only a few of which have been exported.

Israel

FOR INFORMATION: Israel Government Tourist Office, 350 Fifth Avenue, New York, N.Y. 10001

At the Quiet Beach Hotel, I encountered that famous Israeli smorgasbord breakfast. I would definitely classify it as a "beauty" breakfast, because everything is fresh, natural, and wholesome.

One of the principal attractions of Tiberias is the

hot radioactive mineral springs, which are housed in two large buildings—larger by far than the Dead Sea baths.

To my mind, the most interesting treatments were the PILOMA masks and baths. The muds come from the bed of the Jordan and Ein Bokek on the Dead Sea.

The Israeli Government Tourist Office will send you a brochure explaining the therapeutic benefits claimed by both the Dead Sea and Tiberias springs. The Tiberias springs are probably the oldest spa in the world, mentioned in Joshua (19:35) and later named for the Roman Emperor.

These waters emerge from the ground at a very hot 140 degrees—probably from pools approximately one mile below the earth's surface. There are eighteen individual springs, and all the waters have an identical composition. They are officially classified as thermal, radioactive, sulphurated, sodium-calcium-chloride waters.

The advantage of the mud (or PILOMA) packs is that they retain much heat (up to 130 degrees when immersed in the mineral springs), which can be administered to the body at that or an even higher temperature—which cannot be done with water. They dispense their heat to the body slowly, and seem to be useful in treating sore joints and degenerative spinal disorders. One of the best muds is that found at Ein Bokek beach, along the Dead Sea.

Research has shown that the mineral content of these waters actually penetrates the skin in a sort of ionic interchange between the skin and the water. This supposedly stimulates the autonomous nervous system, one's basic metabolism, various endocrine secretions, and the body's regenerative forces generally. Physicians carefully limit treatments to from five to twenty minutes at a time, followed by twenty-minute or half-hour rest periods.

A newly installed carbon dioxide bubble bath has become the favorite of patients suffering from circulatory and heart conditions. Other baths include vaginal douches for gynecological causes. The mud treatments are given both in private cubicles and in common rooms. The massage I had was very brisk, skillful, and just a little bit exhausting. There is also a good physiotherapy staff to administer underwater manipulations, massage, underwater exercises, douche-massages, and orthopedic gymnastics. Inhalations are given through special apparatus or in a general inhalation room.

If Tiberias interests you, reserve your room for October or November, when both the rains and crowds are still absent.

Ein Noit

Israel's best spring for drinking water is Ein Noit at Ein Bokek on the Dead Sea. The water that emerges from a hillside fount compares with the world-famous Mühlbrun spring in Carlsbad in western Czechoslovakia.

Israel's leading balneologist, Dr. Moshe Atlas (of Czech origin, formerly director of the Bardejev springs), found that the blood cholesterol levels of the residents of a Jerusalem old-age home decreased 20 percent after drinking the Ein Noit waters over several weeks.

Ein Bokek itself is a lovely beach resort where you can enjoy yourself for a pittance.

Japan

FOR INFORMATION: Japan National Tourist Organization, 630 Fifth Avenue, New York, N.Y. 10020

There are over 10,000 mineral springs in Japan (of which 1,100 are said to be therapeutic)—more than any other country in the world. The Japanese people are very conscious of and conscientious about hygiene, and relaxed mixed nude bathing is a national pastime.

Noboribetsu

On the island of Hokkaido, and set in a lush ravine, there is an area of mud pools and sulphur baths called Norboribetsu. Its thermal springs contain salt, iron, alum, and radium. The many hotels in this area, ranging from modest to elegant, give you a variety of options on how to enjoy Japanese leisure.

Beppu

A series of spas on the island of Kyushu is found in Beppu, which is virtually a cauldron of steaming hot springs, some of them situated smack in the center of town. Beppu is noted for its boiling mud ponds and steam-warmed sands.

Turkey

FOR INFORMATION: Turkish Government Tourism and Information Office, 821 UN Plaza, New York, N.Y. 10017

The Turks can claim granddaddy status in the spa and curative-bath commerce. They've got to credit the Greeks with the actual construction, but the Moslems perfected the famous Turkish bath and exported it as far west as Spain. By the thirteenth century, the Turkish bath and its myriad corruptions had traveled up the Danube and throughout Western Europe. The early Church fathers anguished over the libido-stirring steambaths and proscribed them except for reasons of health. Lepers (who seemed to be helped by the baths) were always given separate pools or tubs, and Jews were allowed only one Turkish bath a week.

Although many of the Turkish spas have crumbled, there are still nearly three hundred that have been in continuous use since ancient times. There are waters that bubble and boil, waters that chill, waters to imbibe, and waters for cleansing. And the therapeutic mystiques die hard. In southern Turkey, for example, Corycos' "Bath of the Beautiful" has a door inscription that reads: "He who drinks this water will become clever and live long. The ugly will become beautiful."

Bursa

The most popular spa is Bursa, situated in one of the most charming and best preserved of the old Ottoman cities. Justinian built a palace there so that his courtesans would remain comely. You can luxuriate in the waters of the old quarters built for Suleiman the Magnificent's son-in-law. It has cold, warm, and hot rooms with small domes, small pools, and private cubicles.

The pool is filled with warm water gushing from a marble lion's mouth. If you're a sexual segregationist, bear in mind that Monday is Ladies' Day. In Bursa you'll also want to tour the silk bazaars, ski runs, five-centuries-old Turkish homes, stately mosques, charming rose gardens, and sidewalk cafés under old plane trees.

Yalova

Just a short boat ride from Istanbul, on the Sea of Marmara, is Yalova. Once known as Therma Pythia, it still shows relics of ancient Phoenician temples and the Greek, Roman, and Byzantine baths. Reserve well in advance, since only in winter do the crowds begin to disperse from this favorite resort.

Asclepium

Asclepium goes back to the fourth century B.C. It has an interesting assortment of contemplation and consultation chambers, baths, recreation rooms, temples, and eye-boggling alms and POURBOIRES left by Caracalla, Hadrian, and Marcus Aurelius. On the main gate you'll find the legend: "In the name of the Gods, death is forbidden to enter."

Pamukkale

Pamukkale (or ancient Hieropolis) is vaunted for its waters' healing qualities, but glorified for its natural, utterly intoxicating beauty. The flow of mineralized water over the hillside has formed shimmering pools and white terraces. You may find yourself—swimming addict or no—yielding to the impulse to dive into those pools. Visitors have found it worth the price of admission simply to bask in the kaleidoscopic changes in the falls and the wild flowers surrounding the spa.

Turkish baths may not be the best, but I'd say I've never encountered any better.

Australia

FOR INFORMATION: Australian Tourist Commission, 630 Fifth Avenue, New York, N.Y. 10020

Hopewood Health Centre

Hopewood occupies twenty acres of countryside just thirty-seven miles from Sydney and is regarded as a recreational resort for people with health problems who wish to achieve a higher standard of well-being and to extend the span of their active lives.

Meals consist principally of fresh fruit and vegetables from Hopewood's own organic gardens, as well as nuts, grains, seeds, dried fruit, and some cheeses.

Naturopathic remedies include fresh air, sunshine, exercise, quiet relaxation, therapeutic fasting, hydrotherapy, and manipulative treatment. Obesity treatments are the main stock-in-trade. Interested persons can—for a couple of dollars—sample a demonstration smorgasbord health meal on Sunday afternoon.

Warburton Sanitarium

Warburton emphasizes disease prevention rather than cure, a program promoting fitness and serenity. Its modern building contrasts oddly with the stunning foot-of-the-mountains setting. Warburton specialties seem geared to the treatment of modern-day excesses —overweight, over-drinking, over-everything, general stress—though physiotherapy, salt glows, hot-blanket packs and vibra-foam baths. Some sports, no night life, and a highly restful atmosphere.

The "Coronary Prevention Programme" includes a check-up, daily indoor and outdoor exercise, treatments, daily health lectures and films, smog-free air, rest, and relaxation.

Index